A PRACTICAL MANUAL TO LABOR AND DELIVERY FOR MEDICAL STUDENTS AND RESIDENTS

A PRACTICAL MANUAL TO LABOR AND DELIVERY FOR MEDICAL STUDENTS AND RESIDENTS

SHAD DEERING, MD

To order additional copies of this book, contact:
Xlibris Corporation
1-888-795-4274
www.Xlibris.com
Orders@Xlibris.com
47811

CONTENTS

To my wife, Katie, and our three sons, who were the inspiration for this book and the reason it both needed to be written and why it was completed.

It is not the critic who counts: not the man who points out how the strong man stumbles or where the doer of deeds could have done them better. The credit belongs to the man who is actually in the arena, whose face is marred by dust and sweat and blood, who strives valiantly . . . who knows the great enthusiasms, the great devotions, who spends himself for a worthy cause.

—Theodore Roosevelt, 1910

Acknowledgments

Cover art and figures were created and edited by Kimberly Allison.

A Practical Manual to Labor and Delivery for Students and Residents

On obstetric rotations, medical students are placed in a fast-paced environment where there is often minimal time for instruction in the procedures performed and little explanation of why certain treatment plans are made. Similarly, when first working on labor and delivery, residents are expected to be able to perform many basic tasks and examinations for which there are not good teaching references available, or if there are, they are buried in the middle of a large cumbersome reference book. When you add to this the common variations in different attendings' clinical practice patterns, you have the perfect setup for confusion as you try to learn how to take care of laboring patients.

As an attempt to help students and residents learn how to take care of patients during and after labor and ensure the best care for them, this book was written to provide a practical and evidence-based guide to working on the labor and delivery unit.

This book is meant to bridge the gap between small handbooks that do not contain enough material to understand why you are doing certain things and large textbooks that lack the practical information you need for how to do specific procedures, write notes, orders, and dictations. After reading it, you will be prepared to care for an obstetric patient from the moment they arrive in triage until the time they are discharged. You will understand not only how to perform both simple and complicated procedures, but also why they are necessary, and you will have the answers to the most common pimp questions that are asked of students and residents. The most up-to-date literature and evidence-based recommendations have been used to create simple treatment algorithms for the most common issues you will face, and numerous illustrations are included for clarity as well.

Because of its focus, this book is also a valuable resource for staff physicians who need an updated text on current obstetric care as well as for those who regularly interact with and teach medical students and residents.

There are few experiences in medicine that are more emotionally charged than the delivery of a child, and almost nothing in medicine is more rewarding than taking care of a pregnant patient and being able to place a healthy baby into the mother's arms. To do this, however, every person in the labor and delivery unit must do their job. Every student, resident, nurse, and staff play a critical part in ensuring the best outcome possible. You have the opportunity to be part of one of the most important moments in these patients' lives and also the responsibility to do your job well. This text will help you to do just this, and enjoy the experience in the process.

Chapter 1

Introduction and Basic Principles

- Introduction
- General Principles

Introduction

Managing patients on a labor and delivery suite can be a daunting task for any provider, and especially for the junior resident. It is also an intimidating place to a medical student, with decisions being made rapidly and more blood being lost in a shorter amount of time than nearly anywhere else. The physician is charged with taking care of two patients at the same time and must take into account how the care of one affects the other. Add to this the fact that you are dealing with all the expectations that nine months of pregnancy brings to both the new mother and father, and decisions must often be made quickly to ensure a good outcome when emergencies arise, and you have the modern labor and delivery ward.

Too often in obstetric training, the management of laboring patients is learned by being thrust onto labor and delivery without the benefit of adequate preparation for what will be encountered. While there is much that can only be learned by actually doing, such as cervical exams and deliveries, it is imperative that medical students and junior residents understand certain basics of labor and delivery management so that they can take care of patients and improve their skills. This curriculum is meant to provide a simple, structured overview of how to manage laboring and postpartum patients and function on a labor and delivery unit. While senior residents and staff must continue to teach medical students and junior residents how to perform cervical exams, deliveries, and other procedures, this book will provide a solid framework and background to work from.

The following are some general principles and information about labor and delivery that every student and resident should know.

General Principles

1. *Understand the basics.* The goal of this text is to allow you to know the basic definitions you will need to manage laboring patients as well as recognize when problems occur. If you don't understand why a complication occurs, it is difficult to anticipate or correct it. You also need to know what medications, doses, and instruments to ask for during emergencies. This knowledge is critical to responding to urgent situations in a calm and appropriate manner. While nurses are one of the greatest assets on labor and delivery, junior or inexperienced nurses may not know what you need in an emergency, and you must be very specific in terms of medication doses, instruments needed, and where to find them.

2. *Never be afraid to ask for help.* Good senior residents and staff, when they are unsure of what the proper course of action is, will ask for another opinion. When, not if, a situation arises and you do not know what to do, think through the problem and have an idea of what you would like to do, and then ask for guidance. It is a sign of maturity, not weakness, to ask for help and it will protect your patients.

3. *Do not make decisions without examining the patient.* When first starting to work on a labor and delivery ward, it is imperative to look at the patient before making decisions about management. As you progress and your clinical skills improve, you will have an idea of exactly what to do before you see the patient. But if there is ever a question in your mind about what action to take, then go and see the patient. This also applies to the interpretation of fetal heart rate (FHR) tracings. These always look slightly different in at the bedside, sometimes more reassuring, sometimes less.

4. *Know all your nurses.* Nothing you will learn in this curriculum can help you if you don't work well with the nursing staff. Make it a point to know all of their names. Keep them informed when you are expecting patients on labor and delivery, when you decide to admit them, and when you write an order on their patient. Doing these simple things will make your job of managing a busy labor and delivery infinitely easier.

5. *Know where supplies are located.* If you are faced with an emergency, i.e., a postpartum hemorrhage, eclamptic seizure, or fetal bradycardia, and you have an inexperienced nurse or everyone is busy with other patients, it is imperative that you know where to get the appropriate medications, instruments, or forceps in a timely manner.

6. *Assume the worst and hope for the best.* Whenever you evaluate a patient for a complaint, even one as simple as a headache, think of the worst thing it could

be and work backward to the most benign. This will prevent you from missing the diagnosis of something uncommon but serious in favor of a more common and benign problem. An example of this is a headache. While it may be due to lack of sleep, caffeine, or a simple cold, you should think of preeclampsia or a subarachnoid hemorrhage first and convince yourself these are not the cause. It is usually an easy thing to rule out severe problems (in this case for instance, no physical abnormalities or neurologic deficits, normal vital signs, and no risk factors for bleeding or preeclampsia), but at least you will have considered them.

(* An important part of this last basic concept is not to unnecessarily worry the patient. What I mean is not to tell every woman that has a headache, "I just want to make sure you don't have a tumor or bleeding in your head." You must consider everything to be thorough, but you do not need to mention the very serious but rare possibilities if you can rule them out.)

While most labor ends with a vaginal delivery of a healthy infant, there are numerous complications that can arise at any time. This curriculum will prepare you to manage both normal, uncomplicated laboring patients, and to respond quickly and appropriately to common obstetric emergencies.

Chapter 2

Common Exams and Procedures

Introduction

Brief Overview Of Labor

Exams

- Admission History and Physical Exam
- Cervical Exam
- Clinical Pelvimetry
- Fundal Height
- Leopold's Maneuvers
    - Estimating Fetal Weight
- Exam for Patients on Magnesium Sulfate
- Rule out Ruptured Membranes

Procedures

- Amnioinfusion
- Amniotomy
- Contraction Stress test
- External Cephalic Version
- Fetal Fibronectin Collection
- Fetal Scalp Electrode
- Fetal Scalp Sampling
- Fetal Pulse Oximetry
- Intrauterine Pressure Catheter

- Montevideo Units
- Non-Stress Test
- Ultrasound Evaluation
    - Estimated Fetal Weight
    - Amniotic Fluid Index
    - Biophysical Profile

Introduction

Labor and delivery involves numerous examinations and procedures. While many of the examinations are learned only by actually performing them on patients, some basic instruction in how and when to do the examinations and procedures is essential. You must understand not only what to do during an examination, but also when it is necessary and why you are doing it.

Brief Overview of Labor

Central to learning how to take care of laboring patients is understanding exactly what labor is.

Labor is defined as regular uterine contractions that result in the progressive effacement (thinning) and dilation (opening) of the cervix. This is accompanied by the fetus moving down through the birth canal.

Effacement is usually described as a percentage. The cervix is approximately 4 cm long before labor, and this is said to be 0% effaced, or "long." If it shortens to 2 cm then it is described as 50% effaced. This is determined by digital exam and takes practice to become consistent. When the cervix is completely thinned out, it is said to be 100% or completely effaced.

Dilation of the cervix describes how open the internal cervical os is in centimeters between 0 and 10 cm. It is important to note that in multiparous women, the external os may be dilated 1-2cm normally, but the internal os is usually closed until labor begins. At 10 cm, the cervix is completely dilated. This is another skill that is learned through practice.

The term *station* is used to describe how far down in the pelvis the fetal head is. When the leading body part, most often the fetal head, is at the level of the maternal ischial spines, which can be felt on digital exam, the fetus is said to be at zero station. Everything is relative to this landmark and is measured in centimeters with a range of 5 cm in either direction.

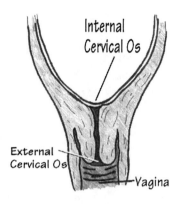

Figure 2-1 Internal and external cervical os

This is important because when certain interventions such as rupturing the amniotic membranes or applying forceps or vacuum devices can be performed safely, they are dependent on the fetal station. (See Chapter 9 "Operative Vaginal Delivery.") A complete description of how to perform a cervical exam is found later in this chapter.

Labor is divided into three stages:

> ***Stage 1:*** This stage begins with regular uterine contractions and ends when the cervix is fully dilated (10 cm) and fully (100%) effaced.
>
> ***Stage 2:*** Begins when the patient is completely dilated and effaced and ends with delivery of the fetus. This is when the patient will push to deliver the infant.
>
> ***Stage 3:*** This stage begins after the fetus is delivered and ends with delivery of the placenta.

Each of these stages, as well as their management, is discussed in detail in subsequent chapters.

Exams

Admission History and Physical Exam

When a patient is admitted to labor and delivery, a thorough physical exam should be performed. While the physical exam of a pregnant patient is essentially the same as for a nonpregnant patient, there are some important differences and findings that are normal that would be abnormal outside of pregnancy. Going through the exam:

History: A thorough history should be taken and include the following:

Patient's age, gravidity, and parity: The patient's current age should be recorded. Gravidity and parity require more of an explanation.

> **Gravidity:** This is the total number of times the patient has been pregnant. This includes all pregnancies, even those that ended in a miscarriage or abortion. This is written as "G__" in the chart. If a patient has been pregnant 3 times, she is a gravida 3, or G3. (Note: If a patient is pregnant with twins or other multiple gestations, this only counts as one pregnancy.)

> **Parity:** The patient's parity refers to the number of births a woman has had, and how far along she was when they occurred. It is written as four numbers, which take into account the following events:

> Full-term births (37 weeks and up)
> Preterm births (20-36 weeks gestation)
> Abortions (This includes spontaneous and elective abortions.)
> Living children (This is the number of children currently living.)

> Note: One part of this nomenclature that is tricky is that, in a woman with twins who delivers, this only counts as one delivery. The following are two examples to demonstrate how to write gravidity and parity.

> **Example 2-1:** A 25 year-old woman is currently pregnant, and this is her third pregnancy. She has had one previous full-term delivery and one spontaneous miscarriage. Her gravidity and parity would be written as G3P1011.

> **Example 2-2:** A 25 year-old woman is currently pregnant, and this is her second pregnancy. She had twins at 35 weeks with the previous pregnancy. Her gravidity and parity would be written as G2P0102. (She has one preterm delivery and two living children.)

Gestational age: It is imperative that the gestational age is recorded accurately as decisions about augmenting or attempting to stop labor are largely based on this.

When writing the gestational age in the chart, it is written as the number of weeks completed plus the number of days of the next week. For instance, if the patient has completed 34 weeks and 4 days of her pregnancy, this is written as "34+4 weeks." A full discussion of how to calculate and check the gestational age can be found in Chapter 4—Management of the First Stage of Labor.

Both the gestational age and the criteria it is based upon should be recorded in the chart. If it based on a sure last menstrual period (LMP) then the chart should say the patient is "____ weeks by a sure LMP." If the patient had an ultrasound that agreed with the estimated date of delivery (EDD), then both the LMP and ultrasound, as well as the gestational age the ultrasound was performed at, should be listed. For example, a patient with an ultrasound done at 8 weeks gestation that agreed with her EDD from her LMP would be recorded in the chart as "____ weeks by sure LMP and 8 week ultrasound." If a patient's EDD was changed based on an ultrasound performed at 8 weeks gestation, then this should be written as, "the patient is ____weeks by 8-week ultrasound."

Chief complaint: Always list the reason that the patient has presented for evaluation.

The 4 OB questions: Every patient who shows up to labor and delivery should be asked the following four questions:

1. Are you having any **BLEEDING?**
2. Are you having any **CONTRACTIONS?** (include time of onset/frequency/intensity)
3. Do you feel like you broke your **WATER?** (include time/color of fluid)
4. Have you felt your baby **MOVING** today? (If not, then how long since the baby moved?)

Prenatal Complications: All complications occurring during this pregnancy should be listed. Some of these may include gestational diabetes, Rh negative status, group B streptococcus (GBS) status, preterm labor, etc.

Past Medical History: All pertinent medical conditions should be listed. While this is no different than in nonpregnant patients some common problems that have obstetric implications include diabetes, hypertension, thrombophilias, and thyroid disease.

Past Surgical History: All previous surgeries must be recorded. Ask specifically regarding abdominal surgery as this can make a cesarean delivery more difficult secondary to adhesions and certain abdominal operations may make a vaginal delivery contraindicated. (See Chapter 10.)

Past GYN History: Make a note of any history of abnormal Pap smears or sexually transmitted diseases. Especially important are HIV and herpes simplex virus (HSV) as they may require a cesarean delivery depending on the situation.

Past OB History: List all previous pregnancies as well as the year they occurred in and what the outcomes were. Include the gestational age at delivery and the infant's birthweight and route of delivery (vaginal, cesarean, forceps, or vacuum). Also note any complications that occurred, such as a shoulder dystocia or postpartum hemorrhage.

Social History: Ask about alcohol or tobacco use in pregnancy as well as other illicit drugs.

Allergies: List all allergies a patient claims as well as what reactions occurred with each.

Family History: Ask about a family history of diabetes, hypertension, preeclampsia, and cancer.

Medications: List all current medications being taken by the patient.

Prenatal Laboratory Results: Make a list of all prenatal laboratory results from the patients chart in your history and physical. These will typically include the following:

Hematocrit	Hemoglobin	Platelets
Pap smear	Rubella	Hepatitis B surface antigen
Blood type	Antibody screen	Gonorrhea/Chlamydia cultures
HIV	GBS culture (See Chapter 14.)	
Urinalysis and culture		

An example outline and sample notes can be found in Appendix B: Sample Notes and Orders.

Physical Examination

Neurologic exam: The patient should be alert and oriented to person, place, and time. She may be in mild distress because of labor, but no focal neurologic deficits should be present.

Head, Eyes, Ears, Nose, and Throat (HEENT): A general inspection is done and any abnormalities noted. Make sure and note any significant facial edema as this can be a sign of preeclampsia. (See Chapter 14.) Often, since you may not have seen the patient yourself, it is easier to simply ask the woman or her partner if they are with them if the patient's face looks swollen.

Lungs: The lungs should be clear to auscultation although at term, there may be slightly decreased breath sounds noted in the bases of both lungs secondary to elevation of the hemidiaphragm by the pregnancy.

Heart: Auscultate the patient's heart. A systolic ejection murmur is a normal finding, and nearly 95% of women will have one at term.

Abdomen: The abdomen will be gravid, which makes palpation of other abdominal organs essentially impossible. The fundal height should be determined and Leopold's maneuvers performed to assess both the position and estimated fetal weight of the fetus, both of these exams are explained later in this chapter.

Genitourinary: The perineum should be visually inspected for evidence of lesions, especially active herpes lesions as these will preclude a vaginal delivery. A digital vaginal exam is performed and the cervix checked to determine dilation, effacement, fetal station, and what the presenting part of the fetus is. (See "Cervical Exam" below.) During the exam, the adequacy of the pelvis is also examined by performing clinical pelvimetry, also explained later in this chapter. A rectal exam is not usually performed as part of the standard admission exam. If collecting a GBS culture is part of your institution's policy, then do this now with a rectal/vaginal swab.

Extremities: Examine the extremities for evidence of edema. Some edema, especially bilaterally in the lower extremities, is common and a normal finding during pregnancy. If unilateral edema is present, especially accompanied by pain, then the diagnosis of a deep-venous thrombosis must be considered and additional studies pursued.

Other: Obviously, if the patient has specific complaints, such as flank pain or breast pain, then the physical examination should focus more attention on these areas.

Outline: A sample outline note of an admission physical exam can be found in Appendix B.

Cervical Exam

Digital cervical exams are performed to assess a patient's labor progress and to help you decide when patients need to be admitted to the hospital. They are performed on almost every patient that will be admitted to labor and delivery, and it takes practice to become consistent in your exams. When students are starting out, it will be easiest to examine laboring patients who have an epidural in place as they are generally more cooperative and less uncomfortable during the exam.

Indications: A cervical exam is indicated during the initial evaluation of a laboring patient, during labor to evaluate progression, and in the presence and evaluation of fetal distress or a nonreassuring fetal heart rate tracing. (See Chapter 3.)

Contraindications: The most important contraindications to a cervical exam are vaginal bleeding and preterm premature rupture of membranes (PPROM).

Bleeding: If a patient presents with vaginal bleeding, then an ultrasound should be performed to determine the location of the placenta. If the placenta is overlying the cervical os, then a cervical exam can cause catastrophic hemorrhage and should not be performed. A transvaginal sonogram is done if the abdominal ultrasound is unclear as to exactly where the placenta is located.

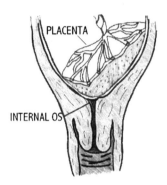

Figure 2-2 Placenta previa

Another possibility is a vasa previa, which occurs when the fetal blood vessels abnormally run through the membranes before inserting into the placenta. If the membranes rupture and the vessels are lacerated, then a fetal hemorrhage occurs, and because of the small fetal blood volume, this is life-threatening to the fetus in a very short period of time.

If you feel the patient has either of these problems, then rapid intervention is imperative to optimize the fetal outcome.

Interventions include monitoring both fetal and maternal vital signs and attempts to stabilize the patient and fetus while being prepared to effect delivery by an urgent cesarean section if necessary.

Premature preterm rupture of membranes (PPROM): This occurs when the membranes rupture before 37 weeks gestation. While there is some controversy about the management of this condition after 34 weeks between expectant management and induction of labor, it is clear that cervical exams can increase the chance of infection. In general, a sterile speculum exam is performed in place of a cervical exam and the effacement and dilation of the cervix are determined visually. PPROM is discussed in more detail in Chapter 14.

Before Performing the Exam:

1. make sure there are no contraindications to the exam,
2. ensure you have a chaperon standing by. (This is sometimes difficult on a busy labor and delivery unit, but is extremely important.)

Performing the Exam: The exam begins by informing the patient that you are going to check her cervix and explaining the indication. After this, position the patient for the exam. If stirrups are available for the feet, then assist the woman in placing her feet into them. If not, then have the patient place her heels together and let her legs fall outward. There are several components that should be evaluated during the exam and then recorded on the patient's chart. These include:

Cervical dilation: The cervix is normally closed prior to the onset of labor. Cervical dilation describes how dilated the internal cervical os is in centimeters, from 0 cm (or closed) to 10 cm. (It is important to recognize that the external os may be several centimeters dilated while the internal os is closed or 1 cm dilated. This is especially true for multiparous patients.) (See figure 2-2.) Ten centimeters means the cervix is fully dilated, and the first stage of labor is complete.

Determining exactly how dilated the cervix is takes practice, and checking a laboring patient after first learning checking after a more senior provider and comparing your exam with theirs will help you to learn this skill. In general, if you can fit one finger into the internal os, the cervix is 1 cm dilated. If your two fingers on top of each other fit tightly into the internal os, this is 2 cm, and if you can insert two fingers side by side, this is 3 cm. (Obviously, these measurements will vary slightly depending on the size of the examiner's hands.) From this point, it becomes slightly more difficult and will take practice to become consistent.

Cervical effacement: Prior to the onset of labor, the cervix is approximately 4 cm long by digital exam. The cervix is usually referred to as being "long" in this case. As the cervix shortens with labor, the effacement is described as a percentage of the remaining length. So if the cervix shortens from 4 cm to 3 cm, it is said to be 25% effaced. When it is only 1cm long, it is 75% effaced, and when it is completely thinned out it is "completely" effaced. This part of the exam also requires significant practice and will seem extremely subjective at first.

Fetal station: The fetal station refers to the leading bony part of the fetal head. The reference point for this measurement is the ischial spines. When the fetal head is at the level of the ischial spines, this is referred to as "zero (0) station." The measurements then go for 5 cm on either side of this, with positive numbers as the fetus is further down into the birth canal and negative numbers when the fetal head is above the level of the ischial spines. (See figures 2-3 and 2-4.) When the fetus is at 0 station, the head is said to be "engaged."

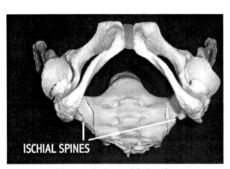

Figure 2-3 Ischial spines

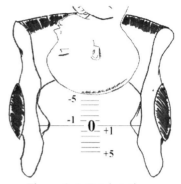

Figure 2-4 Fetal station

This measurement is important because, when the fetus is not engaged, and especially when the head is above -2 station, performing an amniotomy can result in a prolapsed umbilical cord, which requires an urgent cesarean section. (See Chapter 14.) It is also important in determining when an operative vaginal delivery can be safely performed. (See Chapter 9.) In general, an operative vaginal delivery is rarely performed when the fetus is above +2 station.

When starting to perform cervical exams, you may not appreciate the ischial spines at first. Again, performing exams on patients with epidural anesthesia will allow you to do a more thorough exam when starting out to find these landmarks.

Presenting part: Always document what the presenting part is, which will usually be the fetal head. If you are unsure that what you are palpating is the fetal head, then perform an abdominal ultrasound to confirm the presentation.

Fetal head position (if vertex): During the cervical exam, you should always try and determine the fetal head position. This is done by palpation of the fetal sutures. A diagram of the fetal sutures is shown in figure 2-5.

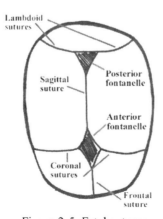

Figure 2-5 Fetal sutures

First, determine the location of the sagittal suture, which will tell you the axis of the fetal head. Then, palpate the fontanels on either side. The anterior fontanel is shaped like a diamond, and the posterior fontanel as a triangle. After determining the axis of the fetal head and where the anterior/posterior fontanels are facing, you can then record the fetal head position.*

The fetal head position is described in terms of the fetal occiput's relationship to the maternal left and right. If the fetus is facing the floor, (figure 2-6a) then it is said to be in the occiput anterior (OA) position. If the fetus is facing up, then it is in the occiput posterior (OP) position (figure 2-6b). If the fetal head is rotated such that the occiput is anterior and to the maternal left, then the fetus is in the left occiput anterior (LOA) position. An example of this, as well as the right occiput posterior positions are shown in figures 2-6c and 2-6d as well. If the sagittal suture runs in a horizontal plane, then the fetus is said to be either left or right occiput transverse (LOT or ROT), depending on which way the fetus is facing. Another diagram demonstrating all the possible head positions is shown in figure 2-7. Always remember that this is in reference to the maternal left and right.

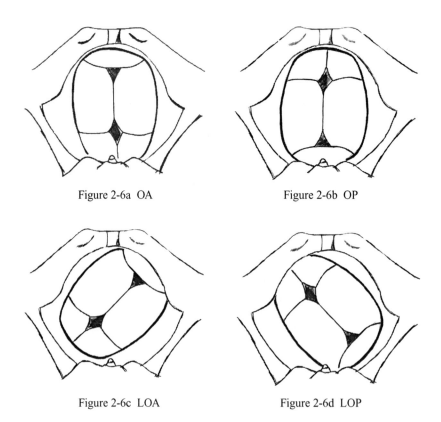

Figure 2-6a OA   Figure 2-6b OP

Figure 2-6c LOA   Figure 2-6d LOP

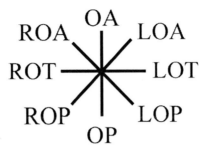

Figure 2-7 Diagram of possible fetal head positions (based on fetal occiput)

It is important to identify the fetal head position early in labor because later on, after a long labor or with pushing, molding and the scalp edema or caput that forms can make this very difficult to determine.

* Note: If caput makes it difficult to define the fontanels, but you can tell which way the sagittal suture is running, then palpation of an ear can assist you by determining which way the fetus is facing.

Recording the Exam

When describing the examination in the chart, it is typically written in shorthand. One common way this is represented is:

Effacement (%) / Dilation (cm) / Station (-5 to +5) / Head Position.

So if a patient was 75% effaced, 4 cm dilated at 0 station, and in the left occiput anterior position, the exam would be recorded in the chart as:

Cervix Exam: 75% / 4 / 0 LOA

If the cervix has not started to efface, it is referred to as "long" in this shorthand. Also, when the cervix is completely effaced or completely dilated, it is characterized as "C" for "complete" in this shorthand. An example of a patient who is 100% effaced, 10 cm dilated, at +1 station in the occiput anterior position would be written as:

Cervix Exam: C / C / +1 OA

* Hint: If you have difficulty reaching the cervix, which will happen at times because of how posterior it can be, then you can have the patient make fists with her hands then lift up her hips and put her hands underneath her hips. Doing this will sometimes make the cervix more accessible by tilting it forward.

Clinical Pelvimetry

During the initial examination on labor and delivery, you should attempt to determine if the patient's pelvis feels "adequate" or large enough to allow for a vaginal delivery. This is not an exact science, and a truly contracted and inadequate pelvis can rarely be determined without a trial of labor. But when a contracted pelvis is suspected, you can monitor more closely for evidence of obstructed labor, and this will also affect your decision to attempt an operative vaginal delivery.

In order to appreciate why this exam matters, and how to perform it, some knowledge of pelvic anatomy and a few basic definitions are necessary.

Anatomy: The important anatomic structures that must be assessed with clinical pelvimetry include the following:

Coccyx
Ischial spines
Pelvic sidewalls
Pubic arch
Sacral prominence

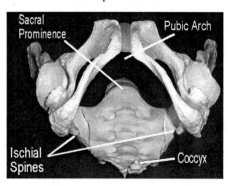

Figure 2-8 Pelvic bony anatomy

Pelvic Shapes: It is also necessary to understand that there are different types of pelvic shapes, some of which can result in obstructed labor, or a baby that will persistently remain in the occiput posterior position. In general, there are four types of pelvic shapes described although most women will have one that falls in between these.

> **Gynecoid:** This is the most common pelvic shape (>50% of women) and is generally compatible with vaginal delivery. The inlet of the pelvis tends to be round, which allows for the fetus to descend and rotate for delivery. The sidewalls are straight and the pubic arch is wide (>90 degrees). The distance between the ischial spines is also usually adequate for vaginal delivery. (Figure 2-9A)

34

Anthropoid: An anthropoid pelvis differs from a gynecoid pelvis in that there is more room for the fetal head in the posterior portion of the pelvis, which can allow for the fetus to engage in the occiput posterior position. The sidewalls may be slightly convergent, and the pubic arch may also be just less than 90 degrees. This type is more common in nonwhite females, and usually allows for a vaginal delivery. (Figure 2-9B)

Android: This type of pelvis is heart-shaped, with the anterior portion being very narrow. The ischial spines are very prominent, and the sidewalls are convergent. The sacrum also tends to be angled anteriorly with very little curve present. The pubic arch is narrow and usually much less than 90 degrees. While vaginal delivery is possible with this type of pelvis, it can be associated with difficult operative vaginal deliveries as well as obstructed labor. (Figure 2-9C)

Platypelloid: A platypelloid pelvis is the least common pelvic shape. The pelvic inlet is very wide in the transverse diameter. The sidewalls are straight and the ischial spines are not prominent. The pubic arch is also very wide. (Figure 2-9D)

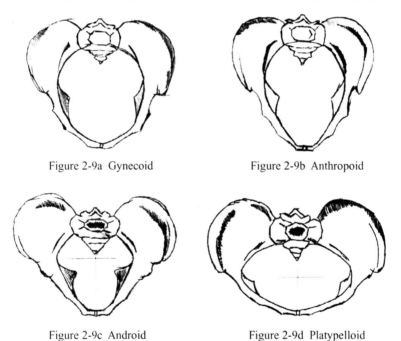

Figure 2-9a Gynecoid

Figure 2-9b Anthropoid

Figure 2-9c Android

Figure 2-9d Platypelloid

Definitions

Diagonal conjugate. This is the distance from symphysis pubis to the sacral promontory (figure 2-10). It can be measured during a vaginal exam by inserting two fingers into the vagina and directing them to the sacral prominence

35

and then measuring how far in your hand was inserted at this point. An adequate diagonal conjugate is 11.5 cm or greater. (The easiest way to do this is, with your hand in the same position as during the exam, measure a distance of 11.5 cm from the tip of your middle finger back toward your hand. When you perform your exam, if the distance is farther than this, it is considered adequate.)

Obstetric conjugate. The diagonal conjugate is not actually the widest diameter available for the fetus to pass through because of the width of the symphysis pubis. To account for this, the obstetric conjugate is calculated by subtracting 1.5 cm from the diagonal conjugate. So an obstetric conjugate of 10.0 cm or greater is generally adequate for a vaginal delivery.

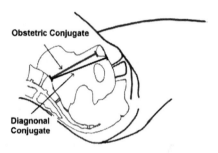

Figure 2-10 Diagonal and Obstetric conjugate

Biischial diameter. This distance is simply the distance between the ischial spines. A normal measurement for this is 8 cm or greater. It is measured by placing a closed fist against the perineum. (The ischial spines will be palpable on either side of the fist. Again, measure your fist prior to performing the exam so you know how wide it is in relation to what a normal biischial diameter should measure. See figure 2-11.)

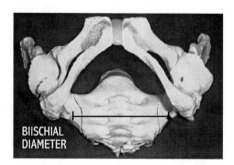

Figure 2-11 Biischial diameter

Pubic arch: The pubic arch is palpated during a vaginal exam. In most women, the arch will be at least 90 degrees, which should be adequate for a vaginal delivery. With certain pelvic shapes, most notably the android pelvis, this arch may be less than 90 degrees. While this does not preclude a vaginal delivery, it should be noted and taken into consideration if an operative vaginal delivery is considered. (See figure 2-12.)

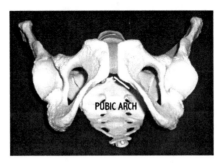

Figure 2-12 Pubic arch

Performing the Measurements: When you perform the exam and measurements, having a mental checklist will help prevent you from omitting any part. The following is a checklist for clinical pelvimetry.

Place the patient in the dorsal lithotomy position and assess the following:

1. Biischial diameter (normal > 8 cm)
2. Pubic arch (> or < 90 degrees)
3. Coccyx mobility (mobile vs. not mobile / prominent vs. not prominent)
4. Sacrum (curved vs. straight)
5. Diagonal conjugate (> or < 11.5 cm)
6. Ischial spines (prominent vs. not prominent)
7. Sidewalls (convergent vs. not convergent)

Recording the Examination: You should note a description of your clinical pelvimetry in your admission physical exam. If the pelvis is adequate by your exam, you can simply state, "Pelvis appears adequate for labor by clinical pelvimetry." If there is an abnormality on exam, it should also be noted, such as a narrow pubic arch or convergent sidewalls.

Fundal Height

The fundal height is checked at each antepartum visit as well as when a patient is admitted in labor. If the fundal height is within 2 cm of the gestational age in weeks (i.e., 34 cm +/- 2 cm at 34 weeks EGA), then the fetus is assumed to be growing appropriately. It is measured from the pubic symphysis to the top of the fundus (figure 2-13). This is obviously easier in some patients as compared to others depending on the body habitus. Some reasons for an increased fundal height include fetal macrosomia, multiple gestation, and polyhydramnios. A fundal height that is lagging can be caused by ruptured membranes, oligohydramnios, a growth-restricted fetus, or labor as the fetus descends into the pelvis.

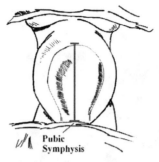

Figure 2-13 Fundal height

On the postpartum ward, the fundal height is checked on a daily basis and is described in relation to the umbilicus. If the top of the fundus is palpable at the umbilicus, it is said to be at "U" whereas if it is 2 cm below, it is at "U-2." If the fundus is above U+2, then you should look for a reason, such as retained clots in the uterus or, more commonly, a distended bladder. Having the patient void and then rechecking will often result in a normal measurement.

Leopold's Maneuvers

At the time of admission, you should perform Leopold's maneuvers to determine both the fetal lie (i.e., vertex, breech, or transverse) as well as to get an estimate of the fetal weight. While it is obviously easier to perform on patients who are not obese, they should still be attempted on every patient. The first three maneuvers are done facing the head of the woman from whichever side of the bed is the easiest for the examiner. For the fourth maneuver it is best to turn and face the woman's feet.

> **1st maneuver:** Using both hands, palpate the fundal portion of the uterus. A head should feel much harder than the buttocks (figure 2-14A). (Don't worry if the fetal position is not completely clear with the first maneuver as the others will usually make things more clear.)

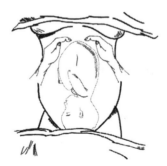

Figure 2-14a 1st maneuver

2nd maneuver: Move your hands from the fundus down on both sides of the uterus. On one side you should feel a firm, relatively straight structure, which corresponds to the fetal back, while the other side should have multiple small and irregular parts, which are the fetal limbs. If the back is directly anterior, then you may not feel any of the fetal extremities. (Figure 2-14B)

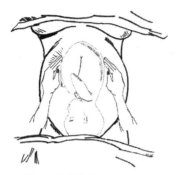

Figure 2-14b 2ⁿᵈ maneuver

3rd maneuver: Using one hand, grasp just superior to the pubic symphysis with the thumb and fingers and determine again what the presenting part is. When the head is palpated, it is noted to be a hard, round mass, and if it is the buttocks, it will be softer and nodular.

If the fetus is not engaged, then the presenting part will be mobile. If this is the case and the fetus is vertex, you can attempt to determine if the head is flexed or extended by determining if the cephalic prominence is on the same side as the extremities (which would imply the head is flexed) or on the same side as the back (which means the head is extended. If the presenting part is deeply engaged, then it will be fixed in the pelvis and not mobile, and you will not be able to determine flexion/extension of the fetal head. (Figure 2-14C)

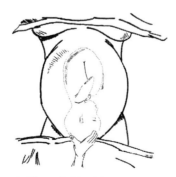

Figure 2-14c 3ʳᵈ maneuver

4th maneuver: Turn and face the patient's feet and place your hands on either side of the presenting part and push down toward the pelvis with your fingers. If the fetus is in a vertex presentation, then the hand on the back of the fetal head should go farther before resistance is encountered as the other hand will be stopped by the cephalic prominence. (See figure 2-14D.) Remember that if the fetus is deeply engaged, this will be difficult or impossible to determine. If the fetus is breech, then you will not palpate the cephalic prominence.

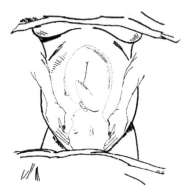

Figure 2-14d 4th maneuver

These maneuvers, while they require practice, will allow you to determine the fetal position with a reasonable degree of certainty. One study reported that abnormal presentations were correctly identified 88% of the time with just these maneuvers (Lydon-Rochelle 1993).

If, after you have performed your maneuvers and the cervical exam, there is any question in your mind as to whether the fetus is vertex or breech, perform an abdominal ultrasound to make sure. There is no harm in looking, but committing a woman to labor with a breech fetus by mistake is something you want to avoid.

Estimating Fetal Weight: While performing the maneuvers and determining the fetal lie, you should attempt to estimate the fetal weight. As you palpate the fetus, imagine that you are palpating 1-liter bags of normal saline and try and decide how many bags would be equal to the fetus. For every 1 liter bag, assume the weight would be 1,000 grams. Keep in mind that the average birth weight at term in the United States is between 3,000 and 3,600 grams. (Williams 2001).

Exam for Patients on Magnesium Sulfate

Whenever patients are on magnesium sulfate, whether for preterm labor or for seizure prophylaxis for preeclampsia (see Chapter 14), they should be examined on a regular basis by a physician to monitor for magnesium toxicity. Check with your institution's policy, but usually a physician should write a note every two hours for patients undergoing treatment with magnesium sulfate. The exam and note should focus on the following:

Vital Signs: These should include the patient's pulse, blood pressure, and temperature and pulse oximeter reading if there is any complaint of shortness of breath.

Urine Output: Since magnesium sulfate is excreted in the urine, a decrease in urine output can result in accumulation of toxic amounts of magnesium sulfate. The amount of urine output over both the past hour and past 6-12 hours should be recorded.

Heart: This part of the exam is usually normal, as cardiovascular collapse occurs only with extreme toxicity.

Lungs: Monitor for evidence of decreased breath sounds as well as crackles that can be the first signs of pulmonary edema.

Reflexes: Deep tendon reflexes (DTR) should be monitored. DTRs disappear when the serum level of magnesium sulfate is 10 mEq/L and since respiratory failure can occur at serum levels of 12 mEq/L, you must be extremely vigilant when DTRs are not present. (See Chapter 14 for a discussion of magnesium sulfate toxicity and treatment.)

Assessment: The note should report whether the patient is stable or unstable.

Plan: The plan should include any changes to the magnesium sulfate regimen being given.

(See Appendix B for a Magnesium Sulfate Sample Note.)

Rule Out Ruptured Membranes (ROM)

This is one of the most common complaints of women who present to labor and delivery for evaluation. After taking a standard history as described earlier in this chapter, if the patient complains of any suspicious leakage of fluid, then a sterile speculum exam should be performed. There are four things you are looking for during the exam:

Pooling: A very sensitive marker of ruptured membranes is pooling of amniotic fluid in the vagina. It can often be seen on the labia and perineum even before placement of the speculum when the membranes are grossly ruptured. (Even if this is seen, the speculum should still be placed to evaluate the rest of the parameters as well as determine cervical dilation.)

Valsalva: With the speculum in place and the cervix in view, have the patient Valsalva. If you see fluid come from the cervical os, this is evidence of ruptured membranes.

Ferning: After obtaining a sample of fluid from the vagina and allowing it to dry on a slide, observe the slide under a microscope. Amniotic fluid will demonstrate a pattern that looks like the leaf of a fern (Like the tree on the back of the Connecticut state quarter!) whereas vaginal fluid will not.

Nitrazine: The normal pH of vaginal fluid is between 4.5 and 5.5 and amniotic fluid usually has a pH of between 7.0 and 7.5. If the fluid obtained from the vagina during the exam demonstrates a pH above 6.5, it will cause the nitrazine paper to change colors, and this is suggestive of ruptured membranes. Some things that can cause a false-positive nitrazine test include blood and semen.

Before starting the exam, make sure you have the following:

1. Sterile speculum
2. Sterile gloves
3. Nitrazine paper
4. Sterile cotton-tipped swab
5. Glass slide
6. Chaperon/Assistant

The steps to performing the exam include the following:

1. Put on sterile gloves and have your assistant open the sterile speculum in a sterile manner so that you can grasp it.
2. Place the speculum into the vagina and visualize the cervix and note how dilated it appears.
3. Look for **pooling** of fluid in the vagina.
4. Take a sterile swab and obtain a sample of whatever fluid is present.
5. Apply the swab to both **nitrazine** paper and the blank slide.
6. Have the patient **valsalva** to see if any fluid comes from the cervix.
7. Remove the speculum.
8. Allow the slide to dry completely and then place it under a microscope to look for **ferning**.

9. Perform an abdominal ultrasound to determine fetal presentation (vertex vs. breech).

After performing the exam, a sterile digital vaginal exam can be performed if the patient is at term, and there was difficulty in visualizing the cervix secondary to a significant amount of amniotic fluid. If, however, the patient is preterm, then you should refrain from performing a digital exam until necessary as you are trying to prevent infection.

If the exam is negative for ruptured membranes, then it is prudent to determine the amniotic fluid index (AFI) to demonstrate a normal level of amniotic fluid.

Recording the Exam: After performing the exam, write a note on the patient's chart and comment on all four of the criteria as well as note how dilated the cervix appeared. It is also important to note the color and consistency of the amniotic fluid, which is usually clear, as meconium or blood may be present and may each require some form of intervention.

Procedures

Amnioinfusion

This refers to the instillation of fluid around the fetus, and it is usually performed during labor when specific situations arise. While in the past, this procedure was performed routinely for any evidence of meconium, more recent evidence has shown that an amnioinfusion is not indicated for oligohydramnios in the absence of fetal heart rate abnormalities and questioned its use with the presence of meconium.

Indications for Amnioinfusion:

Oligohydramnios: When a patient with oligohydramnios is laboring, it is important to monitor for variable decelerations and be ready to perform an amnioinfusion, though doing this prophylactically is probably not indicated (Hofmeyr 2000).

Variable decelerations: When variable decelerations are present during labor, performing an amnioinfusion can decrease the severity of the decelerations by preventing cord compression. It may also decrease the risk for cesarean section for FHR abnormalities by up to 80% (Pitt 2000; Hofmeyr 2000).

Meconium: When meconium staining of the amniotic fluid is noted during labor, an amnioinfusion is often

43

performed, especially if there is thick meconium. The theory behind this procedure is to dilute the meconium in hopes of preventing meconium aspiration syndrome after birth, which can result in significant infant morbidity and mortality. In practice, however, amnioinfusion has been shown to decrease the incidence of meconium below the vocal cords, but not to decrease the risk of meconium aspiration syndrome (Xu 2007). Because of the discrepancy, many physicians will not perform an amnioinfusion for meconium unless there are variable decelerations present as well. The most recent ACOG Committee Opinion on the topic agrees with this and recommends that amnioinfusion be performed in the presence of repetitive variable decelerations regardless of amniotic fluid meconium status (ACOG 2006).

Contraindications for Amnioinfusion: The contraindications to an amnioinfusion are essentially the same contraindications to placement of an intrauterine pressure catheter (IUPC) or any condition that makes amniotomy contraindicated. (See IUPC in this chapter.) Chorioamnionitis is a relative contraindications at some institutions.

Before Performing Amnioinfusion:

1. make sure the nurse has room temperature normal saline available for the infusion.
2. have the equipment and tubing in the room and ready to start the infusion.
3. consider whether there are any contraindications to the procedure.

Procedure: After an IUPC is inserted, either a bolus or continuous infusion of normal saline can be given. The bolus protocol will usually be 500 cc of normal saline (although up to 800 cc may be given) running in at 10 mL to 15 mL/minute. The continuous protocol begins with 10 mL/minute for the first hour, followed by 3 mL/minute after this (ACOG 1995). The nurse should monitor how much fluid leaks out during the labor and whether or not the meconium becomes more diluted if this is part of the reason the amnioinfusion is being given.

Complications: Complications with amnioinfusion are rare, but the most common ones reported are uterine hypertonus and FHR abnormalities (Wentstrom 1995). Overall, the procedure is considered very safe.

Amniotomy – Artificial Rupture of Membranes (AROM)

Indications for AROM: An amniotomy may be performed in order to assist in the progress of labor (see Chapter 7) or to allow for better assessment of fetal status and uterine contraction strength by allowing for internal monitors (intrauterine pressure catheter (IUPC) and fetal scalp electrode (FSE)) to be placed.

Contraindications for AROM:

- **Maternal infection:** In patients with HIV, or those who have active herpes (HSV) lesions, amniotomy should not be performed as it can increase the risk of transmission of the infection to the fetus.
- **Fetal head not engaged:** If the fetal head is not engaged, or well-applied to the cervix, then performing an amniotomy could precipitate a cord prolapse. (See Chapter 14.)
- **Nonvertex presentation:** If the presenting part is a foot, or the fetus is in a transverse lie, then rupturing the membranes is contraindicated as they fetus should not labor in that position, and there is a risk of umbilical cord prolapse.

Before Performing AROM:

1. make sure you have sterile gloves and an amniotomy hook,
2. ensure the patient's nurse or assistant is in the room in case of fetal distress or a cord prolapse,
3. make sure there are no contraindications to the procedure.

A digital cervical exam is performed. During the exam, you should check to make sure the fetal head is either engaged or well-applied and not higher than -2 station and that no portion of the umbilical cord is palpable. If the fetus is -2 station, then having your assistant apply moderate fundal pressure can help keep the head well-applied to the cervix in an attempt to prevent a cord prolapse during the procedure. The amniotomy instrument, often referred to as an "amniohook," is inserted between the index and middle fingers of the hand in the vagina with the sharp hook facing down in order to prevent any trauma to the vagina or cervix. When the amniohook is in place against the fetal vertex, it is rotated 180 degrees and then gently scraped against the membranes until a hole is made, at which point you will both feel and see amniotic fluid.

If internal monitors (FSE or IUPC) need to be placed, this can be done at this time.

Recording the Exam: You should make a note in the chart after performing an AROM and note the cervix examination, the time it was performed, if internal monitors were placed, and the color and amount of amniotic fluid that was seen. If meconium is present, comment on whether it is thin, thick, or particulate.

Complications: The most emergent complication that can result from amniotomy is a prolapsed umbilical cord, which requires immediate cesarean delivery (See Chapter 14). Fortunately, this is a rare occurrence when the fetal head is well-applied to the cervix at the time of amniotomy. As there will be less amniotic fluid around the fetus after amniotomy, variable decelerations may also occur.

Contraction Stress Test (CST)

A contraction stress test (CST) induces contractions in an attempt to determine if the fetus is compromised. A well-oxygenated and normal fetus will be able to tolerate the intermittent stress of contractions without difficulty while a compromised fetus will demonstrate distress with temporarily decreased oxygenation that occurs normally with contractions. The incidence of a stillbirth occurring within a week of a reassuring, or negative, CST is extremely low at 0.3 per 1,000, which is even lower than that for a reassuring NST, which has been reported as 1.9 per 1,000 (Freeman 1992).

Because this test involves inducing contractions, it is rarely used in preterm patients, and because other less invasive tests are now possible on labor and delivery, such as the biophysical profile (BPP), it is not commonly performed. However, when patients come to labor and delivery for evaluation of labor, and they are spontaneously contracting at least three times in 10 minutes, this is essentially a spontaneous CST. If this is the case, it should be noted in the chart as a normal CST is even more reassuring than a reactive NST as stated previously.

Indications for CST: A CST is usually performed after another less invasive test is equivocal regarding fetal status. For instance, if a patient has a nonreactive nonstress test (NST), a CST can be performed as a follow-up test.

Contraindications for CST: Patients who should not labor should not have this test performed. Some of these conditions include the following:

- Preterm premature rupture of membranes (PPROM)
- Placenta previa or vasa previa
- Previous classical uterine incision or other uterine surgery that makes labor contraindicated (See Chapter 10 "Cesarean Section")
- Preterm labor or patients at risk for preterm labor

Before Performing CST:

1. make sure there are no contraindications to the procedure.
2. counsel the patient regarding the possibility of fetal distress and need for urgent delivery.

Procedure: The patient is placed in the recumbent position on her side, and external monitors are placed to continuously monitor both the fetal heart rate and contractions. Peripheral intravenous access is usually obtained even if Pitocin is not used to stimulate contractions. In order for the test to be interpreted, the patient must have at least three contractions in 10 minutes that last at least 40 seconds each and a concurrent tracing of the fetal heart rate. If the patient is spontaneously contracting and meets these criteria, then the test may be interpreted, and no uterine stimulation is required. If the patient is not contracting, or her contractions do not meet these criteria, then contractions must be stimulated. Two available methods are intravenous (IV) Pitocin and nipple stimulation.

> **IV Pitocin:** A dilute solution of IV oxytocin is started at a rate of 0.5 mU/min to stimulate contractions. This rate is doubled every 20 minutes until adequate contractions are achieved.

> **Nipple stimulation:** The patient is instructed to rub one nipple for 2 minutes or until a contraction occurs. If this does not produce adequate contractions, then the stimulation is stopped and then repeated in approximately 5 minutes. If this still does not result in adequate contractions, then IV Pitocin is administered.

Stop the test when either an adequate test has occurred, or there is significant fetal distress.

Interpretation of Results: After adequate contractions and a concurrent tracing of the FHR have been obtained, the results are classified according to the following four categories:

1. **Negative:** No late decelerations or significant variable decelerations are present.
2. **Positive:** Late decelerations are present with at least 50% of contractions.*
3. **Equivocal—suspicious:** Intermittent late or intermittent significant variable decelerations are present.
4. **Equivocal—hyperstimulatory:** Uterine hyperstimulation is present (contractions are lasting > 60 seconds or occur < 2 minutes apart), and decelerations are present as well.

5. **Unsatisfactory:** Fewer than three contractions in 10 minutes or an uninterpretable tracing. (ACOG 1999)

   * Note: If late decelerations are present after more than half of contractions, this is a positive test even when there are not 3 contractions in 10 minutes. (See Chapter 3 "FHR Monitoring" for a discussion/explanation of decelerations.)

Intervention:

If the test is **positive**, then delivery is usually indicated although it is important to remember that a nonreactive NST and a positive CST when seen together can be associated with congenital anomalies and that an ultrasound to evaluate this should be performed if possible.

If the test is **equivocal**, then a biophysical profile can be performed, and uterine hyperstimulation should be corrected if present.

If the test is **negative**, you can reassure the patient that this is very reassuring and that the fetus appears stable at this time.

Complications: When contractions occur in a compromised fetus, then fetal distress may occur, requiring delivery. Uterine hyperstimulation may also occur, and if fetal distress occurs with this, it should be treated in the same manner as if it occurs during spontaneous labor. (See Chapter 14.)

External Cephalic Version (ECV)

An external cephalic version refers to a procedure during which a baby is externally manipulated from a breech or transverse position to a vertex position. There have been multiple studies that have demonstrated that this procedure can reduce the need for cesarean section for malpresentation without increasing perinatal mortality and success rates of up to 76% have been reported though the average success rate is closer to 60% (Hofmeyr 2002; ACOG 2000).

Indications: When the fetus is found to be breech approaching term, an option for avoiding a cesarean section is to attempt to turn the fetus to a vertex position to allow for a vaginal delivery. It is generally attempted at 36 weeks gestation in order to maximize the chances for success, minimize the chance that the fetus will revert to a breech or transverse position if the ECV is successful, and to prevent any problems related to prematurity should an emergency delivery be required. It may be attempted during labor as long as the membranes are intact and there are no contraindications present.

Contraindications: There are several instances in which an ECV should not be attempted. Some of these include the following:

- Other indications for cesarean section that are not changed by a version (such as placenta previa or previous uterine surgery)
- Ruptured membranes
- Nonreassuring fetal heart rate tracing or other evidence of fetal distress
- Hyperextended fetal head
- Placental abruption

Other conditions that are a relative contraindication include the following:

- Maternal obesity
- IUGR
- Previous cesarean delivery
- Oligohydramnios

(Hofmeyr 2003)

Before Performing the Procedure: Prior to attempting an ECV, the following steps should be taken:

1. Ultrasound to assess the following:

   a. Exclude placenta previa.
   b. Determine the AFI (as oligohydramnios is a relative contraindication to ECV).
   c. Confirm fetal position.

2. Nonstress test or biophysical profile to document fetal well-being.
3. Informed consent obtained, signed and placed onto the chart.
4. Ensure that the OR and Anesthesiologist are available in case an emergency cesarean section is needed.
5. Obtain Rhogam if the patient is Rh negative.

Procedure: The patient is placed in a recumbent position after the fetal status has been determined to be reassuring. The uterus must be relaxed, and this is usually accomplished with a single dose of terbutaline 0.25 mg SQ.* The abdomen is lubricated with either ultrasound lubricant, mineral oil, or powder (cornstarch). The breech is disengaged and elevated from the pelvis by pushing the fingertips of one hand behind the symphysis pubis. If the procedure is being done by a single provider, then the free hand is used to push on the fetal back at the same time as the buttocks

49

is manipulated and a forward roll is attempted. If two operators are attempting the ECV, then one physician elevates the breech and the other attempts to move the head and back in the forward roll. The movements should be slow and steady and the fetal heart rate checked at least every two minutes. The attempt is aborted if a prolonged deceleration or fetal bradycardia occurs. In general, no more than four attempts are made and no single attempt should last for more than five minutes. After the procedure, the fetus should be monitored for at least an hour to ensure there is no evidence of fetal distress. If the patient is Rh negative, then anti-D immunoglobulin is administered.

* There is a school of thought that recommends placing an epidural or spinal anesthesia prior to attempting an ECV, but the results of current research are conflicting.

Potential complications: There are no significant maternal risks, except for the potential for an emergent cesarean section should fetal distress occur. In terms of fetal risks, the exact incidence of complications is not well-defined. The fetal heart rate tracing may be nonreactive after the procedure, and a transient bradycardia may also occur. Other rare but reported complications include placental abruption and preterm labor (DeRosa 1991). To date, randomized trials of ECV have not demonstrated any increase in perinatal mortality (Hofmyer 2002). If significant fetal distress does occur, then an emergent cesarean section is performed.

Fetal Fibronectin (fFN) Collection

During the workup of preterm labor, a vaginal swab for fFN is often done for use in the evaluation. While a positive test is associated with an increased risk of preterm delivery, the real value of the test lies in its high *negative* predictive value of up to 99%. It is important to think about doing this test at the beginning of your workup because once you have checked the patient's cervix, you cannot collect a sample for 24 hours.

Indications: During the workup of a patient with preterm labor, a fetal fibronectin (fFN) swab may be done. You should check with your institution about the availability of the test as well as whether it is incorporated into their standard protocol for preterm labor evaluation if they have one.

Contraindications: This test should not be performed when there is active bleeding, ruptured membranes, or within 12-24 hours of a previous vaginal examination when any kind of lubrication was utilized. While some authors list the presence of a cervical cerclage as a contraindication to the procedure, there is now literature to support the use and interpretation of the test when a cerclage is present (Roman 2003).

Complications: There are no expected complications from the procedure.

Procedure: A sterile speculum examination is performed during the evaluation of a patient for preterm labor. Samples are taken from the posterior fornix or external os using the swab from the manufacturer's kit.

Before performing the collection, make sure the following conditions are met:

- Cervical dilation of < 3 cm
- Intact membranes
- Gestational age between 24+0 and 34+6 weeks
- No intercourse in the past 24 hours
- No digital or vaginal ultrasound examination in the past 24 hours
- No use of lubricants for the examination

Results: The results are generally reported as either positive or negative. A positive result is returned when a concentration of fFN is greater than 50 nm/mL.

Intervention: A negative result is very reassuring in that it has a very high negative predictive value (up to 99%) in relation to the risk of preterm delivery (Honest 2002). On the other hand, a positive result implies an increased risk of delivery within the next 7-10 days although the incidence of this is only between 13% and 30% (Honest 2002). Because of this, there are no evidence-based recommendations for exactly how to use a positive test, and the major value of the fetal fibronectin test lies in its high negative predictive value and ability to determine which patients will not deliver in the two weeks after a negative result (Iams 2003). Please refer to Chapter 14 and the section on preterm labor for a discussion of how to interpret the results based on the clinical situation.

Fetal Scalp Electrode (FSE)

During labor, when a fetal heart rate tracing is concerning or difficult to monitor with external fetal monitors, a fetal scalp electrode (FSE) may be placed. The FSE gives a more accurate assessment of the fetal heart rate as well as serving as a fetal electrocardiogram. It allows for interpretation of the short-term variability, which is important in assessing fetal well-being. It can only be placed after the amniotic sac has ruptured, so if the fetus is too high up for the membranes to be ruptured, it should not be placed. An FSE should not be placed if the mother has an infection that could be transmitted to the baby more easily through the small break in the skin created by the FSE. Some examples of this would be HIV or Hepatitis B infection.

Indications for placement of FSE:

- Inability to monitor FHR with external monitors.
- Concerning FHR tracing.

- Twins in labor with difficulty monitoring both twins.

Contraindications to placement:

- HIV-infected mother
- Maternal infection with acute hepatitis B
- Active HSV lesions
- Fetal bleeding disorder
- Contraindications to amniotomy (AROM)

Before placement of an FSE, consider the following questions:

1. What is the indication for placing this? (Complications are extremely rare, but you need to know why you are doing any procedure.)
2. Does the nurse have the cable to hook up the FSE? (It is a different cable than the external fetal monitor.)
3. Are there any contraindications to placement?

Placement: A digital cervical exam is performed with the dominant hand and the fontanelles palpated to determine the fetal head position. The FSE is then inserted into the vagina with the free hand and held between the fingers of the dominant hand. The tip of the FSE is pressed against a bony portion of the fetal skull, and then the end of the probe rotated in a clockwise fashion, which will attach the FSE to the scalp. Care must be taken to avoid placement over a fontanelle or suture as this can injure the fetus.

Complications: Complications of FSE placement are very rare but can result from improper placement, such as injury to an eye or over a fontanelle. The placement site can also become infected and osteomyelitis has been reported (McGregor 1989).

Fetal Scalp Sampling

At times during labor you will have a FHR tracing that is not reassuring and does not respond to conservative measures, such as maternal position changes, discontinuing oxytocin infusion, administering oxygen by face mask to the mother, and fetal scalp stimulation. (See Chapter 3.) When this occurs, and delivery is not imminent, then performing this test can help you determine whether or not the fetus is truly in distress and need of immediate delivery. (Of note, this procedure is not used at many institutions, so you will need to see if this is an option at your hospital.)

Indications for Fetal Scalp Sampling: This procedure is indicated when there is a nonreassuring FHRT that does not respond to conservative measures or scalp stimulation.

Contraindications to Fetal Scalp Sampling:

-   Contraindications to rupture of the membranes.
-   Maternal HSV or HIV infection.
-   Fetal bleeding disorder.
-   Patient not in active labor or fetus not low enough in the pelvis to safely perform the procedure.

Before performing fetal scalp sampling, do the following:

1. Ensure there are no contraindications.
2. If the membranes are not ruptured, then make preparations to rupture the membranes (AROM).
3. Make sure you have a fetal scalp sampling kit.
4. Assign one person to take the blood samples obtained to the lab for immediate analysis.
5. Call and inform the laboratory you are going to perform this procedure.
6. Alert the pediatricians that this is being done and you will inform them should delivery be required.
7. Counsel the patient regarding the procedure.

Procedure:

1. Insert the cylinder that comes in the kit into the vagina and place the tip against the fetal skull.
2. Wipe the scalp clear of blood and amniotic fluid with the sterile swab included in the kit.
3. Coat the area to be incised with the silicone gel from the package. (This will cause the blood to form beads rather than running down the scalp.)
4. Make an incision approximately 2 mm deep in the area you have prepared with the cutting instrument. (This is a long plastic handle with a small blade on the end and is provided in the kit.)
5. Collect the beads of blood immediately into the heparinized capillary tubes and send them to the laboratory.
6. Remove the cylinder from the vagina.

Interpretation and Interventions Based on Results: The pH results from this test are assigned into one of the three categories.

> **< 7.20:** If the pH is in this range, then immediate delivery is indicated by whatever route is most expedient (vaginal or cesarean).

7.20-7.25: If the pH is between these ranges, then the procedure is repeated in 30 minutes and the FHR monitored closely until then for evidence of worsening distress.

> 7.25: When the pH is in this range, labor may continue with close monitoring.

Complications: In general, the bleeding from the small incision stops almost immediately, and complications are rare. There is always a small risk of a scalp infection after delivery, and if the fetus has a bleeding disorder, then the bleeding may be more than normal.

Fetal Pulse Oximetry

This method of fetal monitoring measures the oxygen saturation of arterial hemoglobin by utilizing a sensor in a catheter that is similar in appearance to an IUPC catheter and reflects fetal tissue perfusion. It is based on the principle that O_2Hb and Hb differ in their ability to absorb light at different wavelengths (Yam 2000). If the fetal oxygen saturation falls below 30%, then fetal distress is present, and intervention should be made. This technology is still being investigated, but may be commonplace in the near future. Whether or not it will improve fetal outcomes is yet to be determined, and at this time, it is not in widespread use.

Intrauterine Pressure Catheter (IUPC)

An intrauterine pressure catheter can be used to determine both the timing and intensity of uterine contractions, and also to perform an amnioinfusion during labor. It can only be inserted when the membranes are ruptured.

Indications for IUPC Placement:

- Inability to monitor contractions during labor. (Often secondary to maternal obesity.)
- Protracted labor with need to document contraction strength.
- Need for an amnioinfusion. (i.e., for meconium or variable decelerations)

Contraindications to IUPC Placement:

- Any contraindication to rupturing the membranes. (See AROM.)
- Cervix completely dilated. (Placing the IUPC is nearly impossible at this time although it may be attempted.)

Before placement of IUPC, do the following:

1. Ensure there are no contraindications.
2. If AROM needs to be performed, make preparations for this.
3. Make sure the nurse has the appropriate cables to hook up the IUPC after placement.
4. Get out sterile gloves for the procedure.

Placement of IUPC: Start by putting on a pair of sterile gloves and performing a digital cervical exam. If the membranes need to be ruptured, that is done at this time. After this, insert the tips of the index and middle fingers between the fetal head and the cervix to make room to insert the IUPC. Have your assistant open the IUPC catheter in a sterile fashion and then thread the catheter between the two fingers of the hand that is in the cervix and advance the tip of the catheter to the cervix. The catheter itself will usually have a removable plastic sheath around it that you can insert up the external cervical os. At this point, hold onto the outer plastic sheath and thread the actual catheter between the cervix and the fetal head and up into the uterus. After this is done, carefully remove your hand from the vagina, and the plastic sheath is then removed from around the catheter.

Recording the Exam: Make a note in the patient's chart and describe your cervical exam as well as the fact that you placed an IUPC. If you are starting an amnioinfusion, note this as well.

Complications: Complications of IUPC placement are uncommon, but if it is forced into the placenta, then hemorrhage is possible.

Montevideo Units (MVUs)

This is a way to quantify the actual intensity of contractions. It requires the use of an IUPC because external monitors can only provide information on the timing and duration of contractions, and not their actual strength. To determine how many Montevideo units (MVUs) are present follow this procedure:

1. Count all contractions in a 10-minute period.
2. For each contraction, measure the pressure (listed in mmHg on the tracing) from the baseline to the peak.
3. Add the values for each contraction.

An example of this is seen in figure 2-15.

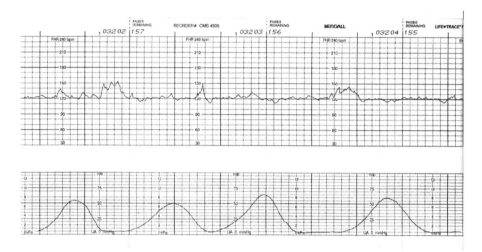

Figure 2-15 Montevideo units

An adequate contraction pattern will have at least 200 MVUs. If this is not the case and the patient is not progressing in labor, then you can consider labor augmentation. (See Chapter 7.)

NonStress Test (NST)

Nearly every patient who comes to labor and delivery will be evaluated with a nonstress test (NST). While much of this will become pattern recognition, it is important to have a systematic method to evaluate this test, which is discussed in detail in Chapter 3. If contractions are present, and at least 3 are present in a 10-minute period, then you have a spontaneous contraction stress test (CST) rather than a nonstress test.

Indications for NST: An NST is performed for all patients who present to labor and delivery after 24 weeks gestation as part of the basic assessment of the fetus. This test is also performed as part of antepartum testing for high-risk pregnancies. The most common patient that will have an NST on labor and delivery is the woman at term (> 37 weeks) who presents to rule out labor.

Contraindications for NST: Because an NST is not invasive, there are no contraindications to performing an NST. In cases where significant fetal distress is noted though, emergent delivery may be indicated and preclude completing the test.

Performing an NST: The patient is placed in either the lateral recumbent or supine position with lateral hip displacement to prevent the gravid uterus from compressing the inferior vena cava, and external monitors are placed on the abdomen to record both the fetal heart rate and uterine activity for 20 to 40 minutes. The FHRT is monitored for accelerations, which are defined as elevations of the FHR of at least 15 bpm above baseline for at least 15 seconds.* If there are at least two accelerations present in the first 20 minutes, the test may be stopped at this time. If accelerations are not present, then the test can be continued up to 40 minutes.

* Note: If the patient is < 32 weeks gestation, then the accelerations must only be 10 bpm above baseline for 10 seconds to meet criteria for a reactive tracing.

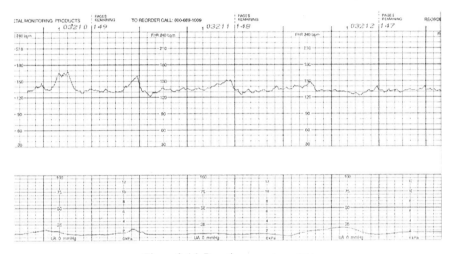

Figure 2-16 Reactive non-stress test

Interpretation of NST: The results of an NST are classified as either *reactive* or *nonreactive*, depending on whether not at least two accelerations of adequate size as stated before are present. It is important to note that this will be dependent on gestational age as up to 50% of noncompromised fetuses between 24 and 28 weeks will have a nonreactive NST (Bishop 1981). This number decreases to only 15% between 28 and 32 weeks gestation, and after this, a reactive NST is expected in nearly all cases (ACOG 1999).

The NST must also be interpreted with consideration given to any decelerations present. If there are late decelerations or significant and repetitive variable decelerations, then the FHRT is nonreassuring even if the test is reactive. Please refer to Chapter 3 for a detailed discussion of FHR interpretation.

Interventions: If the NST is reactive then this is reassuring that the fetus is not felt to be in distress. If during the NST, there are no accelerations in the first twenty minutes, then vibroacoustic stimulation with an artificial larynx may be applied to the maternal abdomen for 1-2 seconds in an attempt to elicit accelerations. After 32 weeks, where a reactive NST is expected, a biophysical profile should be performed if the NST is nonreactive.

Recording the Exam: A note should be made in the patient's chart regarding the exam. The baseline FHR should be noted, and the test should be recorded as either reactive or nonreactive. (These can be abbreviated as RNST and NRNST respectively.) Additional information, such as the presence or absence of decelerations, should be recorded as well as any additional monitoring that is needed.

Ultrasound Evaluation

Estimated Fetal Weight: It is possible to perform measurements utilizing ultrasound to provide an estimated fetal weight. This is more useful with preterm patients who are being admitted for preterm labor where the fetal weight is related to survival in the neonatal intensive care unit (NICU) than for term patients but is an important skill to have.

The three basic measurements that should be taken to calculate an estimated fetal weight on labor and delivery are:

1) **Biparietal diameter:** This measurement should include the thalamus as well as the falx and the cavum septum pelllucidum. The measurement should be taken from the outside edge of the cranium to the internal edge of the skull on the opposite side as shown in figure 2-17a.

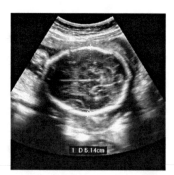

Figure 2-17a Biparietal diameter

2) **Abdominal circumference:** The abdominal circumference is a cross-sectional view of the abdomen and should include the spine as well as the stomach and the portal vein. The measurement encompasses the entire circumference as demonstrated in figure 2-17b. If the fetal heart is visible, then the ultrasound probe is directed too superiorly.

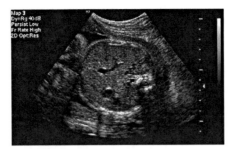

Figure 2-17b   Abdominal circumference

3) **Femur length:** The femur is measured from one end to the other when the femur is visualized in its greatest length. (Figure 2-21c)

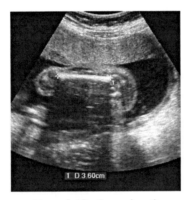

Figure 2-17c Femur length

All ultrasound machines are different, and you must become familiar with the one at your institution and practice obtaining these measurements. It is also important to learn how to record them on the machine and produce an estimation of the fetal weight.

Interpretation of the Exam: It is important to note whether or not fetal macrosomia, which is often defined as a birth weight of > 4,000 grams, is present or if the fetus is growth restricted, which is defined as below the 10th percentile for gestational age. Table 2-1 lists the 10th percentile cutoffs for different gestational ages.

Recording the Exam: In the chart, you should note the position of the fetus as well as the estimated fetal weight based on your measurements. Make sure to comment on the following:

- Fetal lie (vertex, breech, transverse)
- Position of the placenta (anterior, posterior, low-lying, previa)

- Amount of amniotic fluid (AFI)
- Estimated fetal weight

Table 2-1. Cutoff for 10th percentile by gestational age

Gestational Age (wks)	10th percentile (grams)
26	568
27	754
28	765
29	884
30	1,020
31	1,171
32	1,338
33	1,519
34	1,714
35	1,919
36	2,129
37	2,340
38	2,544
39	2,735
40	2,904
41	3,042

—(Adapted from Doubilet 1997)

Amniotic Fluid Index (AFI): The amniotic fluid index is simply an ultrasound assessment of the amount of amniotic fluid around the fetus/fetuses.

Indications for AFI:

- Evaluation of a patient who complains of decreased fetal movement.
- Evaluation of a patient who presents for evaluation of ruptured membranes.
- In conjunction with biophysical profile.

Contraindications for AFI: There are no contraindications to performing an AFI.

Performing an AFI: The AFI is calculated by first dividing the uterus into four quadrants usually using the umbilicus as the center point and drawing an imaginary line vertically and horizontally from there. (See figure 2-18.) An ultrasound is then used to measure the largest vertical pocket of amniotic fluid (in centimeters) in each of these four quadrants, and the AFI is the sum of the four measurements. You must make sure that the pockets of fluid do not contain any sections of the umbilical cord as these cannot be counted in the AFI.

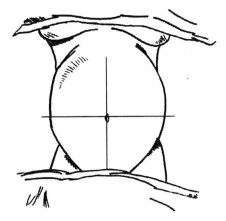

Figure 2-18 Amniotic Fluid Index (AFI) quadrants

Interpretation and Interventions: In general, an AFI of less than 5 cm is classified as oligohydramnios. In the term or post-term patient, oligohydramnios is usually treated with induction of labor. (See Chapter 14 for a discussion of oligohydramnios.) If the patient is preterm, then close monitoring is usually initiated, and an attempt is made to determine the cause, with preterm premature rupture of membranes being one of the more common reasons.

At the other end of the spectrum, polyhydramnios is defined as an AFI of greater than 25 cm. This complication has been associated with maternal diabetes as well as congenital anomalies and warrants further evaluation.

Biophysical Profile (BPP): A biophysical profile is usually performed after an NST is found to be nonreactive or as part of a more intensive antepartum testing regiment. It has five separate components, and a score of 0 or 2 points is given for each part of the test (so it is impossible to have an odd number for a BPP result). It is performed with an ultrasound, with the exception of the NST, and the test continues until either all components are present or when 30 minutes expires.

The five components are:

1. **Nonstress test:** (Reactive or Nonreactive)
2. **Amniotic fluid assessment:** (Largest vertical AF pocket > 2 cm or AFI > 5.0 cm)
3. **Gross fetal body movements:** (at least 3 or more discrete body movements)
4. **Fetal tone:** (At least one episode of rapid flexion/extension of extremity or hand)
5. **Fetal breathing movement:** (at least 30 continuous seconds)

BPP Scores and Interpretations:

8-10: Reassuring and correlates well with a good fetal outcome.

6: Equivocal and repeat testing is indicated within 12-24 hours or consider delivery if the fetus is mature.

2-4: Reflective of fetal compromise and immediate intervention must be considered.

* Of note, with a BPP of 8 or higher, the perinatal mortality rate is only 1.9/1,000, and the risk of cerebral palsy in the infant is only 0.7/1,000 women. These risks increase as the score decreases, with the risk of perinatal mortality going up to as high as 285 per 1,000 live births with a BPP score of 0/10 (Kim 2003).

Table 2-2*

Biophysical Profile Score	Perinatal Mortality (per 1,000 live births)	Risk of Cerebral Palsy (per 1,000 live births)
≥8	1.9	0.7
6	9.8	13.1
4	26.3	22.1
2	94	146.3
0	285.7	333.0

* (Adapted from Kim 2003)

Modified BPP: Sometimes a modified biophysical profile is performed. Rather than looking for fetal tone, movement, and breathing with the ultrasound, an NST and AFI are done. If the NST is reactive and the AFI is > 5 cm, then the test is normal and reassuring. If the NST is not reactive, or the AFI is < 5 cm, then a full BPP is done as a follow-up test.

References:

Amnioinfusion does not prevent meconium aspiration syndrome. ACOG Committee Opinion #346, October 2006.

Antepartum fetal surveillance. ACOG Practice Bulletin #9, October 1999.

Bishop EH. Fetal acceleration test. Am J Obstet Gynecol, 1981; 141:905-909.

DeRosa J, Anderle LJ. External cephalic version of term singleton breech presentations with tocolysis: a retrospective study in a community hospital. J Am Osteopath Assoc 1991; 91(4):351-352, 355-357.

Doubilet PM, Benson CB, Nadel AS, et al. Improved birth weight table for neonates developed from gestations dated by early ultrasonography. J Ultrasound Med 1997; 16:241.

External cephalic version. ACOG Practice Bulletin #13, Feb 2000.

Fetal Heart Rate Patterns: Monitoring, Interpretation, and Management. ACOG Technical Bulletin #207, July 1995.

Freeman RK, Anderson G, Dorchester W. A prospective multi-institutional study of antepartum fetal heart rate monitoring. I. Risk of perinatal mortality and morbidity according to antepartum fetal heart rate test results. Am J Obstet Gynecol, 1982; 143:771-777.

Hofmeyr GJ. External cephalic version. Up To Date, version 11.2, Apr 2003.

Hofmeyr GJ. Amnioinfusion for umbilical cord compression in labour. Cochrane Database Syst Rev 2000: CD000013.

Hofmeyr GJ, Kulier R. External cephalic version for breech presentation at term (Cochrane Review). In: The Cochrane Library, Issue 4, 2002. Oxford: Update Software.

Hofmyer GJ. Prophylactic versus therapeutic amnioinfusion for oligohydramnios in labour. Cochrane Database Syst Rev 2000; CD000176.

Honest H, Bachmann LM, Gupta JK, Kleijen J, Khan KS. Accuracy of cervicovaginal fetal fibronectin in predicting risk of spontaneous preterm birth: systematic review. BJOG, 2002; 325:301.

Iams JK. Prediction and early detection of preterm labor. Obstet Gynecol 2003; 101(2):402-412.

Intrapartum Fetal Heart Rate Monitoring. ACOG Practice Bulletin #70, Dec 2005.

Kim SY, Khandelwal M, Gaughan JP, Agar MH, Reece EA. Is the intrapartum biophysical profile useful? Obstet Gynecol, Sept 2003; 102:471-476.

Lydon-Rochelle M, Albers L, Gorwoda J, Craig E, Qualls C. Accuracy of Leopold maneuvers in screening for malpresentation: A prospective study. Birth, Sept 1993; 20:132-135.

McGregor JA, McFarren T. Neonatal cranial osteomyelitis: A complication of fetal monitoring. Obstet Gynecol Mar 1989; 73(3 Pt 2):490-492.

Pitt C, Sanchez-Ramos L, Kaunitz AM, Gaudier F. Prophylactic amnioinfusion for intrapartum oligohydramnios: A meta-analysis of randomized controlled trials. Obstet Gynecol, Nov 2000; 96(5) Pt. 2:861-866.

Roman AS, Rebarber A, Sfakianaki AK, Mulholland J, Saltzman D, Paidas MJ, Minior V, Lockwood CJ. Vaginal fetal fibronectin as a predictor of spontaneous preterm delivery in the patient with cervical cerclage. Am J Obstet Gynecol, Nov 2003; 189(5): 1368-1373.

Wenstrom K, Andrews WW, Maher JE. Amnioinfusion survey: Prevalence protocols and complications. Obstet Gynecol, Oct 1995; 86(4 Pt 1):572-576.

Williams Obstetrics, 21st edition. Cunningham GF and Gant NF et al. eds. McGraw-Hill, New York, 2001, pg 134.

Xu H, Hofmeyr J, Roy C, Fraser W. Intrapartum amnioinfusion for meconium-stained amniotic fluid: a systematic review of randomized controlled trials. BJOG 2007; 114:383-390.

Yam J, Chua S, Arulkumaran S. Intrapartum Fetal Pulse Oximetry. Part 1: Principles and technical issues. Obstet and Gynecol Survey Mar 2000; 55(3):163-172.

Yam J, Chua S, Arulkumaran S. Intrapartum Fetal Pulse Oximetry. Part 2: Clinical application. Obstet and Gynecol Survey Mar 2000; 55(3):173-183.

Chapter 3

Fetal Heart Rate Monitoring

- Use of Fetal Heart Rate Monitoring
- Basics of Fetal Heart Rate Monitoring
- Indications for Fetal Heart Rate Monitoring
- Interpretation of Fetal Heart Rate Tracings and Interventions
    - Describing the Fetal Heart Rate Tracing
    - Intervention for Nonreassuring Fetal Heart Rate Tracings/
      Decelerations
    - NICHD Workshop Report on Electronic Fetal Monitoring

Use of FHR Monitoring

In an attempt to evaluate fetal well-being both during labor and in the antepartum period, there are several tests that may be performed. The fetal heart rate (FHR) can be monitored externally with Doppler ultrasound, or a traditional abdominal ultrasound can be used to look at other parameters, including the amount of amniotic fluid that is present, to assess the fetus. The most common tests utilized are the nonstress test (NST) and the biophysical profile (BPP), and both of these are defined and explained in Chapter 2, "Common Exams and Procedures."

Continuous fetal heart rate (FHR) monitoring has been in use since the 1970s. During labor, the fetal heart rate is monitored, usually in a continuous manner, with Doppler ultrasound technology, which produces a tracing of the fetal heart rate. The FHR tracing must be closely monitored and evaluated on a regular basis for signs of fetal distress or compromise. While much of fetal heart rate tracing interpretation is pattern recognition, understanding the underlying physiology will allow you to make appropriate and timely interventions to ensure the best outcome for the fetus.

Basics of FHR Monitoring

The FHR is usually recorded in a continuous manner with Doppler ultrasound technology onto standard FHR tracing paper, which can be seen in figure 3-1. This recording paper generally moves at 3 cm/minute. This means that each small block represents 10 seconds, and each large block one minute as demonstrated again in figure 3-1. The top section of the paper is where the FHR is recorded, and the rate is identified by a scale on the paper and ranges from 30 to 240 beats per minute (BPM). The bottom portion of the recording paper is where contractions are recorded. It also has a scale that runs from 0 to 100 mm Hg. This indicates both the timing and magnitude of uterine contractions. (It is important to realize that only an intrauterine pressure catheter [IUPC] can give a real measurement of the strength of contractions. If external monitors are used to trace contractions, then you cannot comment on their strength, only how often they are occurring. This is discussed in more detail later.)

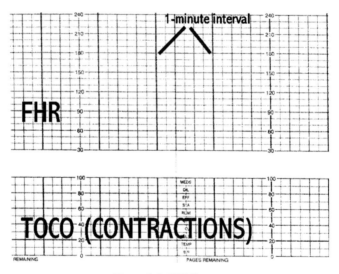

Figure 3-1 FHRT paper

Indications for FHR Monitoring

Antepartum: Testing of the fetus in the antepartum period is done for a multitude of reasons. Some of these include maternal diabetes, multiple gestations, maternal hypertension, and intrauterine growth restriction to name a few. Generally, any condition, maternal or fetal, that places the fetus at increased risk for complications is an indication for antepartum testing. The most commonly performed tests to accomplish this are the nonstress test, biophysical profile, and amniotic fluid index. Because we are focusing on the management of labor and delivery, this text will not go into depth of indications or frequency of antepartum monitoring, but each of these tests is discussed in Chapter 2 in reference to how they are used on labor and delivery.

Intrapartum (during labor): When patients are admitted in labor, FHR monitoring is initiated. Careful evaluation of the initial fetal heart rate tracing (FHRT) is important as one study demonstrated that 50% of all fetuses who eventually required a cesarean delivery for fetal distress could be identified by the first 30 minutes of electronic fetal monitoring (Ingemarsson 1986).

During the first and second stages of labor, the FHR is usually monitored continuously although if a patient desires, they may have intermittent monitoring performed. Intermittent monitoring, when a 1:1 nurse-to-patient ratio is possible, is acceptable in low-risk patients, but ACOG now recommends that those pregnancies with "high-risk conditions" such as fetal growth restriction, preeclampsia, and type 1 diabetes should be continuously monitored during labor (ACOG 2005). Studies between the two types of monitoring have not demonstrated any difference in the risk of cerebral palsy (Thacker 2001). The following are current guidelines for evaluating the FHR during labor:

	High-risk pregnancy	Low-risk pregnancy
1st stage (active labor)	every 15 minutes	every 30 minutes
2nd stage	every 5 minutes	every 15 minutes (ACOG 2005)

When the intermittent auscultation method is used, the FHR should be auscultated/recorded after a contraction for 60 seconds at the time intervals specified above. If at any time during intermittent monitoring the FHR becomes concerning or nonreassuring, then continuous monitoring is usually started and interventions are taken as indicated.

Periodic assessments of the FHRT should be entered into the medical record during labor. See the sample notes for this in Appendix B.

Interpretation of FHR Tracings and Interventions

Describing the Fetal Heart Rate Tracing:

When evaluating an FHR tracing, it is important to have a systematic approach in order to avoid omitting key information either verbally or in the written record. The critical elements to describe are:

1) Identify the patient
2) Internal or external monitors
3) Uterine contractions
4) Baseline FHR
5) Describe FHR variability
6) Presence/absence of accelerations
7) Presence/absence of decelerations (describe any present)
8) Changes or trends of FHR patterns over time
9) Decision and interventions

Each of these elements is discussed in detail in the following sections.

1. **Identify the Patient:** Make sure the fetal heart rate tracing belongs to the appropriate patient. There is nothing worse than looking at the wrong patient's FHRT and making a management decision based on this.
2. **Internal or External monitors:** This is important to note for several reasons. First, short-term variability cannot be evaluated as well with external monitors, and if the FHRT is not reassuring, then internal monitors should be placed. Second, the adequacy of contractions cannot be determined based on external tocodynamometer measurements. Only an IUPC will give actual intrauterine pressure readings, which is helpful when determining if a patient is having strong enough contractions and meets criteria for arrest of dilation.
3. **Contractions:** Comment of the contraction pattern. Is it regular with contractions Q3-4 minutes, or irregular with only 4 contractions an hour? If an IUPC is in place, how many Montevideo units are present? (See Chapter 2 for how to calculate these.) Is there evidence of uterine hyperstimulation present which is defined as any of the following:

    -   A persistent pattern of more than 5 contractions in 10 minutes (averaged over 30 minutes)
    -   Contractions lasting 2 minutes or more
    -   Contractions of normal duration within 1 minute of each other
                                                              (ACOG 1995b)

    Also mention the baseline uterine tone if an IUPC is in place. This will usually be less than 20 mmHg. An elevated resting tone may mean that the uterus is not completely relaxing between contractions or that the dose of oxytocin is too high.

4. **FHR baseline:** This is the average FHR rounded to 5 bpm during a 10-minute tracing. A normal FHR is between 110-160 bpm in the term fetus. If the average FHR changes for > 10 minutes then this is the new baseline and not just an acceleration or deceleration.

Tachycardia is defined as a baseline of > 160 bpm. It is further divided into mild tachycardia (161-180 bpm) and severe tachycardia (>= 181 bpm). Tachycardia may be due to maternal fever, cardiac arrhythmias, intrauterine infection, administration of medications such as terbutaline, and/or fetal distress.

Bradycardia is defined as a baseline FHR of < 110 bpm. It is important to recognize, though, that a baseline FHR of 100-110 is sometimes termed a "relative" bradycardia, and as long as there is good variability and no significant decelerations, a normal fetus will tolerate this baseline without problems.

5. **Variability:** Variability of the fetal heart rate baseline refers to fluctuations in the FHR of two cycles per minute or greater and is due to the fetus's sympathetic/parasympathetic nervous system. Its presence reflects adequate oxygenation and a neurologically intact fetus. A decrease or absence of variability is very concerning and must be evaluated. (Of note, in the past, description of FHR variability was broken down into short-term and long-term components, but this is no longer done.)

    While external fetal monitoring provides a reasonable picture of the FHR variability, it is still best evaluated with an internal monitor (fetal scalp electrode—FSE) which is essentially a fetal electrocardiogram. If there is a question about a FHRT and prolonged periods of absent or minimal variability, then you should consider placing an FSE to evaluate further. (See Chapter 2 for more information on an FSE.) Variability, when present, is very reassuring and very concerning when absent or decreased. The basic definitions applied to baseline variability are listed below:

    - absent : undetectable
    - minimal : <= 5 bpm
    - moderate : 6-25 bpm
    - marked : >25 bpm
                    (ACOG 2005)

Factors that can affect short-term variability include the following:

Increase	Decrease
Fetal breathing	Narcotics/barbiturates/general anesthesia
Fetal movements	Fetal acidemia
	Maternal acidemia
	Fetal sleep cycle
	Magnesium sulfate

Figure 3-2a-b demonstrates examples of minimal and moderate FHR variability.

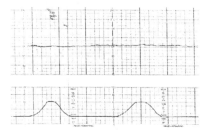
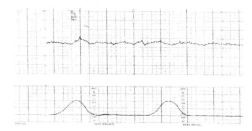

Figure 3-2a Minimal FHR variability   Figure 3-2b Moderate FHR variability

6. **Accelerations:** When the fetal heart rate demonstrates intermittent, abrupt elevations, these are called accelerations. These usually demonstrate a rapid increase from baseline (< 30 seconds from onset to peak) and, when present, are very reassuring and fetal distress or acidemia is very rare. (Note: For a Nonstress test [NST], accelerations must be at least 15 seconds in duration and increase by at least 15 bpm from the baseline to be considered adequate unless the patient is less than 32 weeks gestation at which time a 10 bpm increase for 10 seconds is acceptable.) If the acceleration lasts ≥ 2 minutes it is called a prolonged acceleration. If the increase in the FHR lasts for ≥10 minutes, then this is considered a change in baseline and not an acceleration.

7. **Decelerations:** Decelerations are a common occurrence during labor. It is important to recognize the different types as they have different etiologies and are treated differently. In general, most decelerations last less than one minute. If a deceleration lasts for ≥2 minutes, then it is defined as a prolonged deceleration, which is always something that must be investigated. If the deceleration lasts ≥10 minutes then it is considered a change in baseline and if this baseline is less than 110 bpm, then it is a bradycardia and not a deceleration. The types of decelerations that can occur include early decelerations, variable decelerations, and late decelerations.

   Early decelerations: These are generally the result of fetal head compression. They FHR begins to decrease with the start of a contraction, reaches its lowest point at the peak of the contraction, and then recovers back to normal by the end of the contraction. (See figure 3-3) These decelerations rarely fall more than 30 bpm below the baseline, and are common during active labor. They are not indicative of fetal compromise and do not require intervention. However, if there is any question that the decelerations are actually late decelerations, which are discussed later in this chapter, then internal monitors should be placed.

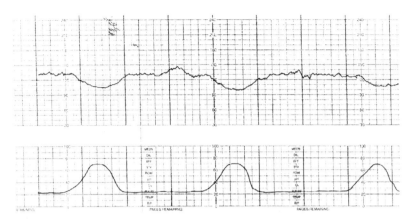

Figure 3-3 Early decelerations

Variable decelerations: Variable decelerations are the most common type of deceleration seen during labor. They appear as abrupt decreases in the FHR from its baseline and are often accompanied by a small acceleration just before and afterward, which are referred to as shoulders. (See figure 3-4) They are a result of cord compression with decreased blood flow to the fetus, usually as a result of uterine contractions. A more urgent cause of variable decelerations is umbilical cord prolapse which is an emergent situation. (This is discussed later in the chapter and in Chapter 14.) Variable decelerations are often associated with contractions, but unlike early decelerations, they do not necessarily begin or end exactly with the contraction. In general, these are a common occurrence and not associated with poor fetal outcome. However, if these decelerations become repetitive (occurring with ≥50% of contractions) and/or prolonged, they can be indicative of fetal compromise. If there are variable decelerations present with less than 50% of contractions, then these are called intermittent variable decelerations.

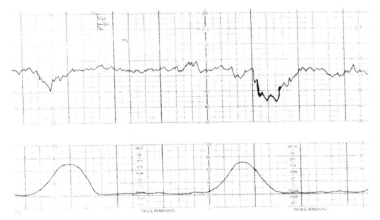

Figure 3-4 Variable decelerations

Other characteristics of variable decelerations that can make them nonreassuring include:

- Slow return to baseline after a contraction
- Decreased variability
- Lack of accelerations
- Tachycardia after decelerations
- Repetitive nature (occurring with ≥50% contractions)
- Duration ≥2 minutes (prolonged decelerations)

If variable decelerations become repetitive and significant with any of the above signs, then intervention should be made to correct the cord compression.

Late decelerations: Late decelerations are similar to early decelerations in appearance in that there is usually a smooth decline (usually ≥ 30 seconds from onset to nadir) in the FHR and a smooth, gradual recovery. What is different is the timing of the deceleration. Late decelerations always begin after the peak of the contraction, and do not recover until after the contraction is over. (See figure 3-5A)

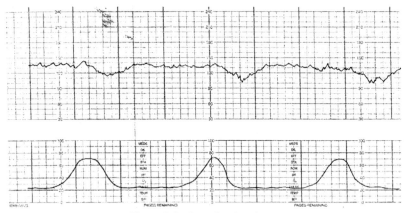

Figure 3-5a Late decelerations

Unlike variable decelerations, the drop in the FHR is usually only 10-20 bpm. These decelerations are the result of uteroplacental insufficiency, which is most commonly caused by either uterine hyperstimulation or maternal hypotension after conduction anesthesia. Other diseases that result in poor placental perfusion, such as hypertension, preeclampsia, or diabetes can also cause late decelerations.

While not often discussed, there are two forms of late decelerations: reflex late decelerations and nonreflex late decelerations. The difference between these is that reflex late decelerations are seen because of a CNS reflex to hypoxia that causes the late deceleration whereas nonreflex late decelerations are a result of a more severe tissue metabolic acidosis and cardiac depression. These have different appearances because reflex late decelerations will generally retain some degree of beat-to-beat variability, and nonreflex late decelerations will not. (See figure 3-5B) Both types of late decelerations are nonreassuring, but the nonreflex late decelerations are even more concerning.

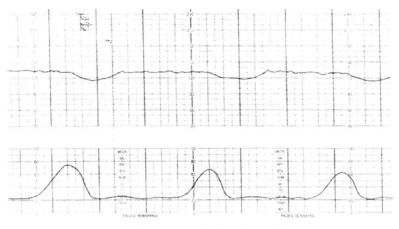

Figure 3-5b Non-reflex late decelerations

While intermittent late decelerations can occur during normal labor, when they occur with most contractions, they are extremely concerning, and intervention must be made to improve uteroplacental blood flow. These interventions are discussed in the next section.

8. **Changes or trends of FHR patterns over time:** Describe how the FHRT has appeared over the time the fetus has been on the monitor. Things that are important to consider are changes in baseline, trends in the FHR variability and any significant changes that have occurred in the past hour.

9. **Decision and Intervention as Needed:** After evaluation of the FHRT, you should classify the tracing as either reassuring or nonreassuring. If the FHRT is reassuring, then you can continue with your current management or augment labor if needed. If you have decided that the FHRT is nonreassuring, then you need to correct the underlying problem. What follows are interventions for these common FHRT abnormalities:

- **Decreased beat-to-beat variability**
- **Fetal tachycardia**
- **Variable decelerations**
- **Late decelerations**
- **Prolonged decelerations/Fetal bradycardia**

Make sure that, after any intervention, you document what you did in the patient's chart as well as the fetal response and current plan. (See Appendix B for sample notes for fetal intervention.)

Decreased beat-to-beat variability. If the beat-to-beat variability is significantly decreased, and there are no spontaneous accelerations noted, then additional steps should be taken to ensure the fetus is not in distress.

1. **Ask if narcotics have been administered:** If narcotics were given, these can result in a decrease in beat-to-beat variability and can be monitored in the absence of tachycardia or significant decelerations. Narcotics can also produce a sinusoidal heart rate, which has decreased variability and cycles within 15 bpm of the baseline 2-5 times per minute and looks like a sine wave. (See figure 3-6.) While this is expected in the presence of narcotics, if these have not been given and the pattern persists for > 20 minutes, it can be an ominous finding associated with severe fetal anemia or acidosis and additional testing, such as scalp stimulation, fetal scalp sampling, and delivery is possibly indicated.

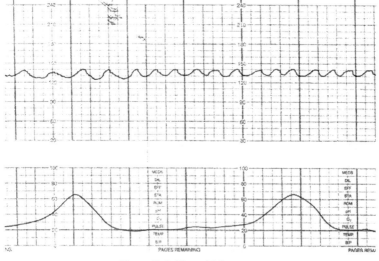

Figure 3-6 Sinusoidal pattern

2. **Turn off Pitocin/oxytocin:** If Pitocin is being administered and the variability is decreased, but without evidence of significant decelerations, then the Pitocin should be stopped and the fetus monitored. If the decreased variability is due to uterine hyperstimulation, then stopping the Pitocin should help to correct

this. If uterine hyperstimulation (see previous definition) is present in the face of significant decelerations, then medications, usually terbutaline, can be given to stop the contractions for a short period of time.

3. **Administer maternal O$_2$:** By administering additional O$_2$ to the mother by a tight-fitting face mask at 8-10 L/min, you will increase the oxygen delivery to the fetus and can help to correct any fetal hypoxia.

4. **Change maternal position:** Changing the maternal position may allow for improved oxygenation of the fetus if cord compression is present. If the patient is supine, then moving her to either side is appropriate. If she is on her left side, have her turn to the other side.

5. **Correct maternal hypotension:** If the mother is hypotensive, especially after an epidural or spinal anesthesia, then correct this with a bolus of intravenous crystalloid (lactated Ringer's or normal saline, 1,000 cc) or by administering ephedrine 2.5-10 mg IV or IM (ACOG 1995a).

6. **Place an FSE:** If the membranes are intact and the fetus is low enough that the membranes can be ruptured, then rupturing the membranes and placing an FSE will allow for a better assessment of the beat-to-beat variability.

7. **Perform scalp stimulation:** Perform a vaginal exam and stroke the fetal scalp with your fingers. If you see an acceleration of at least 10 bpm or greater after 15 seconds of stimulation, then this is very reassuring, and you can continue to monitor the fetus (Elimian 1997). If you do not see acceleration, and your other interventions have not improved the FHRT, then you can consider proceeding to fetal scalp blood sampling.

8. **Consider delivery:** If the variability is minimal to absent after these interventions, and tachycardia or late decelerations are present, then consideration must be given to immediate delivery of the fetus. The route of delivery depends on how far the patient has advanced in labor. If an operative vaginal delivery cannot be safely performed, then a cesarean section may be necessary. (See Chapter 9, "Operative Vaginal Delivery" and Chapter 10, "Cesarean Delivery")

Tachycardia: Common reasons for fetal tachycardia, as well as the interventions required, include the following:

> **Maternal fever:** If the mother is febrile, then the source of the fever should be found. Often in labor, this will be the result of chorioamnionitis. (See Chapter 14) Once the source of the infection is found, then appropriate antibiotics should be started and acetaminophen given to decrease the maternal temperature. Resolution of the fever will usually result in resolution of the tachycardia.

Medications: Terbutaline, given as an intervention for uterine hyperstimulation, and ephedrine, given to correct hypotension from conduction anesthesia, are probably the most common medications that cause fetal tachycardia during labor. If these have been given recently and tachycardia is present, then the fetus may simply be monitored, and as long as significant decelerations are not present, no other intervention is needed.

Fetal Distress: If the tachycardia persists without other identifiable causes, such as chorioamnionitis or medications as mentioned above, is severe (> 180 bpm), or is associated with decreased beat-to-beat variability or significant decelerations (variable or late), then delivery may be required.

Cardiac arrhythmias: Fetal arrhythmias are an uncommon cause of fetal tachycardia, and often appear on the FHRT as intermittent spiking. (See figure 3-7) When these are present, they are usually not a problem in labor and no intervention is required if the FHRT is otherwise reassuring. If they interfere significantly with the interpretation of the FHRT, then a detailed ultrasound echocardiogram of the fetal heart may be indicated if it has not been done previously.

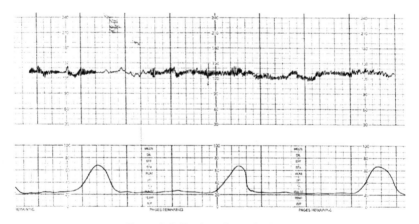

Figure 3-7 Fetal cardiac arrhythmia

Variable decelerations: Because variable decelerations are due to cord compression, the interventions taken to resolve them aim to correct this problem and are indicated when they become recurrent or prolonged in nature. While what follows is a basic algorithm that can be used, note that some of these interventions will occur at the same time. For instance, when you enter the room, you can ask the nurse to turn off the Pitocin, give the patient oxygen by face mask, and cycle the blood pressure cuff while you put on a glove to examine the patient.

1. **Turn off Pitocin/oxytocin:** If pitocin is being administered then it should be stopped as the contractions it causes may be compressing the umbilical cord. When there are significant variable decelerations, especially in the face of uterine hyperstimulation, this should be your first intervention.

2. **Change maternal position:** Changing the maternal position may allow for improved oxygenation of the fetus if cord compression is present. If the patient is supine, then moving her to either side is appropriate. If she is on her side, then move her to her other side.

3. **Administer maternal O_2:** By administering additional O_2 to the mother by a tight-fitting face mask at 8-10L/min, you will increase the oxygen delivery to the fetus and can help to correct any fetal hypoxia.

4. **Check blood pressure and correct maternal hypotension:** Have the patient's blood pressure cuff cycled to take a reading upon entering the room. If the mother is hypotensive or has demonstrated a recent significant drop in her mean arterial pressure (MAP), especially after an epidural or spinal anesthesia, then correct this with a bolus of intravenous crystalloid (lactated Ringer's or normal saline, 1,000 cc) or by administering ephedrine 2.5-10 mg IV or IM. Correcting this is important because, with maternal hypotension, the fetus is less able to tolerate umbilical cord compression with contractions.

5. **Perform vaginal exam:** A vaginal exam will quickly allow you to rule out a prolapsed umbilical cord that can result in significant variable decelerations due to cord compression. If a prolapsed cord is present, you will usually feel a pulsating section of the umbilical cord ahead of the presenting part of the fetus. This complication requires emergency delivery and is discussed in Chapter 14.

   The vaginal exam also allows you to determine if the patient's labor is progressing. Sometimes rapid descent of the fetus through the birth canal will result in variable decelerations or even a prolonged deceleration.

6. **Place an FSE:** If the membranes are intact and the fetus is low enough that the membranes can be ruptured, then rupturing the membranes and placement of an FSE will allow for a better assessment of the beat-to-beat variability.

7. **Place an IUPC:** Placement of an IUPC will allow you to determine the timing of the contractions and the decelerations more accurately.

8. **Give terbutaline:** Administering terbutaline 0.25 mg IV/SQ will decrease contractions for a short period of time, which will hopefully decrease the cord compression that is causing the variable decelerations. (Note: Giving terbutaline IV will result in a much quicker results than SQ. i.e., seconds rather than minutes.)

9. **Consider amnioinfusion:** If the decelerations are not repetitive and prolonged and urgent delivery is not required, then an amnioinfusion can be performed which will provide increased fluid around the fetus and decrease the amount of cord compression that occurs with contractions.

10. **Consider delivery if no resolution:** If the patient continues to have significant, repetitive variable decelerations despite intervention, then delivery will need to be accomplished, especially if a prolonged deceleration or bradycardia develops. If the fetus is low enough in the pelvis and meets criteria for an operative vaginal delivery, this may be done. (See Chapter 9) If not, then an urgent cesarean delivery is performed. (See Chapter 10)

Late Decelerations: Because late decelerations are a result of uteroplacental insufficiency, the interventions taken are meant to correct this issue. The interventions are very similar to those taken for variable decelerations with some small differences, most notably that an amnioinfusion will not help to improve blood flow to the fetus.

- **Turn off Pitocin**
- **Change maternal position**
- **Administer maternal O2**
- **Check blood pressure and correct maternal hypotension**
- **Perform vaginal exam**
- **Place an FSE**
- **Place an IUPC**
- **Give terbutaline if evidence of uterine hyperstimulation**
- **Consider delivery if no resolution**

Prolonged Deceleration or Fetal Bradycardia: When a prolonged deceleration or significant bradycardia develops, immediate intervention is required to resuscitate the fetus. Keep in mind that as you are attempting these actions to resuscitate the baby, you must keep track of how long the deceleration has lasted and make plans for an emergent delivery if the fetus does not recover. The time limits in the following algorithm are estimates of when preparation for emergent delivery should be considered and performed.

Upon entering the room, ask the nurse to do the following:

- Turn off Pitocin
- Administer maternal O2
- Check blood pressure and correct maternal hypotension

Put sterile glove on and:

- perform vaginal exam (rule out a prolapsed umbilical cord)
- place an FSE

After vaginal exam:

Change maternal position: Changing the maternal position may allow for improved oxygenation of the fetus if cord compression is present. If the patient is supine, then moving her to either side is appropriate. If she is on her side, then move her to her other side. If this does not resolve the deceleration, then have the patient move to the "knee-chest position" with her head on a pillow at the head of the bed. (This is often difficult or impossible with a dense epidural block, so keep in mind how much motor control your patient actually has.)

Place the bed in Trendelenburg. Most labor and delivery beds have a mechanism by which the head of the bed can be lowered. This is done in an attempt to move the fetus and resolve any compression of the cord that could be causing the deceleration. After this, proceed by the following algorithm:

Prolonged Deceleration/Fetal Bradycardia

- Turn off Pitocin
- Administer maternal O2 and change maternal position
- Check blood pressure
- Vaginal examination and place FSE

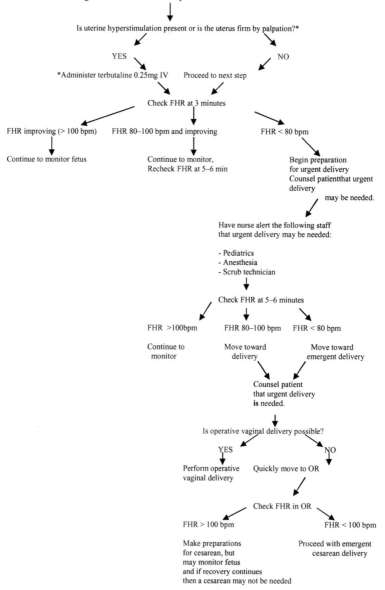

Is uterine hyperstimulation present or is the uterus firm by palpation?*

YES   NO

*Administer terbutaline 0.25mg IV   Proceed to next step

Check FHR at 3 minutes

FHR improving (> 100 bpm)   FHR 80–100 bpm and improving   FHR < 80 bpm

Continue to monitor fetus   Continue to monitor, Recheck FHR at 5–6 min   Begin preparation for urgent delivery Counsel patientthat urgent delivery may be needed.

Have nurse alert the following staff that urgent delivery may be needed:

- Pediatrics
- Anesthesia
- Scrub technician

Check FHR at 5–6 minutes

FHR >100bpm   FHR 80–100 bpm   FHR < 80 bpm

Continue to monitor   Move toward delivery   Move toward emergent delivery

Counsel patient that urgent delivery **is** needed.

Is operative vaginal delivery possible?

YES   NO

Perform operative vaginal delivery   Quickly move to OR

Check FHR in OR

FHR > 100 bpm   FHR < 100 bpm

Make preparations for cesarean, but may monitor fetus and if recovery continues then a cesarean may not be needed   Proceed with emergent cesarean delivery

*   Note: If there is any concern that the decelerations are related to contractions, then terbutaline should be given.

It is important to recognize that intrapartum fetal monitoring has a very high false-positive rate, reported to be between 63% and 99%, which means that you will often be intervening for presumed fetal distress when there is none (Kim 2003). This is not a reason to not take appropriate action when fetal distress or decelerations appear to be present, but rather so that you understand why the fetal outcome is almost always good even when a tracing appears concerning.

NICHD Workshop Report on Electronic Fetal Monitoring:

Recently, the National Institute of Child Health and Human Development Workshop met and published a report on their recommendations for electronic fetal monitoring (Macones, 2008). The guidelines they put forth may well be accepted and integrated into clinical practice in the near future. They are important to be aware of as communication about FHR tracings is central to good management of all laboring patients.

For the most part, the NICHD did not make many changes with regards to the definitions already discussed in this chapter. They do, however, discuss the use of a three-tiered system for categorizing the FHRT. Potential changes from their recommendations include the following:

- No longer using the term "uterine hyperstimulation" and replacing this with "tachysystole" defined as > 5 contractions in 10 minutes averaged over a 30 minute window.
- Use of a three-tiered system as described in Table 10-1.

Table 10-1: Three-Tier Fetal Heart Rate Interpretation System

Category I: Considered reassuring and strongly predictive of normal fetal acid-base status. No specific interventions required.

- Must include ALL of the following:

  o FHR baseline between 110-160bpm
  o Moderate FHR variability
  o No late or variable decelerations

- May or May NOT include either of the following:

  o Early decelerations
  o Accelerations

Category II: Includes all FHR tracings that are not categorized as Category I or III. Require evaluation, continued surveillance and potential intervention.

- Baseline FHR with

  o Bradycardia (< 110bpm with at least minimal variability)
  o Tachycardia (<160bpm)

- FHR Variability with

  o Minimal baseline variability
  o Absent baseline variability without recurrent decelerations
  o Marked baseline variability

- Absence of induced accelerations after fetal stimulation
- Recurrent variable decelerations with minimal or moderate baseline variability
- Prolonged deceleration ≥ 2 minutes but < 10 minutes
- Recurrent late decelerations with moderate baseline variability
- Variable decelerations with other characteristics (i.e. slow return to baseline, reflex tachycardia after the deceleration)

Category III: These FHR tracings are predictive of abnormal fetal acid-base status and require prompt evaluation and intervention.

- Absent FHR variability with any of the following:

  o Recurrent late decelerations
  o Recurrent variable decelerations
  o Bradycardia

- Sinusoidal pattern

References:

ACOG Technical Bulletin #207, July 1995a, Fetal Heart Rate Patterns: Monitoring, Interpretation, and Management.

ACOG Technical Bulletin #215, 1995b, Dystocia and the Augmentation of Labor.

Elimian A, Figueroa R, Tejani N. Intrapartum assessment of fetal well-being: A comparison of scalp stimulation with scalp pH sampling. Obstet Gynecol, Mar 1997; 83(3):373-76.

Ingemarsson I, Arulkumaran S, Ingemarsson E, Tambyraja RL, Ratnam SS. Admission test: a screening test for fetal distress in labor. Obstet Gynecol, 1986; 68:800-806.

Intrapartum Fetal Heart Rate Monitoring, ACOG Practice Bulletin #70, Dec 2005.

Kim SY, Khandelwal M, Gaughan JP, Agar MH, Reece EA. Is the intrapartum biophysical profile useful? Obstet Gynecol, Sept 2003; 102:471-476.

Macones GA, Hankins GDV, Spong CY, Hauth J, Moore T. The 2008 National Institute of Child Health and Human Development Workshop Report on Electronic Fetal Monitoring: Update on definitions, interpretation, and research guidelines. Obstet Gynecol, Sept 2008; 112(3):661-666.

Thacker SB, Stroup DF. Continuous electronic heart rate monitoring versus intermittent auscultation for assessment during labor. In: The Cochrane library, issue 3. Oxford, Update Software, 2001.

Chapter 4

Management of the First Stage of Labor

- Definition and Normal Duration
    - Latent Phase
    - Active Phase
- Labor Triage
    - Triage Decision Analysis
    - Determination of Gestational Age
    - Common Presenting Complaints
        - Decreased Fetal Movement
        - Rule Out Labor
        - Rule Out Ruptured Membranes
        - Rule Out Preeclampsia
- Management of the Latent Phase
    - Prolonged Latent Phase
    - Pain Control
    - Fetal Distress
- Management of the Active Phase
    - Protraction and Arrest Disorders
    - Pain Control
    - Fetal Distress
- Management of Meconium
- Group B Streptococcus Prophylaxis

Definition and Normal Duration

As described in Chapter 2, labor is divided into three stages with the first stage beginning with regular uterine contractions and cervical change (effacement and dilation) and ending when the cervix is completely (100%) effaced and dilated (10 cm). This is the longest stage of labor and often requires some intervention from the physician either to provide analgesia or to augment the progress of labor. The first stage of labor is further divided into a latent and active phase.

Latent Phase

The latent phase of labor begins with regular uterine contractions and cervical dilation and lasts until the cervix is dilated to at least 3-4 cm and almost completely effaced. The length of this stage differs between primiparous and multiparous patients. In the classic paper on this subject by Friedman, the average lengths of the latent phase of labor were reported as:

	Normal	*Prolonged*
Nullipara:	6.4 hrs (+/- 5.1hrs)	>20 hrs
Multipara:	4.8 hrs (+/- 4.9hrs)	>14 hrs

(Friedman 1978)

These definitions are helpful in determining who needs to be admitted to the hospital, which patients can be allowed to go home, which patients may require labor augmentation, and how to counsel patients as to how long they can expect this part of labor to last.*

* (It is important to note that patients who undergo induction of labor will not necessarily follow the same timeline as many will require cervical ripening, which is discussed in Chapter 7.)

Active Phase

The active phase of the first stage of labor begins when the cervix is dilated 3-4 cm and the cervix almost completely effaced. It is typically much shorter in duration than the latent phase. The original work by Friedman has been reevaluated recently, and the average duration of the active phase for both nulliparous and multiparous women is listed below in both a normal population of spontaneously laboring patients (Albers 1996) and in patients undergoing labor induction with an unfavorable cervix (Rinehart 2000):

	Spontaneous Labor		Induction of labor w/ unfavorable cervix
	(Friedman 1978)	*(Albers 1996)*	*(Rinehart 2000)*
Nullipara:	4.6 hrs (+/- 3.6)	7.7 hrs (+/-5.9)	10.3 hrs (+/- 8.0)
Multipara:	2.4 hrs (+/- 2.2)	5.7 hrs (+/-4.0)	7.0 hrs (+/- 6.0)

This is important only in that it appears this phase of labor lasts longer than was previously thought, especially in patients undergoing induction of labor. The American

College of Obstetricians and Gynecologists (ACOG) has published guidelines on how they define abnormal labor patterns and duration, and these are discussed later in the chapter.

Labor Triage

The triage rooms on labor and delivery are usually where patients are first seen and evaluated and a determination is made as to whether or not they require admission to the hospital. Learning to triage patients quickly and appropriately is a valuable skill that is essential to managing laboring patients.

Triage Decision Analysis. When you see patients on labor and delivery, you will eventually take one of three courses of action. The first is to admit the patient for labor or another indication, the second is to perform further monitoring or workup to ensure the mother and fetus are not in distress, and the third is to discharge the patient to home. A diagram of basic triage decisions is presented below:

Triage Decision Analysis:

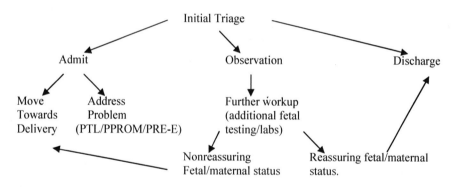

Determination of Gestational Age. One of the most important and crucial things you can do on labor and delivery is to determine the patient's gestational age as accurately as possible. This has implications in both the preterm and term fetus with regard to your management. While most patients who present to labor and delivery will have had prenatal care and an accurate due date, you will, unfortunately, encounter patients who present late in pregnancy with little or no prenatal care and very unsure dates. Knowing how to correctly date a pregnancy will also assist you in deciding on the most accurate gestational age.

One pitfall to avoid, especially when there are no records available, is using an EDC from an ultrasound as reported by the patient. Many patients will be given a due date in the first trimester and then be told a different date after a second trimester screening ultrasound, which they interpret as their "new" due date. A simple way to determine the patient's gestational age is by the following algorithm.

1. Ask the patient what the first day of her last menstrual period (LMP) was and use this to calculate an initial estimated date of confinement (EDC).* Either a pregnancy wheel, which may be obtained from a medical book store, or Naegele's rule, which calculates the EDC by adding seven days to the LMP and then subtracting three months, can be used to determine the initial EDC.

    (*If the patient has a history of irregular menses, then this method is not considered very accurate and is an indication to have a first trimester ultrasound to establish her EDC.)

2. Ask if the patient had an ultrasound early in her pregnancy. If she did, then compare the EDC from the ultrasound with that based on her LMP and determine how different they are. In general, the following rules apply:

    -   If the EDC is off by > 5 days from a first trimester sonogram, change the dates to agree with the ultrasound.
    -   If the EDC is off by > 10 days from a second trimester sonogram, change the dates to agree with the ultrasound.
    -   If there are no ultrasound examinations, but the patient has a sure LMP, use this to determine the EDC.
    -   If the patient has irregular menses and has not had an ultrasound, perform an ultrasound and use the EDC from this.

The important thing to remember is that, once the dates are set by a first trimester ultrasound, they are not changed based on later ultrasounds! The most accurate dating possible is a sonogram between 6-12 weeks that measures the crown-rump length of the fetus.

Common Presenting Complaints. While patients will present with a wide variety of complaints, what follows are some of the more common presenting complaints that patients have when they come for evaluation.

Decreased Fetal Movement. Many patients, especially near term, will present with a complaint of decreased fetal movement. This may be either a subjective decrease in overall movement, or they may not have been able to get 10 kicks/movements in an hour as they were instructed to check for. (Fetal kick counts involve counting movements any time during the day. They are usually started after 28 weeks, and the patient counts movements until she either reaches 10 movements or an hour passes. If the patient does not feel 10 movements, then this is considered decreased fetal movement.) When this occurs, the following actions should be taken:

1. After establishing the patient's gestational age, ask the four basic questions*:

   a. Are you having any **BLEEDING?**
   b. Are you having any **CONTRACTIONS?** (include time of onset/frequency/ intensity)
   c. Do you feel like you broke your **WATER?** (include time/color of fluid)
   d. When was the last time you felt your baby **MOVING?**

   * (The fourth question is slightly modified as the patient's presenting complaint is decreased movement.)

   If the patient answers yes to any of the first three questions, then these issues must also be addressed during her time on labor and delivery. After asking these questions, proceed to steps 2 and 3.

2. Place the fetus on the monitor and obtain a nonstress test (NST). (See Chapter 2.)
3. Perform an abdominal ultrasound to determine the amniotic fluid index (AFI). (See Chapter 2.)

Interventions. If the patient has a reactive NST and a normal AFI, and is not in labor, she may be reassured that her fetus demonstrates no evidence of distress and then discharged to home to follow up with her regular physician.

If the patient has a nonreassuring fetal heart rate tracing (FHRT), then she should not be discharged until the reason for this is found or she is delivered. There are different levels of fetal distress and additional tests that may be performed and these are discussed in detail in Chapter 3.

If the patient has an AFI of less than 5, then this is classified as oligohydramnios. (See Chapter 14.) If oligohydramnios is present in a term patient, induction or augmentation of labor is usually undertaken. It is also important to note that oligohydramnios may result from spontaneous rupture of membranes with a slow leak that the patient did not notice. Because of this, when oligohydramnios is present, you should perform an examination to rule out ruptured membranes, which is discussed later in this section.

Rule out Labor. This is probably the most common reason that women come to labor and delivery. It is not uncommon, especially for a primigravida, to be evaluated multiple times before they actually go into active labor and are admitted. The following steps are taken to rule out labor:

1. After establishing the patient's gestational age, ask the four basic questions:

   a. Are you having any **BLEEDING?**
   b. How often are you having **CONTRACTIONS?** (include time of onset/frequency/intensity)
   c. Do you feel like you broke you **WATER?** (include time/color of fluid)
   d. When was the last time you felt your baby **MOVING?**

2. Place the fetus on the monitor and obtain a non-stress test (NST). (See Chapter 2.)
3. Perform a digital cervical examination (or a sterile speculum examination if there is a possibility of ruptured membranes.)

   Interventions. The two key things to evaluate when a patient presents for evaluation of possible labor are fetal status and the presence or absence of cervical change. In general, only the patient with a reassuring FHRT who is not in labor will be discharged, while all others will be at least kept for observation.

It is important to realize that the actual cervical dilation or effacement that physicians use to determine if a patient is in labor and requires admission to labor and delivery may vary significantly. It is dependent on both the patient's parity as well as other factors, such as the amount of pain they are experiencing, whether or not they have a history of rapid labor, and how far away they live. Some general guidelines for labor triage are as follows:

- If the patient does not have regular contractions (at least every 5-7 minutes) and is < 3cm dilated, she may be discharged to home with labor precautions. These precautions should include instructions to call back or return if she feels that her membranes rupture, she experiences significant vaginal bleeding, or the contractions become more frequent and painful. If the patient has significant pain, but is not in labor, she may be given medications for the pain to go home with, assuming the fetal status is reassuring. (See Chapter 8.)
- If the patient has regular contractions (at least every 5-7 minutes) and is 2-3 cm dilated, she may be offered the option of walking for 1-2 hours and then

having her cervix checked again to determine if she is progressing in labor. If the patient makes cervical change when rechecked, she is admitted.

(Also, if the patient has a history of rapid labor, is in significant pain, or lives more than 30 minutes from the hospital, it is reasonable to have them walk even if they are only 1-2 cm dilated.)

- If the patient has regular contractions and is > 3cm dilated, she will usually be admitted to labor and delivery.

* (Note: All of these assume a term patient and a reactive NST with no evidence of fetal distress!)

Remember that these are just guidelines and there will be circumstances where patients will be kept for observation or given pain medication for latent labor and monitored to see if they progress in labor.

Rule out Ruptured Membranes. Many women will call labor and delivery and report that they have experienced a large "gush" of fluid. Regardless of their gestational age, the patient should be advised to come in to labor and delivery for evaluation.

1. After establishing the patient's gestational age, ask the four basic questions:

   a. Are you having any **BLEEDING?**
   b. How often are you having **CONTRACTIONS?** (Include time of onset/ frequency/intensity.)
   c. What time do you feel like you broke you **WATER?** (Include color of fluid and if they are continuing to leak fluid.)
   d. When was the last time you felt your baby **MOVING?**

2. After asking these questions, perform a sterile speculum examination and observe the cervical os. There are four different parameters you will observe for during your exam. First, look for evidence of POOLING of amniotic fluid in the vagina as well as for fluid coming from the os as the patient bears down with a VALSALVA maneuver. Obtain a small amount of fluid from the posterior vaginal fornix or lateral sidewall with a sterile cotton swab and smear this on a slide. Allow the slide to dry and then look for evidence of a FERNING pattern. (Ferning will often not appear until the slide is *completely* dry.) Also, place some of the vaginal secretions collected with the swab on NITRAZINE paper to see if the color changes because of an increased vaginal pH, which is seen with amniotic fluid. (This will usually turn nitrazine paper blue.)

False-positive results may occur for the following reasons:

Nitrazine: Contamination with blood, semen, alkaline antiseptics, or bacterial vaginosis (Mercer 2003).

Ferning: Cervical mucus may demonstrate some degree of ferning

False-negative results may occur in the following situations:

Nitrazine/Ferning: Prolonged leakage of a small amount of fluid or minimal fluid present in the vagina.

If the patient has a good history for ruptured membranes, i.e., a large gush of fluid with continuing leakage, but the four tests above are normal, then an ultrasound should be performed. If the amniotic fluid volume is normal (AFI between 5 and 25 at term—see Chapter 2), then ruptured membranes is very unlikely. If, on the other hand, the AFI is low or low-normal (between 5 and 8), then the speculum examination may be repeated after having the patient lie down for several hours. (If this does not confirm or rule-out the diagnosis, then an ultrasound-guided amniocentesis with instillation of indigo carmine [1 mL in 9 mL of sterile saline] may be done with observation for passage of blue fluid from the vagina. This procedure, however, is not generally performed unless there is a very high index of suspicion for ruptured membranes in a preterm patient.)

Interventions

If the patient is term and found to have ruptured membranes, you may perform a digital examination to determine how dilated the cervix is if you could not see this on the speculum examination. If you could see the cervix well, then perform an abdominal ultrasound quickly to confirm that the fetus is in a vertex position and admit the patient to labor and delivery.

If, however, the patient is preterm, especially less than 34 weeks, please refer to the section on PPROM (preterm premature rupture of membranes) in Chapter 14 for a discussion of how to proceed with these patients.

There has been a debate for some time regarding whether or not the term patient with ruptured membranes who is not in labor should undergo labor induction or just conservative monitoring as the majority of term patients will enter labor spontaneously within 24 hours of rupture of membranes. There are now multiple studies, however, that have demonstrated a significant decrease in the risk of both maternal infection (chorioamnionitis and endometritis postpartum) and neonatal NICU admissions and overall morbidity (Hannah 1996; Tan 2000). These studies also did not demonstrate an increase in the risk of cesarean section with induction compared to conservative management. Because of these recommendations, especially in patients who are known to have a positive culture for group B streptococcus (see GBS later in this chapter), admission and induction of labor is recommended.

Make a note in the chart and admission history and physical of the time at which the patient believes the membranes ruptured, as well as the color of the fluid.

Rule out Preeclampsia. Patients may be referred to labor and delivery for evaluation of possible preeclampsia after 20 weeks gestation, or they may call with complaints of worsening edema, a severe headache, or visual disturbances. This is not an uncommon reason to see a patient after a clinic visit where the patient is found to have new onset hypertension. In these cases, the initial approach should be the same, beginning with the standard four questions about bleeding, contractions, ROM, and fetal movement. In addition to these, you should inquire about symptoms that may be associated with preeclampsia. These questions include the following:

a. Are you having any swelling? (Edema is common in preeclampsia but will often be in the upper extremities and the face rather than just in the lower extremities, which may occur with normal pregnancy.)

b. Are you having any headaches? (Severe headaches may be a sign of severe preeclampsia and CNS irritation and should be noted.)

c. Are you experiencing any right upper quadrant pain? (Another possible component of severe preeclampsia is severe right upper quadrant pain from an expanding liver hematoma.)

d. Have you been seeing any flashing lights? (Scotomata is another sign of CNS irritation and possible severe preeclampsia.)

After asking these questions, you should send some basic laboratory tests. These tests include:

- Urinalysis (for evidence of proteinuria) or Urine protein/creatinine ratio
- CBC
- Chemistries (with particular attention to the creatinine)
- Uric acid
- AST/ALT
- LDH

During the time you are waiting for these results, the fetus should be placed on the monitor to obtain an NST and the patient should have serial blood pressure readings taken.

Interventions. Please refer to Chapter 14 for a thorough discussion of the diagnosis of preeclampsia, including risk factors, laboratory results, and management.

Management of the Latent Phase

The latent phase of labor begins with regular uterine contractions and cervical change and ends when the cervix is almost completely effaced and 3 to 4 cm dilated. While many patients will not be admitted until they are in active labor, patients may present with ruptured membranes or be admitted for delivery for other indications while in the latent phase. If the patient progresses in labor and enters the active phase, then no intervention is required. Some patients, however, will not make cervical change over several hours and have a prolonged latent phase of labor.

Prolonged Latent Phase

A prolonged latent phase of labor is defined as >20 hours in nulliparous patients and >14 hours in multiparous patients. This complication occurs in between 4%-6% of labors (Satin 2007). An unfavorable cervix at the onset of labor and epidural anesthesia are risk factors for a prolonged latent phase. While women with a prolonged latent phase are at increased risk of eventual cesarean delivery and longer hospital stays, perinatal mortality does not appear to be affected (Friedman 1978; Chelmow 1993).

When a patient has a prolonged latent phase, then consideration must be given to how best to augment labor. Options for treatment include the following:

- **Therapeutic rest:** This involves administering narcotics to the patient and is discussed in the next section.
- **Amniotomy:** If the patient is a candidate for artificial rupture of membranes (AROM), then this intervention may be performed. It has been shown to decrease the duration of the first stage of labor and is more effective when used in conjunction with oxytocin augmentation (Fraser 2000).
- **Labor augmentation:** The latent phase may be augmented with one of two methods. First, if the cervix is unfavorable, then cervical ripening may be attempted. (See Chapter 7.) If the cervix is favorable, then oxytocin augmentation of labor may be used. Success rates (i.e., getting patients to transition from latent to active labor) of up to 85% have been reported with the use of oxytocin (Friedman 1978). (See Chapter 7.)

You will probably notice that cesarean delivery is not listed as a treatment option for a prolonged latent phase of labor. This is because there is no increase in perinatal mortality associated with a protracted latent phase as long as the fetal status remains reassuring (Satin 2007). In general, a cesarean section in the latent phase should be reserved for fetal distress or other indications such as presentation in labor with a breech fetus or for a repeat cesarean delivery.

Pain Control. When patients present with regular uterine contractions and you determine they are in the latent phase of labor, pain is often a significant concern. Especially in the nulliparous patient experiencing labor for the first time, this early labor can be extremely uncomfortable. Also, when patients are admitted for labor induction and are in the latent phase, contractions from Pitocin or other induction agents can be very painful as well. Options for pain control during the latent phase of labor include narcotics and epidural anesthesia.

Narcotics:. A good rule of thumb when administering narcotics during labor is to ask yourself what the are chances of the patient delivering within 2 hours. (This is where understanding the normal length of labor is important.) If a significant amount of the narcotic is present in the fetal system at the time of delivery, then the infant can be significantly depressed and require resuscitation. This complication, fortunately, rarely occurs with narcotics given in latent labor.*

* For example, the half-life of meperidine is 63 hours in the neonate, which is why it is generally not used for analgesia during labor.

A kind and appropriate intervention for the patient in pain during latent labor who desires relief is to administer narcotics for therapeutic rest. You can reassure the patient that the medication will not stop labor, but will provide them pain relief. One study reported that after therapeutic rest, 85% of women will wake up in active labor, 10% will not be in labor, and 5% will continue to have continued contractions without being in labor (Koontz 1982). Because of their effects on the FHRT, which includes decreased variability, narcotics should only be administered after obtaining reassuring fetal testing, usually in the form of a reactive nonstress test (RNST). If the patient is only in latent labor and fetal testing is reassuring, then the patient can be discharged to home with PO medication for pain if she has not demonstrated cervical change. If, however, PO pain medication has not been successful, or the woman is extremely uncomfortable, they can be given IV medication and monitored on labor and delivery to ensure it is effective. (See Chapter 8 "Obstetric Analgesia/Anesthesia," for doses of narcotics used for therapeutic rest.)

Epidural: This is not the first choice for latent labor as it is may prolong the latent phase. However, there are cases in which this is a reasonable thing to pursue during latent labor. ACOG does not recommend that a woman be required to achieve a certain degree of cervical dilation before an epidural is administered and clarifies that patient comfort is an important consideration. (ACOG 2004). Some indications for an epidural in the latent phase of labor include the following:

- Induction for intrauterine fetal demise (IUFD)
- Inability to control pain with adequate doses of IV/IM narcotics
- Maternal cardiac or CNS conditions for which pain may cause maternal or fetal compromise

Fetal Distress. Whenever a patient is evaluated for labor at the hospital, you must evaluate the FHR tracing. If a patient is in the latent phase of labor and there is fetal distress, the first thing to do is determine the etiology and correct it if possible. (See Chapter 3 "Fetal Heart Rate Monitoring, Intervention" for nonreassuring testing) If you cannot correct the underlying cause, or a nonreassuring FHR tracing persists despite appropriate interventions, the only option for a timely delivery is a cesarean section.

Management of the Active Phase

The active phase of labor begins when the cervix is almost completely effaced and dilated 3-4 cm and ends when the cervix is completely dilated. In contrast to the latent phase of labor, patients in the active phase are expected to make cervical change every hour. If they do not, then they may have either a protraction or arrest disorder, and their labor may require augmentation in an attempt to accomplish a vaginal delivery.

Protraction and Arrest Disorders

The overall incidence of protraction and arrest disorders in the first stage of labor is around 13% (Satin 1992). A protraction disorder simply implies that the patient has continued to make cervical change, just at a much slower rate than anticipated while an arrest disorder means they have ceased to make progress at all.

Protraction disorders. A nulliparous patient has a protracted active phase of labor when they fail to dilate at least 1.2 cm/hr and a multiparous patient if they dilate < 1.5 cm/hr. These rates are two standard deviations below what is normally expected. When this occurs, there are two interventions that may be attempted. These are amniotomy and oxytocin augmentation, which were discussed in the previous section. If a patient has a protracted active phase of labor, you should also consider the placement of an intrauterine pressure catheter to better assess the adequacy of the patient's contractions.

Arrest disorders. A patient is diagnosed with arrest of dilation when they have demonstrated no cervical change for at least 2 hours with adequate uterine contractions.

Adequate uterine contractions are measured with an intrauterine pressure catheter (IUPC) and defined as >200 Montevideo units. If the patient meets these criteria, then a cesarean section may be performed. Part of the reasoning behind performing a cesarean section for an arrest of dilation is the absence of any change over this time period may imply that either the fetus is too large or the patient's pelvis too small to permit a vaginal delivery.

There is, however, recent data that suggests, in the absence of fetal distress, you may wait up to four hours with adequate contractions and no cervical change before performing a cesarean section. When this was done in a trial of over 540 women, 88% of multiparous women and 56% of nulliparous women who had been diagnosed with arrest of dilation went on to have a vaginal delivery (Rouse 1999). In this situation where the fetal status is reassuring, it appears to be reasonable to continue augmentation of labor, especially in multiparous patients who desire to avoid a cesarean delivery.

An algorithm for the management of the active phase of labor can be seen in figure 4-1.

For the indications, contraindications, and standard dose regimens for oxytocin augmentation of labor, please refer to Chapter 7 "Induction and Augmentation of Labor."

Figure 4-1: Labor management—Active phase

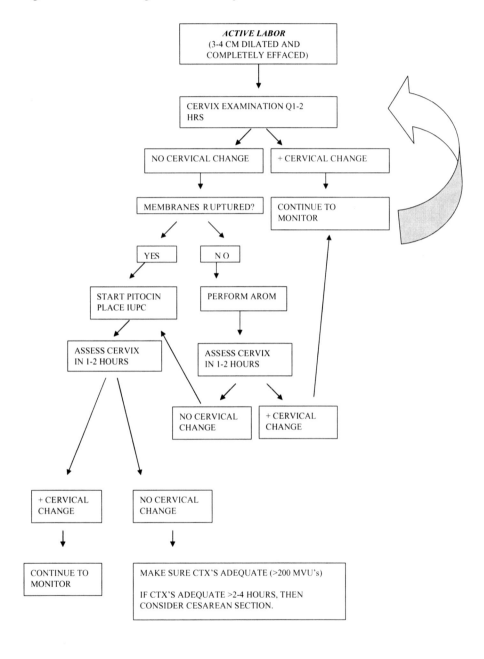

Pain Control. Options for pain control during the active phase of labor are similar to those available during latent labor. The difference is that intravenous narcotics should not be administered if you believe the patient may deliver within the next two hours. For this reason, narcotics are rarely given after a patient reaches approximately 6 cm, and some form of conduction anesthesia (epidural or spinal) is generally the recommended option at this time. (See Chapter 8 "Obstetric Analgesia/Anesthesia.")

Fetal distress. Similar to the latent phase, if fetal distress occurs, you must attempt to determine the reason and correct it if possible. (See Chapter 3.) If you cannot accomplish this in a timely fashion, then you must perform a cesarean delivery as an operative vaginal delivery is not possible during the first stage of labor.

Management of Meconium

Meconium passage prior to birth occurs in approximately 12% of all births (Wiswell 1990). If a patient has meconium in the latent phase of labor, this implies that they have ruptured membranes and will therefore be admitted to labor and delivery. More often, this complication is not seen until the active phase of labor, which is when most patients will spontaneously rupture their membranes.

When noting meconium passage in the chart, you should write both the time it was noted as well as whether it appeared thin, thick, or particulate. (If you see extremely thick meconium, consider the possibility of a breech fetus that is passing meconium directly into the cervix.) It is also very important to notify your pediatricians and whoever will be resuscitating the baby of the timing, presence, and provide a description (thin, thick, particulate, etc.) of the meconium and ensure they are present for the delivery.

While there is some controversy regarding the use of an amnioinfusion when meconium is present during labor in the absence of variable decelerations (which is another common indication for amnioinfusion), there are several trials that have demonstrated a reduction in the rate of meconium aspiration syndrome and fetal distress when an amnioinfusion is performed for patients found to have meconium-stained amniotic fluid as well as a trend toward reduced perinatal mortality (Macri 1992; Pierce 2000; Hofmeyr 2000). The current recommendation from ACOG at this time, however, is to consider an amnioinfusion when there are variable decelerations present, regardless of the presence or absence of meconium (ACOG 2006).

Group B Streptococcus Prophylaxis

Group B streptococcus, or *streptococcus agalactiae*, is an encapsulated gram positive organism that is the most common bacterial pathogen found in newborns. These bacteria can be found in 10%-30% of pregnant women, and because of this, it is important to administer antibiotics during labor to prevent the occurrence of early neonatal sepsis from this organism (Regan 1996). Over the past several years either a strategy of treating patients based on risk factors for GBS (such as gestational age < 37 weeks, ruptured membranes for > 18 hours, or a previously affected baby) or by screening every pregnant patient during the third trimester and treating only those women who had a positive culture was utilized. Recently, though, new guidelines for screening and treating patients for GBS during pregnancy have been published by the Centers for Disease Control and Prevention (CDC) in response to an article that demonstrated routine screening of all patients to be superior (50% more effective) to the risk-factor approach (Schrag 2002). These recommendations include the screening of all pregnant patients between 35 and 37 weeks gestation and the treatment of all patients during labor who have positive cultures. See figure 4-2 for an algorithm for term patients and figure 4-3 for preterm patients.

Figure 4-2. GBS screening and treatment in term patients (all patient should be screened between 35-37 weeks.*)

GBS status at presentation:

	Positive	Negative	Unknown
Treatment:	Treat with antibiotics (See Fig 4-3)	No treatment	No treatment unless any of the following occur: labor at <37 wks; ruptured membranes for > 18 hours; intrapartum temperature of ≥ 100.4°F or ≥ 38.0°C

* Note: If the patient had GBS bacteruria during this pregnancy, or she previously had a child affected by GBS sepsis, then she should be treated with intrapartum antibiotic prophylaxis (IAP) regardless, and a culture is not necessary.

Figure 4-3: GBS screening and treatment in preterm patients (For patients presenting in labor or with PPROM at <37 weeks gestation)

	Unknown GBS	*+ GBS (previous culture) (or + GBS in urine)*	*-GBS culture*
Initial Care:	Obtain culture and start PCN G IV	Start PCN G IV for at least 48 hours.	No prophylaxis
Followup:	If negative culture, stop PCN G.	If undelivered and PTL stops, then stop PCN and treat at delivery.	
	If positive culture, continue for at least 48 hrs		

(Adapted from CDC, 2002)

The first line of antibiotic treatment is penicillin G, with ampicillin being used if this is not available. If the patient is allergic to penicillin, then their allergy should be investigated further, and either a cephalosporin or another antibiotic used. See figure 4-4 for an algorithm to determine what antibiotic to use in the penicillin-allergic patient.

Figure 4-4: GBS antibiotic prophylaxis, choice of antibiotic

	Medication	*Dose*
1st Choice:	Penicillin G	5 million units IV, then 2.5 million units Q4 hrs until delivery
2nd Choice:	Ampicillin	2gm IV, then 1gm IV Q6 hrs until delivery

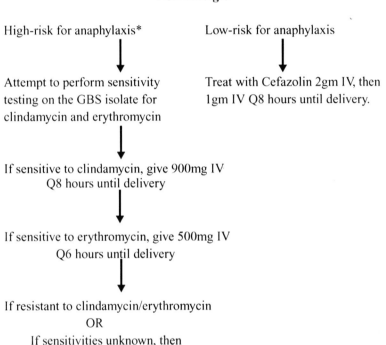

PCN-Allergic

High-risk for anaphylaxis*

Attempt to perform sensitivity testing on the GBS isolate for clindamycin and erythromycin

If sensitive to clindamycin, give 900mg IV Q8 hours until delivery

If sensitive to erythromycin, give 500mg IV Q6 hours until delivery

If resistant to clindamycin/erythromycin
OR
If sensitivities unknown, then

Vancomycin 1gm IV Q12 hours until delivery

Low-risk for anaphylaxis

Treat with Cefazolin 2gm IV, then 1gm IV Q8 hours until delivery.

*Patients at high risk for anaphylaxis are those who have had an anaphylactic reaction to penicillin, asthma, or who are taking a beta-blocker (which can make anaphylaxis very difficult to treat should a reaction occur.)

(Adapted from CDC, 2002)

The goal of antibiotic prophylaxis is to have the patient not deliver for at least four hours after the medication has been administered. At times, this may mean not rupturing a patient's membranes or augmenting labor as aggressively as you might in a GBS-negative patient, especially a multiparous patient who presents in active labor that you expect to deliver quickly.

A positive GBS culture in a previous pregnancy is not an indication for antibiotic prophylaxis during the current pregnancy unless the previous child was infected as well. Also, if a patient has demonstrated GBS in their urine during pregnancy, they should receive antibiotic prophylaxis during labor and screening between 35-37 weeks is not necessary.

It is important to note that antibiotic treatment does not reduce the incidence of late-onset GBS infections, which are those that occur between 7-89 days of life (Schrag 2000). Also, patients who have a planned cesarean delivery and do not labor or have ruptured membranes prior to the procedure, do not require GBS prophylaxis regardless of the GBS cultures.

Currently, there is work being done, as well as clinical trials, to develop a vaccination for GBS. In the near future, these may become available and reduce or obviate the need for patients to receive antibiotic prophylaxis during labor.

References:

Albers LL, Schiff M, Gorwoda JG. The length of active labor in normal pregnancies. Obstet Gynecol 1996; 87:355-359.

Amnioinfusion does not prevent meconium aspiration syndrome. ACOG Committee Opinion #346, October 2006.

Chelmow D, Kilpatrick SJ, Laros RK Jr. Management and neonatal outcomes after prolonged latent phase. Obstet Gynecol 1993; 81:486-491.

Dystocia and the Augmentation of Labor. ACOG Practice Bulletin #49, Dec 2003.

Fraser WK, Turcot L, Krauss I, Brisson-Carrol G. Amniotomy for shortening spontaneous labor. Cochrane Database Syst Rev 2000;:CD000015.

Friedman EA: Labor: Clinical Evaluation and Management. 2nd ed. New York, Appleton-Century-Crofts, 1978.

Hannah ME, Ohlsson A, Farine D, et al. Induction of labor compared with expectant management for prelabor rupture of the membranes at term. TERMPROM Study Group. NEJM 1996; 334:1005.

Hofmeyr GJ. Amnioinfusion for meconium-stained liquor in labour. Cochrane Database Syst Rev 2000; CD000014.

Koontz WL, Bishop EH. Management of the latent phase of labor. Clin Obstet Gynecol 1982; 25:111-114.

Macri CJ, Schrimmer DB, Leung A, et al. Prophylactic amnioinfusion improves outcome of pregnancy complicated by thick meconium and oligohydramnios. Am J Obstet Gynecol 1992; 167:117-121.

Mercer BM. Preterm premature rupture of the membranes. Obstet Gynecol 2003 Jan; 101(1):178-193.

Pain relief during labor. ACOG Committee Opinion #295, July 2004.

Pierce J, Gaudier FL, Sanchez-Ranchez L. Intrapartum amnioinfusion for meconium-stained fluid: meta-analysis of prospective clinical trials. Obstet Gynecol 2000; 95:1051-1056.

Prevention of perinatal group B streptococcal disease: Revised guidelines from CDC. Morbidity and Mortality Weekly Report Aug 2002; 51: No. RR-11.

Regan JA, Klebanoff MA, Nugent RP, et al. Colonization with group B streptococci in pregnancy and adverse outcome. Am J Obstet Gynecol 1996; 174:1354-1360.

Rinehart BK, Terrone DA, Hudson C, Isler CM, Larmon JE, Perry KG Jr. Lack of utility of standard labor curves in the prediction of progression during labor induction. Am J Obstet Gynecol June 2000; 182(6):1520-1526.

Rouse DJ, Owen J, Hauth JC. Active-phase labor arrest: oxytocin augmentation for at least 4 hours. Obstet Gynecol 1999; 93:323-328.

Satin AJ. Prolonged latent phase of labor. Up To Date, Version 16.1, 2008.

Satin AJ, Leveno KJ, Sherman ML, et al. High versus low-dose oxytocin for labor stimulation. Obstet Gynecol 1992; 80:111-116.

Schrag SJ, Zywiki S, Farley MM, et al. Group B streptococcal disease in the era of intrapartum antibiotic prophylaxis. NEJM 2000; 342:15-20.

Schrag SJ, Zell ER, Lynfield R, et al. A population-based comparison of strategies to prevent early-onset group B streptococcal disease in neonates. NEJM 2002; 347:233-239.

Tan BP, Hannah ME. Oxytocin for prelabour rupture of membranes at or near term. Cochrane Database Syst Rev 2000; CD000157.

Wiswell TE, Tuggle JM, Turner BS. Meconium aspiration syndrome: have we made a difference? Pediatrics 1990; 85:715-721.

Chapter 5

Management of the Second Stage Management

- Definition
- Normal Duration
- Management of the Second Stage
    - Fetal Monitoring
    - Anesthesia
    - Pediatric Involvement
    - Pushing
    - Spontaneous Vaginal Delivery
        - Episiotomy
    - Breech Vaginal Delivery
- Potential Second Stage Complications
    - Fetal Distress
    - Labor Dystocia

Definition

The second stage of labor begins when the woman's cervix is completely dilated and completely effaced (usually reported as "complete/complete" or "C/C" in the chart). It is during this stage that the patient will push to deliver the fetus, and it ends with the delivery of the fetus.

Normal duration

The normal duration of the second stage of labor is dependent on whether or not the patient has had a previous vaginal delivery. For nulliparous patients, the duration of the second stage of labor is approximately 50 minutes while it is only 20 minutes for multiparous patients.

Multiple factors can affect the length of the second stage of labor. Some of these include epidural use, fetal and maternal weight, and the station of the fetal head when the patient enters the second stage. ACOG recommends that the second stage should be allowed to progress without operative intervention as long as the FHRT remains reassuring and the fetus demonstrates some descent during pushing until the patient meets criteria for dystocia, which is defined later in this chapter (ACOG 2003). If fetal distress develops during this stage, then an operative intervention, either forceps, vacuum extraction, or a cesarean section, is indicated.

Management of the Second Stage

Fetal Monitoring. While pushing, the FHR is usually monitored in a continuous fashion, with attention to any decelerations and their timing related to contractions. If the patient has been using intermittent monitoring during labor or desires this while pushing, then the FHR must be recorded every 15 minutes after a contraction in a low-risk patient and every 5 minutes after a contraction in any patient considered to be "high-risk"* (ACOG 1995).

*(The term "high-risk" is not well defined, but should include patients with preterm labor, preeclampsia, bleeding, significant maternal medical conditions, or patients whose fetus has demonstrated signs of distress.)

If you have difficulty in monitoring the fetus with external monitors, which often need to be adjusted inferiorly during pushing as the baby descends, then you may place a fetal scalp electrode in order to better assess fetal status. (See Chapter 2 "FSE Placement.")

Anesthesia. Most commonly, if a patient desired an epidural for pain relief, it will already be in place by the time they enter the second stage of labor. In general, an epidural is not administered this late in labor. In certain patients, however, such as a nulliparous woman with a fetus at zero station who is in extreme pain, it may be possible to have either a spinal or even an epidural placed for analgesia. The advantage of the spinal in this situation is in its rapid onset of analgesia. A combined spinal/epidural technique, discussed in Chapter 8, may also be of benefit as it provides rapid pain relief with the spinal component but also allows for additional boluses through the epidural catheter that is left in place if needed. In a multiparous patient with a history of rapid deliveries, it may be impossible to place either a spinal or epidural prior to delivery. Whether or not conduction anesthesia (i.e., spinal or epidural) may be administered at this stage is dependent on the clinical situation as well as the anesthesiologist. Before calling the anesthesiologist, it is prudent to perform a cervical examination so that you know exactly what the fetal station and cervical dilation are so you can communicate this to the provider.

Narcotics should generally not be used during the 2nd stage of labor as delivery will likely occur soon enough that the fetus could be affected. If any narcotics have been given within 2 hours of delivery, then you should notify the pediatrician and have naloxone hydrochloride hydrochloride (0.1mg/kg) drawn up in case there is significant neonatal depression. (See table 5-1 for doses based on fetal weight.)

Table 5-1. Doses of Naloxone Hydrochloride

Fetal Weight (gms)	*Dose (mL of 0.4 mg/mL concentration)*
4,000	1.0 mL
3,000	0.75 mL
2,000	0.5 mL

A pudendal nerve block is another option during the second stage of labor. It is performed by inserting a needle through the vagina and injecting the pudendal nerves with a local anesthetic. When performed correctly, this technique provides anesthesia that is adequate for operative vaginal delivery. This technique is discussed in detail in Chapter 8.

Pediatric Involvement. There are certain situations where it is prudent to have a pediatrician attend a delivery. In general, these situations are those where you anticipate there is some risk that the fetus will require immediate attention and possibly resuscitation (Primhak 1984). Some of these situations include the following:

- Cesarean section
- Meconium
- Forceps or vacuum delivery
- Breech vaginal delivery
- Umbilical cord prolapse
- Delivery after significant hemorrhage (placental abruption/vasa previa)
- Chorioamnionitis
- Maternal history of substance abuse
- Recent administration of narcotics or the use of general anesthesia
- Multiple pregnancy
- Fetal distress/Nonreassuring fetal heart rate tracing
- Preterm delivery (<37 weeks)
- Known/suspected fetal anomaly

By keeping these situations in mind, you will be able to call the pediatricians prior to delivery to notify them you would like them to be in attendance. This will save you time and reassure the parents should the baby require immediate resuscitation after delivery.

Pushing. Much is written in the lay press about how and when to push during labor. While there is some science involved in the process, much of this phase is an art, especially in teaching and coaching the patient in pushing, and there is much you can learn from experienced delivery nurses.

> **Pushing Position and Coaching:** In general, whatever position the patient desires to assume that still allows you to adequately monitor the fetus is acceptable. Some women will feel more comfortable on their back while others will want to push on their side or use a "squatting bar" to support themselves while they bear down. When patients begin pushing, especially nulliparous patients or those with a dense epidural, it is sometimes helpful to place your fingers into the vagina and push posteriorly to assist them in knowing where to push. This will also allow you to determine if they are pushing effectively as you will feel the fetal head applying pressure to your fingers when they bear down in the correct manner.*

> * (Once the patient is pushing in the correct manner, you do not need to continue this with every push as the increased manipulation will only result in additional tissue edema or a laceration.)

When coaching, or explaining pushing to patients, many physicians and nurses will have the patient take a deep breath as the contraction begins to build (which can be seen on the monitor if you are using either external or internal monitors) and then hold their breath and bear down in a similar manner to having a bowel movement while the coach (father, nurse, birthing assistant, or physician) counts to ten. At this point, the patient exhales and quickly takes another deep breath and bears down again while the coach counts. Usually, patients will do three sets of pushes with each contraction. Remember again that this is something of an art rather than a science, and women may want to push differently, and some providers will not have the patient hold their breath and rather use an "open glottis" technique. Your goal in this process is to help patients push effectively while doing your best to respect their desires for the delivery.

When to begin pushing. Recently, there have been several studies that have examined whether women need to begin pushing as soon as they are completely dilated or if they can wait either a specified amount of time or until they feel the urge to push.

One study randomized 252 patients with epidurals to either beginning to push as soon as they were completely effaced and dilated or to wait to push until either the head appeared at the introitus or for a specified length of time (120 minutes for nulliparous patients and 60 minutes for multiparous patient) (Hansen 2002). This study found that the group of women who delayed pushing had a longer second stage overall, but pushed for a shorter time and had fewer fetal heart rate decelerations than those patients that began pushing immediately. They also found no evidence of an increase in lower APGAR scores, severe lacerations, operative vaginal delivery, or infection between the groups.

Another study of 1,862 nulliparous women with epidural analgesia randomized the participants to either immediate pushing versus waiting 2 hours or until the head was visible at the perineum (Fraser 2000). This report found that, similar to Hansen's study, the overall length of the second stage was longer (187 minutes versus 123 minutes, P = 0.0001) with delayed pushing, but the actual time pushing was shorter (68 minutes versus 110 minutes, P = 0.0001). There was also no increase in the risk of episiotomy, lacerations, postpartum fever, or blood loss of greater than 500 mL at delivery, and the neonatal outcomes were the same between the groups.

What these studies show is that when a patient enters the second stage of labor, it is not necessary to begin pushing immediately. Some patients may be very tired from a long labor or may have a very dense epidural block from an infusion that may need to be decreased so that they can feel enough pressure to push adequately. If the fetal heart rate tracing is reassuring, then a delay in pushing may decrease the actual amount of pushing required and does not appear to be associated with adverse fetal outcomes. At the same time, the overall length of the second stage will be shorter with immediate pushing, and this strategy is acceptable as well.

Spontaneous Vaginal Delivery. The majority of deliveries are uncomplicated. What follows is a description of how to perform an uncomplicated vaginal delivery as well as notes for different times when complications may occur. Delivery of a breech presentation is discussed separately in Chapter 14.

Delivery of Head

As the mother bears down with contractions, the fetal head will cause the perineum to bulge. When this occurs, place one hand at the inferior vaginal opening (see figure 5-1). The other hand is placed on the anterior portion of the head. The goal is to protect the perineum by applying slight pressure with the posterior hand while at the same time not letting the head cause a significant anterior tear. If you have to err on one side, the long-term morbidity is much less from anterior lacerations.

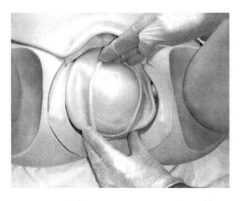

Figure 5-1 Hand position at the time of vaginal
delivery and supporting perineum

If an episiotomy is cut, it will almost always be just prior to delivery of the fetal head. Please refer to the following section and Chapter 11 for further discussion of this procedure.

Allow the head to deliver and then have the mother stop pushing and pant. (Some women, especially those without an epidural, may not be able to stop pushing, and you will simply proceed with the delivery.) After the head delivers, it will restitute/turn to one side or the other.

If there has been any meconium-stained fluid present during labor, then you should have a DeLee suction device set up, which you will first place down each nostril and deep suction, then into the mouth, again performing deep suctioning. While the goal is for the baby not to cry before giving the child to the waiting pediatrician so they can evaluate for meconium below the vocal cords, there is no need to place a finger in the mouth in an attempt to prevent this. If there is no meconium present, then use a bulb syringe to suction the infant's nares and mouth.

After suctioning, palpate the fetal neck to determine if there is a nuchal cord present. Nuchal cords occur in approximately 5% of all deliveries (Dhar 1999). If one is present, then reduce it by pulling it gently over the fetal head. If it is too tight to allow this, then place two Kelly clamps on the cord and cut in-between with bandage scissors.*

* (The presence or absence of a nuchal cord as well as the manner in which it is reduced should be included in the delivery summary. Also, be careful not to accidentally cut the baby when you have a tight nuchal cord, and you are "surgically reducing" it with clamps and scissors.)

Delivery of the Shoulders

Place your hands on the fetal head with the fingers pointing toward the fetal nose and have the mother begin to push again. (See figure 5-2.) As you apply gentle downward traction to deliver the anterior shoulder, you will see it appear at the introitus. If it does not come with relative ease, then you have a shoulder dystocia and must take immediate action to reduce the shoulder. (See Chapter 14 "Shoulder Dystocia.")

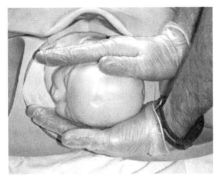

Figure 5-2 Hand position for shoulder delivery

After the anterior shoulder appears at the introitus, change the direction of traction upward, and the posterior shoulder will deliver.*

* (If you have cut an episiotomy, or are concerned about a perineal laceration, you or your assistant can attempt to support the perineum with a hand.)

Delivery of the Body and Clamping of the Cord

After the shoulders have delivered, the rest of the baby will rapidly deliver. The most important thing to remember here is to not drop the child as they are quite slippery when then come out! You can use your arms and body to cradle the child if needed. (Do *anything* but drop a baby!) You may continue to use bulb suction to clear any secretions from the infant's mouth and nose.

At this time, take two clamps and clamp the umbilical cord. Exactly where you do this is not terribly important as another plastic clamp will be placed by the delivery room nurse and the cord trimmed to the appropriate length. In general, doubly clamping and cutting the cord around 12-16 inches from the umbilical cord insertion is adequate. (If the delivery has been uncomplicated, some fathers may want to cut the cord. This is something you can discuss with the parents prior to delivery. If you allow them to do this, make sure that you clearly show them where to cut and keep all fetal extremities and other parts away from the scissors.)

After the cord is cut, the infant may be placed on the mother's abdomen if it has good color, respirations, and no evidence of distress. If additional resuscitation is needed, then the newborn is given to the labor and delivery nurse and taken over to the warmer.

At this point, the second stage of labor is over and the third stage begins.

Episiotomy. An episiotomy is an incision made in the perineum during delivery to provide additional room for the fetus to deliver. While an episiotomy is performed in approximately 40% of deliveries in the United States, it is not a procedure that should be performed as a standard part of every delivery as there may be significant short and long-term morbidity to the mother (Weeks 2001). Types of episiotomies, indications, repair techniques, and complications are discussed in detail in Chapter 11.

Potential Second Stage Complications

Fetal Distress. During pushing, it is not uncommon to have FHR decelerations. Early decelerations, caused by compression of the fetal head during contractions, are not associated with fetal distress and may be watched and the patient reassured. Variable decelerations, however, may become more severe with pushing and must be monitored closely. Between pushes, the fetus should recover from these decelerations back to a normal baseline. When moderate to severe variable decelerations are present with pushing, having the patient push with every other contraction will sometimes allow the fetus enough time to recover between pushes to allow for a vaginal delivery. Late decelerations may occur intermittently, but if they become repetitive, then some action should be taken.

If normal conservative interventions are not able to correct fetal distress during the second stage of labor, then a decision must be made as to what the best route of delivery will be. If the fetus is at an appropriate station (+2 or lower) and meets the criteria listed in Chapter 8 ("Operative Vaginal Delivery"), then either forceps or a vacuum device may be used to facilitate the delivery.

If, on the other hand, the fetus is not close enough to delivery to perform an operative delivery, then a cesarean section must be performed. The speed at which this is accomplished depends on the degree of fetal distress. If there is a prolonged deceleration or fetal bradycardia, then an urgent cesarean is indicated. If this is the case, the following steps need to be taken and personnel mobilized in a rapid fashion:

1. Quickly counsel the patient on the need for an urgent C/S delivery.
2. Call the chief resident/staff as appropriate.
3. Inform the charge nurse you are calling an urgent C/S.
4. Alert the anesthesiologist.
5. Unhook the patient's bed from the wall and any monitor cords.
6. Call the scrub tech to the OR.
7. Call the NICU/Pediatrics and alert them of the situation.
8. Ask for antibiotics in the OR. (Chapter 10 "Cesarean Section")

Labor Dystocia. Dystocia is defined as difficult labor. In the second stage of labor, dystocia may result from any of the following:

- **Cephalopelvic disproportion:** This simply means that the fetus is too large to fit through the maternal pelvis. Unfortunately, this is not a diagnosis that can often be predicted secondary to the poor ability to accurately determine fetal weight prior to birth as well as our limited ability to clinically judge which women have an adequate pelvis for childbirth. While there are specific cases when a cesarean section for fetal macrosomia is indicated, in general, prophylactic cesarean delivery for a fetus that is "too large" has not been shown to be a reasonable or cost-effective intervention (Rouse 1996).
- **Malpresentation:** Approximately 5% of fetuses will remain in a persistent occiput posterior or transverse position during the second stage of labor (Satin 2002). These patients tend to have a longer second stage of labor and are at increased risk of requiring some form of operative intervention (Sizer 2000; Fitzpatrick 2001).
- **Epidural use:** The use of epidurals has been associated with an increased risk in the duration of the second stage of labor as well as the need for an operative vaginal delivery (Howell 2000). It has not, however, been associated with an increased risk of cesarean section or operative vaginal delivery for dystocia (Howell 2000; Halpern 1998).
- **Uterine hypocontractility:** There are times when, even in the second stage of labor, uterine contractions may space out to the point where adequate progress is not made. In this situation, it is reasonable to begin oxytocin in order to help labor along.

Interventions that can be taken if the patient is not making good progress with pushing efforts and the fetal heart rate tracing is reassuring include the following:

- Delayed pushing (discussed earlier in this chapter)
- Decreasing the epidural infusion rate if there is a very dense block in order to allow the patient to push more effectively

- Change maternal pushing position
- Administering oxytocin if uterine contractions are not frequent enough

During the second stage of labor, ACOG criteria for dystocia depend on whether or not the patient is nulliparous or multiparous and if she has an epidural for anesthesia. The criteria are summarized in Table 5-2

Table 5-2. ACOG definitions of second stage dystocia (arrest of descent)

	Epidural	*No Epidural*
Nulliparous	*3 hours*	*2 hours*
Multiparous	*2 hours*	*1 hour*

(ACOG 2003)

When patients do not progress well during the second stage of labor and meet the criteria listed in above for dystocia, then there are several options that may be considered. These are: continued observation, operative vaginal delivery, or cesarean section.

Continued observation. If a patient has been making steady progress during pushing and the FHRT has remained reassuring, then the time limits set in table 5-2 are not absolute indications for operative intervention. Interventions mentioned previously, such as decreasing the epidural rate, changing the maternal position, or administering oxytocin may be attempted with continued close monitoring of the fetal status.

- **Operative vaginal delivery:** If the fetus is felt to be an appropriate candidate for operative vaginal delivery and has met the criteria listed above, then this option may be discussed with the patient. If the patient has not exceeded these time limits, but has become exhausted from pushing, then operative intervention may also be offered.
- **Cesarean delivery:** If the fetus is not felt to be a candidate for operative vaginal delivery for whatever reason, and continued observation is not desired by the patient or there is evidence of fetal distress, then a cesarean delivery may be offered to the patient.

References:

Amnioinfusion does not prevent meconium aspiration syndrome. ACOG Committee Opinion #346, October 2006.

Dhar KK, Ray SN, Dhall GI. Significance of nuchal cord. J Indian Med Assoc. 1995 Dec;93(12):451-453.

Dystocia and the Augmentation of Labor. ACOG Practice Bulletin #49, Dec 2003.

Fetal Heart Rate Patterns: Monitoring, Interpretation, and Management. ACOG Technical Bulletin #207, July 1995.

Fitzpatrick M, McQuillan K, O'Herlihy C. Persistent occiput posterior position and delivery outcome. Obstet Gynecol 2001; 96:1027-1031.

Fraser WD, Marcoux S, Krauss I, Douglas J, Goulet C, Moulvain M. Multicenter, randomized, controlled trial of delayed pushing for nulliparous women in the second stage of labor with continuous epidural analgesia. Am J Obstet Gynecol May 2000; 182(5):1165-1172.

Halpern SH, Leighton BL, Ohisson A et al. Effect of epidural vs parental opioid analgesia on the progress of labor: a meta-analysis, 1998, JAMA; 280:2105-2110.

Hansen SL, Clark SL, Foster JC. Active pushing versus passive fetal descent in the second stage of labor: A randomized controlled trial. Obstet Gynecol 2002; 99:29-34.

Howell CJ. Epidural versus non-epidural analgesia for pain relief in labor. Cochrane Database Syst Rev 2000; CD000331.

Primhak RA, Herber SM, Whincup G, et al. Which deliveries require pediatricians in attendance? Br Med J 1984; 289:16-18.

Rouse DJ, Owen J, Goldenberg RL, Oliver SP. The effectiveness and costs of cesarean delivery for fetal macrosomia diagnosed by ultrasound. JAMA 1996; 276:1480-1486.

Satin AJ, Macedonia C. Abnormal labor: Protraction and arrest disorders. Up to Date version 10.3, Aug 2002.

Sizer AR, Nirmal DM. Occiputoposterior position: associated factors and obstetric outcome in nulliparas. Obstet Gynecol 2000; 96:749-752.

Weeks JD, Kozak LJ. Trends in the use of episiotomy in the United States: 1980-1998. Birth 2001; 28:152-160.

Chapter 6

Management of the Third Stage of Labor

- Definition
- Normal Duration
- Management
- Potential Complications
    - Retained Placenta
    - Avulsion of Umbilical Cord
    - Postpartum Hemorrhage
    - Uterine Inversion

Definition

The third stage of labor begins after the delivery of the fetus and ends when the placenta and membranes have been removed. While this may seem anticlimactic compared to the actual delivery of the baby, you must remember to be vigilant as significant complications, including catastrophic hemorrhage can occur either before or after the placenta delivers. In fact, at times a large amount of blood may build up behind the placenta and surprise you as the placenta delivers.

Normal Duration

In general, the placenta will deliver within approximately ten minutes although it may take up to 30 minutes in some cases. If it has not delivered within 30 minutes of delivery, then the third stage of labor is considered prolonged, and it may be necessary to manually remove the placenta. In patients who have the third stage managed actively, which is defined and discussed in the next section, the placenta tends to deliver around 9 minutes earlier than with conservative management (Prendiville 2000).

Management

After the baby is delivered, the cord clamped and cut, and the infant given to the mother or pediatrician, the removal of the placenta may be managed in either an active or passive manner. Passive management generally means simply awaiting the spontaneous delivery of the placenta while active management involves early cord clamping, the use of uterotonics (such as oxytocin), and gentle traction on the umbilical cord. When active management is done, the blood loss during the third stage of labor is significantly decreased by almost 80 mL and the risk of postpartum hemorrhage is decreased with a relative risk of 0.38 (95% confidence interval 0.32-0.46) as compared to passive management (Prendiville 2000). A recent meta-analysis of over 4,500 deliveries reported that active management of the third stage can prevent approximately 60% of postpartum hemorrhages and decrease the risk of requiring a transfusion by almost 65% (Bukowski 2001). As a prophylactic measure, oxytocin appears to be superior to both ergot alkaloids, which are associated with an increased risk of retained placenta, and misoprostol (Elbourne 2001; Villar 2002). Because of all the evidence that demonstrates the benefits of active management of the third stage of labor, it is recommended that this be done for all deliveries.

To actively manage the third stage of labor, after delivery of the infant when the cord has been clamped and cut and the infant given to either the mother or nurse, place a sterile towel on the maternal abdomen and keep one hand on the uterus, applying mild pressure in the suprapubic region. (See figure 6-1.)

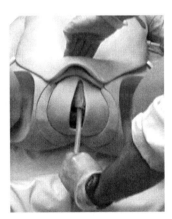

Figure 6-1 Hand on maternal abdomen to prevent uterine inversion

This is done to assess uterine tone and monitor for evidence of atony. With the other hand, apply gentle downward traction on the cord. It is imperative that you do not apply excessive force on the cord as it is possible to both avulse the cord, which results in bleeding and the need to manually extract the uterus, and to cause a uterine inversion,

117

which is an emergency and associated with severe hemorrhage. The following are signs that the placenta is separating from the uterus:

1. The uterus becomes more firm
2. A sudden gush of blood will occur
3. The umbilical cord will descend or lengthen

As these occur, you can have the mother gently bear down to assist with delivery of the placenta. As the placenta delivers, take care not to leave the membranes behind as they can cause problems with bleeding later. In order to prevent this, you can either take ring forceps and gently tease out any that remain attached or twist the placenta in a clockwise direction to ensure they are removed. Once the placenta and membranes are out, ask the nurse to start the Pitocin (oxytocin) infusion, if it is not already running, and inspect the placenta. A standard routine for oxytocin after delivery is 20 units in 1,000 mL of lactated Ringer's (LR) or normal saline (NS) at 10 mL/min. (There have been studies that have evaluated whether or not it makes a difference if the Pitocin is given before or after delivery of the placenta, and there appears to be no significant difference in blood loss with either method at this time [Prendiville 2000; Jackson, 2001].)

Upon inspection of the placenta, you should make a note of the following things:

1. How many vessels are in the cord? (Normal is three, two arteries and one vein. If there are only two vessels, then you should alert the pediatricians to this fact as it can be associated with other congenital anomalies.)
2. Is the cord insertion normal? (The umbilical cord usually inserts into the center of the placenta. Two common variations of this are a marginal insertion, which is where the cord inserts into the edge of the placenta and occurs in 7% of term deliveries, or a velamentous insertion where the umbilical vessels separate in the membranes away from the placenta [Benirschke 2000]).
3. Is the placenta intact? (This is important in preventing hemorrhage from retained placenta. If there is a large area that appears to be missing, an ultrasound may be performed to look for any retained portion of the placenta or membranes.)

Potential Complications

Retained Placenta. If the placenta has not delivered within approximately 30 minutes, it is considered to be a retained placenta and manual removal is generally indicated. (Also, if there is significant bleeding prior to the placenta delivering, then manual removal may also be required to enable the uterus to contract.) This complication occurs in approximately 0.5%-3% of vaginal deliveries (Weeks 2002).

If the patient requires manual removal of the placenta, first ensure the patient has adequate anesthesia. If the epidural is functioning, this will almost always suffice. If not, then it may be necessary to administer IV narcotics, such as fentanyl, as long as the patient is hemodynamically stable. If pain control is an issue or the patient is becoming unstable, then contact your anesthesiologist early in the process rather than later.

After the patient is comfortable, use one hand to grasp the uterine fundus abdominally, and then place the other hand into the uterus through the vagina. Once your hand is inside the uterus, find the edge of the placenta and then create a cleavage plane between the uterine wall and the placenta with your fingers. You will continue to extend this plane until you have separated the placenta from the uterine wall and then grasp the placenta in your hand and gently remove it through the vagina. Any trailing membranes are grasped with ring forceps in the same manner as with spontaneous delivery of the placenta. If there is any question that there may be retained membranes or part of the placenta still in the uterus, take a sponge and insert it with your hand back into the uterus and wipe the uterine cavity to remove any remaining debris. (*Make sure you do not leave a sponge in the uterus as it can cause continued bleeding and become a nidus for infection.)

If you have any question about whether or not you removed all of the placenta, an abdominal ultrasound can quickly be done to determine if there is any remaining placental tissue in the uterus as it will often show up as a hyperechoic (bright) area rather than a thin endometrial stripe. In a study by Carlan et al. they found that the ultrasound appearance of retained placental tissue was variable, and the examination was most reassuring if there was a thin endometrial stripe and no hyperechoic areas as the negative predictive value (i.e., there is no retained placental tissue) when this is seen is 87% (Carlan 1997). Another study reported that, when the uterus appeared empty on ultrasound, that 17 of 18 patients did not have any pathologic evidence of placental tissue after dilation and curettage (Shen 2003).

If you are unable to completely remove the placenta at this point, you may use a banjo curette in order to attempt to remove any remaining placental tissue. Doing this under ultrasound guidance may be helpful in locating any retained tissue as well. To perform this procedure, take the following steps:

1. Ensure adequate anesthesia (may use epidural if they have this or IV narcotics)
2. Notify anesthesia support as you may need them to go to the OR to help with this
3. Counsel the patient on the procedure
4. Grasp the anterior cervix with a ring forceps

5. Gently insert the banjo curette into the uterus and perform a curettage (have an assistant monitor with an abdominal sonogram if available)
6. Be prepared for additional bleeding
7. Monitor urine output closely after the procedure
8. Consider sending a CBC 4-6 hours after the procedure if there was significant blood loss

Some physicians will place patients on prophylactic antibiotics for 24 hours after manual removal of the placenta if the patient had chorioamnionitis during her labor. There is no data to support or refute this practice at this time and this decision is left up to the preference of the provider.

Avulsion of the umbilical cord. If the umbilical cord detaches while you are applying gentle traction (and this can occur easily if you do not supervise medical students or junior residents closely) then it is important to proceed quickly to perform a manual removal of the placenta to prevent a significant hemorrhage. This complication seems to occur more often with very preterm deliveries as the placenta does not separate as easily after a term delivery and extra care should be taken in these cases. The procedure for manual removal is the same as described in the previous section.

Postpartum hemorrhage. This complication occurs in approximately 4% of vaginal deliveries and 6% of cesarean deliveries. It is a significant problem that can rapidly cause a patient to become hemodynamically unstable and requires quick intervention to correct. A thorough discussion of this problem is found in Chapter 14 Common Obstetric Emergencies.

Uterine inversion. This complication occurs in approximately 1:2,500 deliveries (ACOG 1998). It is often associated with an abnormally implanted placenta, such as a placenta accreta, increta, or percreta, although excessive traction on the umbilical cord has also been implicated. When this occurs it is an obstetric emergency and must be dealt with quickly to avoid significant maternal morbidity and mortality. This complication is discussed in detail in Chapter 14 as well.

References:

Benirschke K, Kaufmann P. Pathology of the Human Placenta, 4th ed. New York, Springer-Verlag, 2000.

Bukowski R, Hankins, GDV. Managing postpartum hemorrhage. Contemporary OB/GYN 2001 Sept:92-102.

Carlan SJ, Scott WT, Pollack R, Harris K. Appearance of the uterus by ultrasound immediately after placental delivery with pathologic correlation. J Clin Ultrasound 1997 Jul-Aug; 25(6):301-308.

Elbourne DR, Prendiville WJ, Carroli G, Wood J, McDonald S. Prophylactic use of oxytocin in the third stage of labor. Cochrane Database Syst Rev. 2001; (4): CD001808.

Jackson KW Jr, Allbert JR, Schemmer GK, Elliot M, Humphrey A, Taylor J. A randomized controlled trial comparing oxytocin administration before and after placental delivery in the prevention of postpartum hemorrhage. Am J Obstet Gynecol, Oct 2001; 185(4): 873-877.

Postpartum Hemorrhage. ACOG Educational Bulletin #243, January 1998.

Postpartum hemorrhage. ACOG Practice Bulletin #76, Oct 2006.

Prendiville WJ, Elbourne D, McDonald S. Active versus expectant management in the third stage of labor. (Cochrane Review). Cochrane Database Syst Rev 2000;3: CD000007.

Shen O, Rabinowitz R, Eisenberg VH, Samueloff A. Transabdominal sonography before uterine exploration as a predictor of retained placental fragments. J Ultrasound Med 2003; 22:561-564.

Villar J, Gülmezoglu AM, Hofmeyr GJ, Forna F. Systemic review of randomized controlled trials of misoprostol to prevent postpartum hemorrhage. Obstet Gynecol, Dec 2002; 100(6):1301-1312.

Weeks AD, Mirembe FM. The retained placenta—new insights into an old problem. Eur J Obstet Gynecol and Reprod Biology, May 2002; 102(2):109-110.

Chapter 7

Induction and Augmentation of Labor

Introduction

Making a decision to influence labor is central to any obstetrician's practice. It is a common practice in obstetrics, but one that can cause fetal distress and increase a mother's chance of requiring a cesarean delivery and must, therefore, be handled carefully. In general, labor may be induced or augmented. The difference is that with induction the patient has not yet begun to labor and demonstrate cervical change, and with augmentation, the labor is simply being assisted.

Induction of Labor

Background. Labor induction is a commonplace occurrence in today's obstetrical practice. From 1990 to 1998, the rate of labor induction in the United States increased from 9.5% to 19.4% of all births (Zhang 2002). As induction has become much more common, it is imperative for OB/GYN physicians to understand both the indications and potential complications that can occur.

Indications for labor induction. A decision to induce labor must take into consideration both the maternal and fetal conditions. When contemplating induction, you must be able to clearly state in the medical record why you are intervening. This is important because the incidence of both chorioamnionitis and cesarean delivery are increased when labor is induced. Induction of labor is indicated when the benefits of delivery, to either the mother or fetus, outweigh the risks of prolonging the pregnancy. Some commonly accepted indications for induction of labor are:

- Chorioamnionitis
- Fetal demise
- Pregnancy-induced hypertension
- Preeclampsia/Eclampsia
- Postterm pregnancy (usually defined as >42 weeks*)
- Premature rupture of membranes (at > 34 weeks)
- Fetal compromise (i.e., IUGR, oligohydramnios, isoimmunization)
- Maternal medical conditions (i.e., diabetes, chronic hypertension, renal disease)
- History of rapid labors (when the patient lives a significant distance from the hospital)

* While a true post term pregnancy is defined as one lasting 42 weeks or more, the American College of Obstetricians and Gynecologists do not currently recommend a specific upper limit for gestational age for expectant management of pregnancy (ACOG 1997). However, there is a good deal of literature, including a meta-analysis of 19 trials of routine care versus selective induction after 41 weeks, that has demonstrated induction of labor at 41 weeks does not result in an increase in the cesarean section rate and may even lower the perinatal mortality rate (Hannah 1992; Crowley 1999).

Contraindications to labor induction

The following are contraindications to labor induction:

1. *FETAL*

   a. Evidence of significant fetal compromise (i.e., an ominous FHRT or BPP of 4 or less (if this is the case, immediate delivery, not induction, is required.)
   b. Malpresentation (i.e., transverse lie, incomplete breech)
   c. Placenta previa or vasa previa
   d. Fetal anomalies (such as severe hydrocephalus that would not allow for passage of the fetal head.)

2. *MATERNAL*

   a. Inadequate pelvis (determined by clinical pelvimetry to be too small for vaginal delivery)
   b. Active genital herpes infection
   c. Medical conditions that make labor dangerous for the mother
   d. Maternal cardiac disease or CNS lesions

3. *UTERINE*

   a. Previous classical uterine incision or "T" or "J" uterine incision
   b. Prior myomectomy with entrance into the uterine cavity
   c. *Two previous cesarean sections without a prior vaginal delivery (ACOG 2004)

* There is currently some controversy regarding induction of labor for patients who have had a previous cesarean section. While the most current recommendations from ACOG do state that if a patient has had two previous cesarean sections and no vaginal deliveries they should have a repeat cesarean section, there is debate about the risks involved with induction of labor in patients with a single previous cesarean.

The baseline risk of uterine rupture for patients with a previous cesarean section who have spontaneous labor is only 0.5% (Lydon-Rochelle 2001). For patients who undergo induction of labor without a prostaglandin (as this is contraindicated), the risk of uterine rupture increases to approximately 1%. Even though this rate is higher, ACOG states that "induction of labor remains a reasonable option, but the potentially increased risk of uterine rupture associated with any induction should ᴄᴄ discussed with the patient and documented in the medical record" (ACOG 2006). Additionally, in these patients the indication for induction must be clearly stated in the chart.

Timing of labor induction. When labor induction is undertaken for either logistic reasons or electively and not for fetal or maternal disease states listed above, then the American College of OB/GYN recommends that either fetal lung maturity be documented by amniocentesis or one of the following criteria be met:

- Fetal heart tones documented for at least 30 weeks by Doppler.
- It has been at least 36 weeks since the patient had a positive urine or serum pregnancy test performed at a laboratory.
- A 6-12 week ultrasound of the crown-rump length confirms a gestational age of at least 39 weeks.
- A 13-20 week ultrasound supports a gestational age of at least 39 weeks and is consistent with the physical exam.

(ACOG 1999)

Other things that must be considered prior to induction of labor include an assessment of the following:

1. Gestational age: (as mentioned above)
2. Fetal size: Induction of labor for presumed macrosomia has not been shown to decrease the risk of shoulder dystocia, but in certain situations, a cesarean section may be offered for an extremely macrosomic fetus. (See Chapter 10: Cesarean Section.)
3. Fetal presentation: Induction should not be performed if the fetus is breech or transverse. In this situation, an external cephalic version may be attempted if appropriate. (See Chapter 2: Common Exams and Procedures.)
4. Clinical pelvimetry: An assessment of the patient's pelvis should be performed and induction of labor is not recommended if the patient has a significantly contracted pelvis.
5. Cervical examination: Examination of the cervix will help you to both determine what method to use for induction, as well as allow you to counsel the patient on the anticipated success rate. (See Bishop Score below.)

Labor Induction. After the decision has been made to proceed with induction of labor, then attention is turned to how to proceed. The method of induction will depend on the cervical examination and whether or not cervical ripening is felt to be needed prior to the administration of oxytocin.

Cervical Ripening

When the cervix is not prepared for regular labor, it is often referred to as "unfavorable." The goal of cervical ripening is to make the cervix more "favorable" for labor and thus increase the chances of having a vaginal delivery. One method used to grade the cervix in terms of how "favorable" it is at the beginning of an induction is the Bishop score, which grades cervical dilation, effacement, station of the fetal vertex, consistency of the cervix, and the position of the cervix. With a Bishop's score of ≥ 8, induction of labor will usually be successful, or at least as successful as normal spontaneous labor and oxytocin is often started without cervical ripening in these cases (Bishop 1964). (See table 7-1 for how to calculate the score.)

Table 7-1. Bishop Score

BISHOP SCORE

	0	1	2	3
Dilation: (cm)	Closed (0)	1-2	3-4	5-6
Effacement: (%)	0-30	40-50	60-70	80+
Station:	-3	-2	-1,0	+1,+2
Cervix:	Firm	Medium	Soft	—
Position:	Posterior	Midposition	Anterior	—

* Notes: Station is on a +3 to -3 Scale
"Position" refers to the position of the cervix in the vagina
"Cervix" refers to the consistency of the cervix on exam

It is also important to note that success rates are dependent on parity as well, with multiparous patients who have had a vaginal delivery being much more likely to have a successful induction than nulliparous patients. (See table 7-2 for the risk of cesarean section depending on the initial bishop score based on parity.)

Table 7-2. Incidence of cesarean section for failed induction based on Bishop score

Initial Bishop Score	Nullipara	Multipara
0-3	45%	8%
4-6	10%	4%
7-10	1%	1%

(*Adapted from Wing 2003)

When it comes to which agent to use, much of this is based on staff preference. It is important, however, to understand how each method works, the potential complications, and what the fetal monitoring requirements are for the different medications.

Medications Available for Cervical Ripening

Prostaglandin E2. This is also called dinoprostone (see the medication database for additional information). It can be applied either as a gel, or as a vaginal insert which is called Cervidil. The price for a single application of this is approximately $75. A general protocol for the insertion of either is as follows:

- Confirm patient's EDC
- Confirm that fetus is vertex by ultrasound (it's embarrassing to induce a breech!)
- Ensure the FHRT is reassuring
- Insert either gel (intravaginal or intracervical) or vaginal insert
- Have the patient remain recumbent for 30 minutes after placement

If gel inserted: Monitor FHR for 2 hours, if the FHR is reassuring and there is no change in uterine activity, you can discontinue monitoring.

If Cervidil placed: Continuously monitor FHR while in place until 15 minutes after it is removed.

It is recommended that Pitocin not be started for at least 6-12 hours after these medications are used. (Note: There are reports of concurrent use of dinoprostone and pitocin, but the most recent study, while it demonstrated a significantly shorter time interval from induction to delivery, was too small to detect a significant difference in potential side effects such as uterine hyperstimulation (Christensen 2002).)

Prostaglandin E1. Misoprostol, or Cytotec, is a synthetic prostaglandin E1 that is marketed for prevention of peptic ulcers. It is extremely inexpensive at around $1 for 100 mcg, but cannot be used in patients who have had a previous cesarean section because of a significant increase in the risk of uterine rupture (Plaut 1999). It has been shown in several studies to be as good as or better than prostaglandin E2, but should be used in doses of 25mcg Q3-6 hours to minimize the occurrence of uterine hyperstimulation and fetal distress. If the patient is contracting more than three times in 10 minutes when it is time for subsequent doses, then the next dose is usually not placed in an attempt to avoid uterine hyperstimulation. The procedure is the same as for prostaglandin E2, but the patient must be continuously monitored after this is used.

Pitocin should not be started until at least 4 hours after the last dose of misoprostol.

Other Methods for Cervical Ripening

Foley Balloon. Using this method, a Foley catheter, with a 30 cc balloon and not the standard smaller 10cc balloon, is inserted into the cervical os and then inflated. It can be placed either during a speculum exam using ring forceps to place the catheter, although you must be careful where you grasp the catheter as you can make a hole in the balloon doing this, or during a digital vaginal exam. (If it is difficult to place through the cervix, then it is possible to place a urologic sound through the catheter to assist in the placement.) The catheter is then taped to the patient's leg and oxytocin is often started. It is not necessary to place a weight on the end of the catheter. This procedure has been shown to be as effective as misoprostol and prostaglandin E2 gel for labor induction (St Onge 1995; Sciscione 2001).

In some institutions, sterile normal saline is then infused through the catheter at a rate of 30 mL/hr. This is referred to as an extra-amniotic saline infusion. When compared to misoprostol, this procedure has been shown in some studies to result in the same or shorter induction-to-vaginal delivery time, while a Cochrane analysis of the technique recently reported that use of extra-amniotic saline infusion was less likely to result in delivery within 24 hours and increased the risk of cesarean section (Vengalil 1998; Mullin 2002; Boulvain 2001).

Hygroscopic Cervical Dilators. These may be placed into the cervical os in the same manner as a foley catheter balloon. They are generally very safe, although rare cases of anaphylaxis have been reported after their insertion. These work by slowly expanding in the cervix and may be used concurrently with oxytocin.

Membrane Stripping. This involves performing a vigorous cervical exam and rotating the examining finger 360 degrees once your finger is through the internal os in an attempt to separate the membranes from the lower uterine segment. This will increase the level of prostaglandins present, which is important for the stimulation of labor. This is generally not performed until 38 or 39 weeks gestation, and will result in approximately two thirds of patients going into spontaneous labor within the next 72 hours. In a recent meta-analysis, membrane stripping reduced the chances of prolonged pregnancy (both >41 weeks and > 42 weeks) and reduced the risk of labor induction (Boulvain 2001). It is important to explain to your patients that the procedure does not increase the risk of maternal or neonatal infection, and it will also probably not cause the membranes to rupture earlier (Boulvain 1999).

Complications of Labor Induction

The major complications associated with labor induction are an increased risk of cesarean delivery and operative vaginal delivery. It is the increased risk of cesarean delivery when induction is undertaken as compared to spontaneous labor that has led to the use of the different methods of cervical ripening previously discussed.

Another complication that can occur with any of the prostaglandins or Pitocin is uterine hyperstimulation leading to fetal distress. The relative potential for this complication to occur is the reason for the different monitoring requirements for pitocin versus the various prostaglandins. This complication is discussed in detail later in this chapter.

An unlikely, but potentially catastrophic complication of labor induction is uterine rupture, where a full thickness defect in the uterine wall can result in massive hemorrhage and a compromised fetus. This is fortunately a rare occurrence (see table 7-3) but because prostaglandins have been associated with an increased risk of uterine rupture in patients with a previous cesarean delivery, they are not used in that population. This complication is discussed in detail in Chapter 14.

Table 7-3. Incidence of uterine rupture in patients who have had a previous cesarean delivery

Risk of Uterine Rupture

Spontaneous labor 0.4%-0.5%

Induced with pitocin 0.7%-1.1%

Induced with prostaglandins 1.4%-2.4%

(ACOG 2006)

Augmentation of Labor

Augmentation of labor refers to "stimulation of uterine contractions when spontaneous contractions have failed to result in progressive cervical dilation or descent of the fetus" (ACOG 2003).

Indications for Labor Augmentation. If a patient has a labor protraction disorder then augmentation of labor is indicated if the fetal status is reassuring.

Contraindications to Labor Augmentation. Contraindications to labor augmentation are essentially the same as contraindications for labor induction. One additional note is that if a fetus demonstrates an intolerance to contractions with spontaneous labor, and has a non-reassuring FHRT, then labor cannot be augmented at that time as it will likely worsen the fetal condition by causing additional stress and decreased uterine perfusion with more frequent and intense contractions.

Methods of Augmentation. When labor augmentation is considered, there are generally two options, medications and amniotomy and both of these are discussed here.

Medications Available. In general, oxytocin (Pitocin) is almost always the medication utilized for labor augmentation, although rarely with a very unfavorable cervix, misoprostol is sometimes utilized at the same doses as previously discussed.

Oxytocin. This is a synthetic version of the natural hormone oxytocin. When given intravenously, it will stimulate uterine contractions by acting on oxytocin receptors in the myometrium. (See the medication database for additional information on Pitocin.)

Preparation. Pitocin is diluted in a lactated Ringer's (LR) solution, usually with 10-20 units pitocin per 1,000 mL of LR. This will result in a concentration of either 10 mU/mL or 20 mU/mL.

Dosage. Pitocin is always given IV, and the dosage varies. It is always started slowly, and then titrated up to achieve adequate contractions. (*Note: When external toco is used to record contractions, only the duration and timing and not the actual strength of the contraction is measured. When an IUPC is used, then the pressure of each contraction can be measured. This is important when attempting to define "adequate" contractions.)

Pitocin is usually given in either a "low-dose" or "high-dose" protocol. There are many studies which have demonstrated that the high-dose protocols result in a shorter duration of labor and fewer cesarean deliveries for dystocia, but an increased incidence of uterine hyperstimulation. Importantly, there appears to be no adverse neonatal effects when high-dose protocols are used (Satin 1992). In general, the high-dose protocols are not used in patients with a prior cesarean delivery. Also, most institutions have a written protocol for what regimens are acceptable, so check where you work. Some common protocols are listed below:

	Starting Dose	*Maximum Dose*	*Dose Increase*	*Interval*
High dose	6 mU/min	42 mU/min	*6 mU/min	15-40 min
Low dose	1-2 mU/min	20-40 mU/min	1-2 mU/min	15-40 min

(Note: The dosage increase of 6 mU/min in the high dose regimen should be changed to 3 mU/min if significant uterine hyperstimulation occurs.)

While there is no maximum dose established for Pitocin, most institutions do not run infusions at more than 40 mU/min. At high doses for long periods of time, there is a risk of water intoxication, which is discussed later in this chapter.

Please refer to Appendix B: Sample Notes and Orders to see an example for how to write orders for each of these pitocin protocols.

Contraindications:

- Abnormal fetal presentation (i.e., other than vertex)
- Multiple gestation (relative contraindication)
- Pathologic hydramnios
- Excessively large fetus
- High parity (6 or more deliveries)

(*Note: Some institutions do not give Pitocin to patients who have had a cesarean delivery. Check on your institution's policy for induction of labor with VBAC patients.)

Fetal Monitoring. Continuous fetal monitoring is recommended while Pitocin is given.

Complications. There are several potential complications with IV oxytocin administration. Some common problems are listed below.

Acute hypotension. If the IV pump used to administer the dilute oxytocin malfunctions, an accidental bolus can cause sudden maternal hypotension. The treatment for this is to immediately discontinue the infusion and correct the hypotension as needed.

Water intoxication. When Pitocin is administered in doses of 20 mU/min or greater, it exerts a powerful antidiuretic action. This is because oxytocin is similar in its molecular structure to vasopressin. If additional IV fluids are given to patients on high doses of pitocin (for things such as maternal hypotension or prior to an epidural being placed) then water intoxication may develop which can lead to convulsions, coma, and even death. Monitoring fluid intake is a must when patients are receiving high doses of Pitocin for a long period of time.

Uterine hyperstimulation. Even at normal doses given for labor augmentation, uterine hyperstimulation and resulting fetal distress secondary to decreased perfusion may develop. The mechanism is simple, with each contraction the blood flow to the fetus decreases and if contractions are too strong, too frequent, or too long in duration, the fetus cannot tolerate the decrease in perfusion.

Uterine hyperstimulation is defined as any of the following:

- A persistent pattern of more than 5 contractions in 10 minutes
- Contractions lasting 2 minutes or more
- Contractions of normal duration within 1 minute of each other
(ACOG 2003)

In the presence of uterine hyperstimulation, the intervention depends on the fetal response. If the fetus is tolerating the increased uterine activity, then the dose of oxytocin can simply be decreased to correct it. If, however, the fetus is demonstrating distress in the form of variable or late decelerations, or even worse, bradycardia, then the oxytocin must be stopped and immediate interventions made which often include the administration of terbutaline to cause the uterine muscle to relax and improve perfusion. (See Chapter 3 "FHR Monitoring" for a protocol for intervention.)

Uterine rupture. While this is a rare event, and almost always occurs in women with a previous uterine scar, the use of Pitocin can increase the risk of this happening. This complication is discussed in detail in Chapter 13: Obstetric Emergencies.

Amniotomy. This involves the artificial rupture of the amniotic membranes. It is often used in when the latent phase is prolonged or there are inadequate contractions during the active phase. Performing this prior to starting oxytocin is a reasonable intervention, and it also allows you to place an IUPC to determine the strength of the patient's contractions or a fetal scalp electrode (FSE) if you need to monitor the fetal heart rate tracing more closely. It has been shown that amniotomy during the active phase of labor will shorten the duration of labor and can decrease the need for oxytocin augmentation (Garite 1993; Fraser 1993). A recent meta-analysis demonstrated that early amniotomy (which means it is performed as soon as it is safe with the fetal head being well engaged at -2 station or lower and no contraindications exist rather than waiting until advanced labor) reduces the duration of the first stage of labor by 60 to 120 minutes (Fraser 2002). This intervention may also decrease the need for oxytocin augmentation of labor (Lopez-Zeno 1992; ACOG 2003).

References:

Allot HA, Palmer CR. Sweeping the membranes: A valid procedure in stimulating the onset of labour? Br J Obstet Gynaecol, 1993; 100:898-903.

Bishop EH. Pelvic scoring for elective induction. Obstet Gynecol 1964; 24:266-268.

Boulvain M, Irion O, Marcoux S, Fraser W. Sweeping of the membranes to prevent post-term pregnancy and to induce labour: A systematic review. Br J Obstet Gynaecol, 1999; 106:481-485.

Boulvain M, Kelly A, Lohse C, et al. Mechanical methods for induction of labour (Cochrane Review). Cochrane Database Syst Rev 2001; 2:CD000451.

Boulvain M, Stan C, Irion O. Membrane sweeping for induction of labour (Cochrane Review). Cochrane Database Rev 2001; 2:CD000451.

Christensen FC, Tehranifar M, Gonzalez JL, Qualls CR, Rappaport VJ, Rayburn WF. Randomized trial of concurrent oxytocin with a sustained-release dinoprostone vaginal insert for labor induction at term. Am J OB/GYN, Jan 2002; 186(1):61-65.

Dystocia and the Augmentation of Labor. ACOG Practice Bulletin #49, Dec 2003.

Crowley, P. Interventions for preventing or improving the outcome of delivery at or beyond term (Cochrane review). In: The Cochrane Library, Issue 1, 1999. Oxford: Update Software.

Garite TJ, Porto M, Carlson NJ, Rumney PJ, Reimbold PA. The influence of elective amniotomy on fetal heart rate patterns and the course of labor in term patients: A randomized study. Am J Obstet Gynecol 1993; 168:1827-1832.

Fraser WD, Turcot L, Krauss I et al. Amniotomy for shortening spontaneous labor (Cochrane Review). In: The Cochrane Library, issue 1, 2002, Oxford: Update Software.

Fraser WD, Marcoux S, Moutquin J-M, Christen A, and the Canadian Early Amniotomy Study Group. Effect of early amniotomy on the risk of dystocia in nulliparous women. N Engl J Med 1993; 328(16):1145-1149.

Hannah ME, Hannah WJ, Hellmann J, et al. Induction of labor as compared with serial antenatal monitoring in postterm pregnancy. A randomized controlled trial. The Canadian Multicenter Post-term Pregnancy Trial Group. NEJM 1992; 326:1587-1592.

Induction of Labor. ACOG Practice Bulletin #10, November 1999.

Induction of Labor for Vaginal Birth After Cesarean Delivery. ACOG Committee Opinion #342, Aug 2006.

Induction and Augmentation of Labor. In Williams Obstetrics, 21st edition. Cunningham GF and Gant NF et al eds. McGraw-Hill, New York, 2001.

Lopez-Zeno JA, Peaceman AM, Adashak JA, Socol ML. A controlled trial of a program for the active management of labor. NEJM 1992; 326:450-454.

Lyndon-Rochelle M, Holt VL, Easterling TR, Martin DP. Risk of uterine rupture during labor among women with a prior cesarean delivery. NEJM 2001; 345:3.

Management of Postterm Pregnancy. ACOG Practice Bulletin #55, 2004.

Mullin PM, House M, Paul RH, Wing DA. A comparison of vaginally administered misoprostol with extra-amniotic saline infusion for cervical ripening and labor induction. Am J Obstet Gynecol 2002; 187:847-852.

Plaut MM, Schwartz ML, Lubarsky SL. Uterine rupture associated with the use of misoprostol in the gravid patient with a previous cesarean section. Am J Obstet Gynecol, 1999 Jun; 180(6 Pt 1)1535-1542.

Satin AJ, Leveno KJ, Sherman ML, Brewster DS, Cunningham FG. High-versus low-dose oxytocin for labor stimulation. Obstet Gynecol 1992; 80(1):111-116.

Sciscione, AC, McCullough H, Manley JS, Shlossman PA, Pollock M, Colmorgen GHC. A prospective, randomized comparison of foley catheter insertion versus intracervical prostaglandin E2 gel for preinduction cervical ripening. Am J Obstet Gynecol 1999 Jan, 180(1 Pt 1):55-60.

Sciscione AC, Nguyen L, Manley J, et al. A randomized comparison of transcervical foley catheter to intravaginal misoprostol for preinduction cervical ripening. Obstet Gynecol 2001; 97:603-607.

St Onge RD, Connors GT. Preinduction cervical ripening: a comparison of intracervical prostaglandin E2 gel versus the foley catheter. Am J Obstet Gynecol 1995; 172:687-690.

Vaginal birth after previous cesarean delivery, ACOG Practice Bulletin #54, July 2004.

Vengalil SR, Guinn DA, Olabi NF, Burd LI, Owen J. A randomized trial of misoprostal and extra-amniotic saline infusion for cervical ripening and labor induction. Obstet Gynecol 1998 May, 91(5 Pt 1):774-779.

Wing D. Induction of labor: Indications, techniques, and complications. Up To Date, April 2003; version 11.2.

Zhang J, Yancy MK, Henderson CE. U.S. National trends in labor induction, 1989-1998. J Reprod Med, Feb 2002; 47(2):120-124.

Chapter 8

Obstetric Analgesia/Anesthesia

Principles of Pain Relief During Labor

Whereas in the past many women gave birth under heavy sedation and may barely remember the experience, in modern obstetrics the objective now is to provide adequate relief from the pain of childbirth while allowing the woman to fully participate in her delivery.

When counseling patients about options for anesthesia during labor, it is important to know what services are available at your particular facility. Also, if support is available for epidural/spinal anesthesia, make sure you check with the anesthesiologist on call before you promise a laboring patient that they will receive their pain relief "right away." This is important in that the anesthesiologist often is responsible for many patients (including those undergoing cesarean section) and may not be available for this non-emergent procedure immediately.

Some women will request to go through labor without the assistance of analgesia. If this is their desire, make it clear to them that you will fully support their decision and that, if they should change their mind, you will make whatever you can available to them depending on where they are in labor.

A common question that many women ask regarding all types of analgesia is "Is this safe for my baby?" After reading this chapter, you will be able to confidently answer this question and speak about specific medications and techniques available, which will go a long ways toward reassuring the patient.

Anesthesia Consultation

When evaluating a patient on labor and delivery, it is important to determine if they have any significant anesthetic risk factors for which an anesthesiologist should see the patient early in labor in case any emergencies arise. Some situations in which this would be appropriate are listed in table 8-1.

Table 8-1. Conditions requiring anesthesiology consultation

- Morbid obesity
- Severe preeclampsia
- Known bleeding disorder or thrombocytopenia
- Previous history of anesthetic complications (malignant hyperthermia)
- Multiple gestation
- History of neck or spine trauma or surgery
- Severe scoliosis
- Significant maternal cardiac, pulmonary, or neurologic disease
- Placenta previa or accreta
- Placental abruption
- History of multiple abdominal operations
- Patients with a spinal cord lesion above T6 (at risk for autonomic hyperreflexia)

By notifying the anesthesiologist of these patients so they can be seen early in their labor and a plan made for analgesia, you can avoid many complications should an emergency occur.

Options for Pain Relief During Latent Labor

For patients who are experiencing latent labor, narcotics are often used to make the patient more comfortable. If the patient does not meet criteria for admission to labor and delivery, then narcotics are often given to relieve the pain of contractions. This is sometimes referred to as therapeutic rest. It is extremely important to ensure that fetal testing, usually in the form of a reactive NST, is reassuring prior to giving a patient any of these medications. If the patient is admitted to the hospital, but has not yet entered active labor, either intravenous or intramuscular narcotics may also be used for pain control in latent labor as well.

Medications utilized during latent labor for analgesia are usually opioid agonists-antagonists and mainly work by sedating the patient (Olofsson 1996). Benzodiazepines, on the other hand, are not recommended during labor because they can cause significant neonatal depression, hypotonia, and problems with neonatal temperature regulation.

It is important to realize that, unlike conduction anesthesia (epidural or spinal techniques) which is discussed later in this chapter, all parenteral medications can cross the placenta and have some effect on the fetus and the fetal heart rate tracing (Hawkins 2000). In fact, high doses of meperidine increase the risk of needing to administer naloxone (an agent that reverses the effects of narcotics) for respiratory depression to the infant nearly fourfold (Sharma 1997). When choosing to give narcotics during labor, you must take into account how quickly the medication will provide some pain relief to the patient, how long it is until you anticipate the patient will deliver, and what the half-life of the medication is in the neonate. A good rule of thumb is to not give parenteral narcotics after the patient is 4-5 cm dilated, which means the patient has entered the active phase of labor. While narcotics can be given after this, they should not be given if you expect the patient to deliver within two to three hours of the dose due to the increased risk of neonatal respiratory depression.

Despite these possible complications, and the specific ones listed with each agent in the next section, the American College of Obstetrics and Gynecology (ACOG) recommends that epidural analgesia not be placed until the patient is at least 4 cm dilated (ACOG 2002). This is because there is conflicting evidence about whether placement of an epidural early in labor increases the cesarean section rate, especially in nulliparous patients (Chestnut 1994; Thorp 1991; Lieberman 1996). Despite this concern, ACOG does also state that circumstances, including parity, should be taken into account and women in labor "should not be required" to be 4 cm dilated before receiving an epidural, especially if parenteral medications do not adequately control their pain.

It is a reasonable strategy to attempt to utilize parenteral narcotics during the latent phase of labor in an attempt to make the patient more comfortable and then an epidural when they enter the active phase. If you cannot adequately control their pain with IV/IM narcotics until the patient enters active labor, then you can discuss the risks and benefits of an early epidural and proceed with that course of action. Listed next is an overview of narcotic usage in labor and a list of common narcotics utilized on labor and delivery.

NOTE: Because all narcotics can cause maternal nausea/vomiting, an antiemetic, most often promethazine 12.5-25 mg IV, can be given along with the narcotic. This not only decreases the nausea, but also provides additional sedation.

Narcotics

Indications:
Relief of pain during the first stage of labor
Therapeutic rest for patients in latent labor
Need for additional analgesia when repairing vaginal lacerations

Contraindications:
Known allergy to specific medication
Imminent delivery (i.e., within approx. 2 hrs)

Procedure:
IV or IM administration as per medication specification
Monitor FHR (external or internal monitors)
Monitor maternal vital signs and watch for respiratory depression

Complications:
Maternal respiratory depression
Fetal respiratory depression
Decreased FHR variability
Sinusoidal FHR pattern
Nausea/vomiting
Pruritis
Loss of gag reflex (with inability to protect airway)

There are many options available and some of the most common are listed below as well as in the medication database. Table 8-2 contains a comparison of these medications with regard to their onset of action and neonatal half-life.

Butorphanol: A synthetic opiod agonist-antagonist with rapid onset of both analgesia and sedation.

Dosage: 1-2 mg IV or IM. May be repeated Q4 hours as needed.

Onset of action: 1-2 min (IV)
                  10-30 min (IM)

Neonatal half-life: The neonatal half-life is unknown, but is similar to that of nalbuphine in adults.

Notes: This medication has been reported to actually increase blood pressure and should be avoided in patients with chronic hypertension or preeclampsia. It may also produce a temporary sinusoidal fetal heart rate pattern.

Fentanyl: A synthetic opiod with rapid onset of action but short duration (20-30 minutes).

Dosage: 50-100mcg IV every hour as needed.

Onset of action: 1 minute

Neonatal half-life: 5.3 hours

Notes: This medication is a rapidly acting narcotic that is also cleared relatively quickly. It may, however, require an anesthesiologist to administer depending on the monitoring requirements of your hospital.

Morphine sulfate: This is a systemic opiod which is very sedating.

Dosage: Typical doses are 2-5mg IV or 10mg IM every 4 hours as needed.

Onset of action: 5 min (IV)
                 30-40 min (IM)

Neonatal half-life: 7 hours

Notes: This medication is often used for therapeutic rest and less commonly for patients actually in labor. It is very sedating but has a much shorter half-life than meperidine.

Meperidine: This is an opiod which is very lipid soluble and rapidly crosses the placenta.

Dosage: 25-50mg IV every 1-2 hours OR 50-100mg IM every 2-4 hours.

Onset of action: 5 min (IV)
30-45 min (IM)

Neonatal half-life: **63 hours**

Notes: This medication can be found in the fetal circulation within 2 minutes of administration to the mother and, by 2-3 hours after administration, the fetal levels are actually higher than the mother's. (Norris, 2000) High doses, which are often required to achieve adequate pain control in active labor, have been associated with a significant increase in the need to intervene at the time of delivery for neonatal respiratory depression. (Sharma, 1997)

Nalbuphine: A synthetic opiod agonist-antagonist with rapid onset of both analgesia and sedation.

Dosage: 10mg IV or IM. May be repeated every 3 hours

Onset of action: 2-3 min (IV)
15 min (IM)

Neonatal half-life: 4.1 hours

Notes: This medication may produce a transient sinusoidal fetal heart rate pattern.

Table 8-2. Narcotic Table: Onset of action and neonatal half-life

MEDICATION	*ONSET OF ACTION*	*NEONATAL HALF-LIFE*
Butorphanol	1-2 min (IV) 10-30 min (IM)	Unknown (similar to nalbuphine in adults)
Fentanyl	1 min (IV)	5.3 hours
Meperidine	5 min (IV) 30-45 min (IM)	63 hours
Morphine	5 min (IV) 30-40 min (IM)	7.1 hours
Nalbuphine	2-3 min (IV) 15 min (IM)	4.1 hours

(*Adapted from ACOG 2002)

141

Options for Pain Relief During Active Labor

During active labor, intravenous or intramuscular narcotics can still be administered. However, care must be taken to not administer too many repeat doses, especially intramuscularly with the delayed release and effect, and not to give them too close to delivery as they can cause significant neonatal depression as previously discussed. When the patient enters active labor and the contraction pain becomes more intense, many women request either an epidural or spinal anesthesia, with over 85% of patients receiving one of these in labor at some institutions.

There is significant debate about what effect an epidural has on the length of labor, the incidence of operative vaginal delivery, the risk of cesarean section, and how it may affect breastfeeding.

With regards to the timing of an epidural, as previously discussed, most physicians attempt to wait until the patient is in active labor (at least 4 cm) to administer an epidural during labor. This is not, however, an absolute requirement.

Many studies have been done to evaluate the effect of epidural anesthesia on labor duration and delivery. A published review on these studies reported that their use resulted in an increased length of both the first and second stages of labor as well as an increase in the need for oxytocin and operative vaginal delivery (Howell 2001). A separate meta-analysis of 10 trials reported that, while the risk of requiring an operative vaginal delivery is increased (OR 2.19, 95% CI 1.32-7.78), the chance that a patient will require an operative vaginal delivery for dystocia (see Chapter 9) is not*(Halpern 1998). This study also noted that patient satisfaction and neonatal outcomes were significantly better with an epidural when compared with parenteral narcotic analgesia.

* (It is important to note that the study by Howell, which involved over 3100 women, did not find a significant difference in the risk of cesarean section when epidural analgesia was used [Howell 2001].)

Epidural anesthesia during labor has also not been shown to decrease the success of breastfeeding and this fear should not deter women from receiving an epidural if they desire one during labor (Halpern 1999).

Indications and contraindications for both epidural and spinal anesthesia, as well as the technique and potential complications, are as follows:

Epidural Anesthesia

Indications:
- Anesthesia during labor
- Multiple gestation attempting vaginal delivery
- Maternal cardiac, pulmonary, or neurologic disease

Contraindications:
- Patient refusal/inability to remain still and cooperate
- Infection at site of needle placement
- *Chorioamnionitis
- **Coagulopathy (i.e., platelets < 100,000, DIC, hemophilia, etc)
- Increased intracranial pressure from mass lesions
- Maternal hypovolemia

Procedure:

A 16- or 18-gauge needle is inserted into the epidural space through the ligamentum flavum in the region of L2-5 and a small catheter is then threaded into this space.

Potential Complications:
- Potential complications of an epidural include:
- Post-epidural placement headache (2%)
- Failure to provide adequate pain relief (10%, Beilin 1998)
- Maternal hypotension (up to 30%)
- Maternal fever (up to 24% of nulliparous women, Philip 1999)
- Fetal heart rate decelerations
- Pruritis

* Chorioamnionitis is listed as a contraindication to epidural/spinal anesthesia in anesthesia texts, but this is usually only in cases where the patient appears septic and the risk of bacetermia is felt to be high (Norris 2000). Antibiotics should be started as soon as chorioamnionitis is diagnosed and the case discussed with the anesthesiologist on call if an epidural is desired.

** Although many anesthesiologists have a set threshold of a platelet count of at least 100,000/uL for placement of an epidural or spinal, there have been several studies reporting that the procedure is safe during labor with counts as low as 50,000/uL (ACOG 2002). Even though this evidence exists, if an anesthesiologist does not feel comfortable with the patient's platelet count and the risk of an epidural hematoma, they may still refuse to place it.

Spinal Anesthesia

Indications: Anesthesia during labor

Contraindications:
- Patient refusal/inability to remain still and cooperate
- Infection at site of needle placement
- Chorioamnionitis
- Coagulopathy (i.e., platelets < 100,000, DIC, hemophilia,etc.)
- Increased intracranial pressure
- Maternal hypovolemia

Procedure:
A spinal needle is inserted through the arachnoid and dura and opioids and/or local anesthetics are injected intrathecally.

Potential Complications:
- Post-placement "spinal" headache (1%-3%)
- Maternal hypotension (25%-67%, Vercauteren 2000; Park 1996)
- Fetal heart rate decelerations
- Pruritis
- Failure to provide adequate pain relief (or the effect wears off prior to delivery)

Combined Spinal/Epidural

This technique is becoming more popular as it allows for both the rapid onset of analgesia from the spinal component, with the ability to continue to provide continuing pain relief with the epidural catheter that is placed during the procedure. It is also effective in providing postoperative pain control after cesarean section with the epidural component. One reported side effect has been a small increased risk of profound fetal bradycardia and even emergency cesarean delivery in 1.5% of cases in one study (Gambling 1998).

Other options for pain relief during active labor include the pudendal nerve block and the paracervical block.

Pudendal Nerve Block

The pudendal nerve includes fibers from S2-4 and innervates the vagina, vulva, and perineum. It also has motor fibers going to the pelvic floor and perineum. Descent of the fetal vertex in the second stage of labor can result in significant pain through the stretching of the pelvic floor. By performing an anesthetic block of this nerve, pain relief for the second stage of labor, and even an operative vaginal delivery, can be obtained.

Indications:
- 2nd stage anesthesia
- Operative vaginal delivery
- Augmentation of an epidural that did not cover the sacral nerves

Contraindications:
- Allergy to local anesthetic agent to be used

Procedure:

A pudendal nerve block kit comes with a needle guide that is inserted into the vagina and directed just posterior to the ischial spines. When injecting the patient's left pudendal nerve, place the needle guide with your left hand, and when injecting the right side, use your right hand to place the needle guide. The needle is then inserted through the needle guide and into the vaginal mucosa until it touches the sacrospinous ligament. Prior to injecting approximately 10 mL of 1% lidocaine or 1% mepivacaine on each side, you must aspirate to ensure you are not directly injecting the pudendal vessels, which are in close proximity to the nerves.

Potential Complications:
- Systemic lidocaine toxicity with convulsions may occur with intravascular injection.
- Hematoma formation
- Infection (very rare)

Paracervical Block

This technique can be used in the first stage of labor, but only provides relief for a relatively short period of time, i.e., 45-60 minutes (ACOG 1996). It is rarely used in current practice because of the potential for serious fetal side-effects and the frequent occurrence of fetal bradycardia. This technique is more helpful for the repair of cervical lacerations or uterine curettage.

Indications:
- Analgesia in the active phase of labor
- Repair of cervical lacerations

Contraindications:
- Allergy to local anesthetic

Procedure:

> This involves injection of 5-10 mL of local anesthetic (usually 1% lidocaine) just below the vaginal mucosa at both the 4- and 8-o'clock positions adjacent to the cervix for a total of 10 to 20 mL. It is important to aspirate frequently to ensure the injections are not intravascular.

Potential Complications:
- Fetal bradycardia
- Fetal distress
- Fetal death

Anesthesia Options for Procedures

Cesarean Delivery

In preparing for a cesarean delivery, either an epidural or spinal anesthesia is normally placed. An epidural takes longer to achieve an adequate level of anesthesia than a spinal anesthetic, but is less likely to cause maternal hypotension. If a patient has been laboring and has a functioning epidural in place, additional medication may be administered through the catheter to obtain a surgical anesthesia level. In cases where the delivery is more urgent and there is not time for conduction anesthesia, a general anesthesia is administered. The decision to administer a general anesthesia should not be taken lightly as the risk of maternal complications is much higher than with either a spinal or epidural. This is discussed in more detail later in this chapter.

Operative Vaginal Delivery

Often, when time comes to consider an operative delivery, the patient will have already received either a spinal or epidural, which should provide sufficient analgesia. If the epidural is not adequate, then it may be redosed by anesthesia as long as there is no pressing fetal distress. If the patient does not have any anesthesia and an operative delivery is required, then some form of pain relief is usually necessary. This is one instance where a vacuum device is advantageous over forceps. The vacuum needs only to be placed on the fetal vertex and does not cause as much maternal discomfort as the placement of forceps. Even in this case, though, anesthesia is usually required. Options for anesthesia with an operative delivery include:

Epidural: This is rarely chosen at the time a decision is made for an operative delivery, because of the relatively long time it takes to place and then take effect.

Spinal: This may be performed relatively rapidly and the onset of pain relief is also very quick. However, if there is evidence of fetal compromise or distress, then there is usually not time for this method. It does, however, provide excellent analgesia when forceps are to be used.

Pudendal block: This can be performed in patients without any other anesthesia, or in those whom an epidural/spinal is not providing adequate relief to allow for an operative delivery. It can be performed rapidly in the presence of fetal distress, and when placed properly, provides excellent pain relief for either a vacuum or forceps delivery. See the previous section for instruction on how to perform the procedure and potential complications.

Perineal infiltration: This method involves local infiltration of the perineal area with a local anesthetic. It is not generally adequate for a forceps delivery, but may provide some relief if an episiotomy must be made during an operative delivery.

Repair of Vaginal Lacerations

For most first- and second-degree lacerations, injections of local anesthetic are usually sufficient to complete the repair with adequate pain relief for the mother. Typically, 1% lidocaine is used for this purpose. It is drawn up into a 5cc-10cc syringe and injected into and around the area to be sutured using a small, usually 21-23 gauge needle. If the patient has a working epidural or pudendal block, then these are almost always adequate as well. (If the epidural is not adequate, it can be redosed by the anesthesiologist for the repair.) The maximum doses of two common local anesthetics that are used are as follows:

1% Lidocaine   4.5 mg/kg
1% Lidocaine w/epinephrine   7 mg/kg

For third- and fourth-degree lacerations, greater visualization is required as well as more time for the repair. If the patient does not have a working regional anesthetic, then IV narcotics and local anesthetics may be required. Some common narcotics used for this include morphine sulfate, meperidine, and fentanyl, all of which have been previously described. In those cases where adequate analgesia cannot be obtained with these measures and the patient is hemodynamically stable, you can consult your anesthesiologist regarding regional anesthesia.

Obstetric Emergencies

Antepartum. When the situation arises and urgent delivery is required, the choice of anesthesia must ensure the ability to rapidly deliver the fetus while making sure the mother remains stable. The type of anesthesia depends on both the fetal status and the proposed route of delivery.

If the fetus meets criteria for an operative vaginal delivery, then analgesia needs to be adequate for the procedure. If the patient has a functioning epidural or spinal anesthesia, then this is usually adequate. If they do not, then a pudendal block may be attempted. In general, vacuum devices require less analgesia than do forceps, which should be taken into account depending on the situation.

If labor has not progressed to the point where an operative vaginal delivery is possible and fetal distress is present, then a cesarean delivery is performed. If the patient has a functioning epidural, then this can usually be used to administer additional medications and achieve an adequate level of analgesia for cesarean section. This does, however, depend on the degree of fetal distress. If severe distress exists, such as a profound bradycardia without recovery, then you may not have time to wait the 10-15 minutes it takes to augment an epidural or place a spinal anesthetic. In this case, a general anesthetic is required. This should not be undertaken lightly as the risk of complications with general anesthesia is significantly higher than with conduction anesthesia. In fact, in pregnancy the risk of maternal death from general anesthesia is 16.7 times greater than with regional anesthesia and the incidence of failed intubation is tenfold higher than in the nonpregnant population (Hawkins 1997; Barnardo 2000).

This is sometimes a difficult thing to decide, and the decision should be made in conjunction with the anesthesiologist as you inform him or her of exactly what level of distress is present and how quickly you need to effect delivery. They will tell you how long it will take for either conduction or general anesthesia to achieve an adequate surgical level. An anesthesiologist will usually recommend general anesthesia if delivery must occur in less than 5-10 minutes.

In extreme emergencies, a cesarean section can be started with local anesthesia while the patient is being intubated or the spinal/epidural anesthesia is becoming adequate. Conditions where this may be necessary include a failed (or contraindicated) regional anesthesia with an inaccessible airway, failed intubation with significant fetal distress, an inadequate regional anesthesia, or no trained personnel available for other types of anesthesia (Norris 2000). A large syringe is filled with local anesthetic and injected subcutaneously where the incision will be made (usually 200-300 mL of 0.5% lidocaine with epinephrine). The incision is then made and successive layers injected as needed until the peritoneal cavity is entered. (You must take into account the maximum doses of local anesthetic that can be used, which were listed earlier in this chapter.) By this time, the anesthesiologist should have the patient asleep or additional intravenous medications can be given after the baby is delivered. Fortunately, this is a very rare occurrence.

Postpartum: In the postpartum patient, the most common emergency requiring anesthesia is postpartum hemorrhage. It is often necessary to make the patient more comfortable in order to manually explore the uterus or repair lacerations that are causing the bleeding. If the bleeding is secondary to uterine inversion, then anesthetic consultation is urgently needed to facilitate replacement of the uterus.

Anesthetic options for postpartum hemorrhage, which usually involves manually exploring the uterus, include the following:

For manual uterine exploration (retained placenta/uterine atony):

- Bolus through an existing epidural catheter
- Intravenous opioids (meperidine, fentanyl, morphine)
- Inhalational nitrous oxide (50% in O2)
- General anesthesia

For vaginal/cervical lacerations:

- Infiltration with local anesthetic
- Bolus through an existing epidural catheter
- Intravenous opioids (meperidine, fentanyl, morphine)
- Inhalational nitrous oxide (50% mixture)

For uterine inversion:

- Nitroglycerin (50-100ug IV)

References:

ACOG Practice Bulletin #36, Obstetric analgesia and anesthesia, July 2002.

Barnardo PD, Jenkins JG. Failed tracheal intubation in obstetrics: a 6-year review in the UK region. Anaesthesia 2000; 55:690-694.

Beilin Y, Zahn J, Bernstein HH, Zucker-Pinchoff B, Zenzen WJ, Andres LA. Treatment of incomplete analgesia after placement of an epidural catheter and administration of local anesthesia for women in labor. Anesthesiology 1998; 88:1502-1506.

Bowes WA. Clinical aspects of normal and abnormal labor. In Maternal Fetal Medicine, 4th ed. Creasy & Resnik eds. W.B. Saunders Co. Philadelphia, 1999.

Chestnut DH, McGrath JM, Vincent RD Jr, Penning DH, Choi WW, Bates JN, et al. Does early administration of epidural analgesia affect obstetric outcome in nulliparous women who are in spontaneous labor? Anesthesiology 1994; 80:1201-1208.

Gambling DR, Sharma SK, Ramin SM, Lucas JM, Leveno KJ, Wiley J, et al. A randomized study of combined spinal-epidural analgesia versus intravenous meperidine during labor: impact on cesarean delivery rate. Anesthesiology 1998; 89:1336-1344.

Halpern SH, Leighton BL, Ohisson A et al. Effect of epidural vs parental opioid analgesia on the progress of labor: a meta-analysis, 1998, JAMA; 280:2105-2110.

Halpern SH, Levine T, Wilson DB, et al. Effect of labor analgesia on breastfeeding success. Birth, 1999; 26:83-88.

Handbook of Obstetric Anesthesia, ed Norris M., Lippincott Williams & Wilkins, Philadelphia, 2000, pages 147, 437.

Hawkins JL, Koonin LM, Palmer SK, Gibbs CP. Anesthesia related deaths during obstetric delivery in the United States 1979-1990. Anesthesiology 1997; 86:277-284.

Hawkins JL. Obstetric anesthesia and analgesia. In Precis: Obstetrics, 2nd ed. Mitchell JL ed, ACOG, Washington, DC, 2000.

Howell CJ. Epidural versus non-epidural analgesia for pain relief in labor. Cochrane Database Syst Rev 2000; CD000331.

Lieberman E, Lang JM, Cohen A, D'Agostino R Jr, Datta S, Frigoletto FD Jr. Association of epidural analgesia with cesarean delivery in nulliparas. Obstet Gynecol 1996; 88:993-1000.

Norris MC. Anesthesia and the compromised fetus. In Handbook of Obstetric Anesthesia. Norris MC ed. Lippencott, Williams & Wilkins, Baltimore, MD, 2000.

Olofsson C, Ekblom A, Ekman-Ordeberg G, Hjelm A, Irestedt L. Lack of analgesic effect systemically administered morphine or pethidine on labour pain. Br J Obstet Gynaecol 1996; 103:968-972.

Park GE, Hauch MA, Curlin F, Datta S, Bader AM. The effects of varying volumes of crystalloid administration before cesarean delivery on maternal hemodynamics and colloid osmotic pressure. Anesth Analg 1996; 83:299-303.

Philip J, Alexander JM, Sharma SK, Leveno KJ, McIntire DD, Wiley J. Epidural analgesia during labor and maternal fever. Anesthesiology 1999; 90:1271-1275.

Sharma SK, Sidawi JE, Ramin SM, Lucas MJ, Leveno KJ, Cunningham FG. Cesarean delivery: a randomized trial of epidural versus patient-controlled meperidine analgesia during labor. Anesthesiology 1997; 87:487-494.

Stephens MB, Fenton LA, Fields SC. Obstetric anesthesia. Prim Care. Mar 2000; 27(1): 203-220.

Thorp JA, Eckert LO, Ang MS, Johnston DA, Peaceman AM, Parisi VM. Epidural analgesia and cesarean section for dystocia: risk factors in nulliparas. Am J Perinatol 1991; 8:402-410.

Vercauteren MP, Coppejans HC, Hoffmann VH, Mertens E, Adriaensen HA. Prevention of hypotension by a single 5-mg dose of ephedrine during small-dose spinal anesthesia in prehydrated cesarean delivery patients. Anesth Analg 2000; 90:324-327.

Wakefield ML. Systemic analgesia: Opiods, ketamine and inhalational agents. In Chestnut DH(ed):Obstetric Anesthesia Priniciples and Practice. St Louis, Mosby-Year Book, 1994, pp 340-352.

Chapter 9

Operative Vaginal Delivery

Indications for Operative Vaginal Delivery

The most recent ACOG Practice Bulletin on this subject states that "no indication for operative vaginal delivery is absolute" (ACOG 2000). This being said, in the right hands, these procedures can allow you to deliver a fetus safely and rapidly, and they are an essential part of any obstetrician's training. Indications for an operative vaginal delivery according to ACOG include:

- Presumed or imminent fetal compromise (example—severe variable decelerations or repetitive late decelerations with pushing)
- Maternal indication for shortened/passive 2nd stage (example—severe maternal cardiac disease or CNS disease)

- Prolonged 2nd stage of labor (see below for definitions as they differ for nulliparous/multiparous patients)
- Aftercoming head of a vaginal breech delivery

Essential Criteria. Having stated the common indications for an operative delivery, there are other criteria that must be met prior to performing an operative delivery. These include the following:

- Size of the baby (EFW, either from sonogram of estimated by Leopold's maneuvers)
- Leading part of fetal skull at +2 station or lower
- Adequate pelvis
- Adequate pain control
- Cervix is completely dilated
- Known fetal head position (i.e., OA, OP, LOA, etc)
- Ruptured membranes

Acronym: **SLAACKR**

Size of baby. The first parameter you must consider is whether or not you believe this infant is small enough to be delivered vaginally. This is why performing Leopold's maneuvers at the time of admission is important in establishing an estimated fetal weight. If you feel that the child is large (fetal weight > 4,000 gms) then, although you may attempt the delivery if you feel the pelvis is adequate (or large enough to allow passage of the fetus), there is a higher chance of a shoulder dystocia and you must be prepared for this complication.

Leading part of fetal skull at +2 station or lower. If the fetus is not at least at +2 station, then you are performing a midforceps delivery, which is only rarely used when it is felt that the fetus can be more rapidly delivered by this method than by cesarean. A mid forceps delivery also requires a physician who has been trained and is comfortable with the procedure as the risks to the mother and fetus are increased over low or outlet forceps deliveries.

Adequate pelvis. If, on clinical pelvimetry, you determine that the patient has a contracted pelvis, then performing an operative delivery is contraindicated. Regardless of how much traction you apply, if the space is too small, the baby still won't fit. (Clinical pelvimetry is described in Chapter 2.)

Adequate pain control. In general, some form of conduction anesthesia (spinal/epidural) is required to perform a forceps delivery. The pressure from the application can be very painful. With a vacuum device, less anesthesia is needed for the application, which is one reason this device is often used. If the patient does not have conduction anesthesia, then a pudendal nerve block may be attempted. (See Chapter 8 for a discussion of these options.)

Cervix completely dilated. Unless the cervix is completely dilated, an operative vaginal delivery should generally not be attempted. If any part of the cervix is caught in the forceps or vacuum device then significant cervical lacerations and hemorrhage can occur.

Known fetal head position. In order to appropriately apply either forceps or a vacuum device, it is imperative that you know the baby's head's position. This can be very difficult after a patient has been pushing for several hours and developed caput, which is why is it important that you check the fetal head position on every labor check and document it in the record.

Ruptured membranes. You cannot place the instruments with the membranes still intact. If the membranes are still intact, which is unlikely when they are completely effaced and dilated, then perform an artificial rupture of membranes (AROM).

Contraindications for Operative Vaginal Delivery

Just as important as knowing the indications and prerequisites for performing an operative vaginal delivery is understanding the conditions when you should not attempt it. These situations include:

General Contraindications:

- Bone demineralization condition (Osteogenesis imperfecta)
- Bleeding disorders (hemophilia, von Willebrand's, etc)
- Fetal head is not engaged
- Head position is not known

Specific for Vacuum:

- Preterm status (< 34 wks gestation) (because of risk of fetal IVH)
- Face presentation

Forceps Delivery

There are multiple texts written on this subject and some of these are listed in the reference section for this chapter as there is too much to cover in this brief text. What this portion will cover are what types of forceps to choose for different deliveries as well as basic instructions on how to apply them in the occiput anterior (OA) position and then checks to perform before applying traction. In order to really learn this, you must get a pair in your hands and practice. This is something that can be done on labor and delivery in any free minutes you have.

Parts of a Forcep

Blades—The blades of the forceps are applied to the fetal head. There are different variations which can be seen in figures 9-2 A-E.

Shank—The shanks connect the handles of the forceps to the blades. Depending on the type of forceps, these may be overlapping or parallel.

Handles—The handles also vary according to the type of forceps. They usually incorporate different locking mechanisms into the design of the forceps.

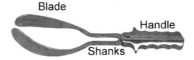

Figure 9-1 Parts of a forcep

Types of Forceps and Indications

Simpson forceps: These are a classic instrument with parallel shanks to allow the blades to fit around any molding that occurs with labor. They are typically used in nulliparous patients when the fetus has a significant amount of molding present.

Elliot forceps: The Elliot forceps are similar in appearance to Simpson forceps, but the shanks are overlapping and not parallel. They are used for delivery of a fetus with minimal molding, usually in multiparous patients.

Keilland forceps: These are the forceps of choice for rotations, especially those of greater than 45 degrees. The reason for this is the absence of a significant pelvic curve, which makes rotation easier through a smaller arc of movement. After rotation, the infant can be delivered with these forceps, although the angle of traction will be different than with the classic instruments such as Simpson or Elliot forceps,

Piper forceps: These forceps are used to deliver the aftercoming head of a breech presentation during vaginal delivery. They are applied after the arms of the fetus are delivered and used to prevent the fetal neck from being hyperextended during delivery.

Luikart modification: This modification is often seen with Simpson forceps (making the Simpson-Luikart forceps) and is notable for the solid blades rather than the fenestrated ones on the classic Simpsons. The advantage of this modification is that vaginal tissue is less likely to be caught in the fenestrations during application and hopefully this will decrease the incidence of vaginal lacerations.

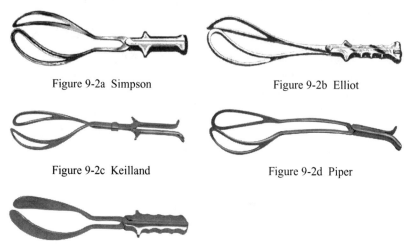

Figure 9-2a Simpson   Figure 9-2b Elliot

Figure 9-2c Keilland   Figure 9-2d Piper

Figure 9-2e Luikart-Simpson

After you have gone through the acronym **SLAACKR**, you are ready to apply the forceps. When placing forceps, the steps are as follows:

1. Counsel the patient
2. Choose appropriate forceps (see above)
3. Check forceps to ensure they match (sometimes after sterilization they are not packaged together correctly)
4. Empty the bladder (or remove the foley catheter)
5. Remove IUPC
6. Remove FSE if it interferes with placement (which it often will)
7. Confirm fetal head position
8. Begin application between contractions
9. Check placement with 3 checks (see below)
10. Apply traction with next contraction
11. Monitor the fetal heart rate between pushes

Application of Forceps

When the fetus is in the occiput anterior (OA) position, the left blade is applied first. (*Note that the LEFT blade is referring to the blade that will be on the fetus's LEFT and not yours.) If the fetus is rotated to either side, then the posterior blade is placed first as it will act as a splint when the anterior blade is placed (Hale 2001). In the OA position, the left blade is held in the right hand, with the left hand holding the handle. The blade of the forcep is held vertically and inserted into the vagina, with the right hand between the vaginal sidewall and the blade. The right hand then guides the blade into place with gentle pressure as the left hand guides the handle through a wide arc in a counter-clockwise fashion. (See figures 9-3 and 9-4.) The left hand does NOT force the forcep in place, but guides it. Grasping the handle with only the thumb and two fingers will help to avoid any temptation to use the left hand too aggressively. The right blade is grasped in the left hand and applied in the same manner, but the arc is in a clockwise direction. (See figure 9-5.)

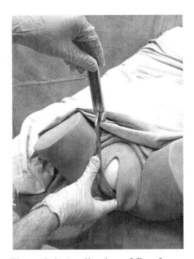

Figure 9-3 Application of first forcep

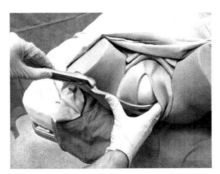

Figure 9-4 Insertion of first forcep and arc

157

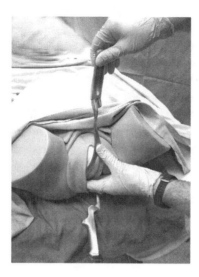

Figure 9-5 Application of second forcep

After both blades are placed, the handles are articulated, or put together, you will perform three checks. If placement is not adequate, they may be disarticulated and small adjustments made.

Checking Placement of Forceps

1. Ensure the saggital suture is centered between the blades and running perpendicular to the plane of the shanks.
2. Be able to place no more than one finger between the fenestrations of each blade and the fetal skull. The amount of the fenestration felt on both sides should be equal.
3. The posterior fontanelle should be midway between the sides of the blades and only one finger's breadth above the shanks.

(Hale 2001)

Applying traction

When applying traction, it is important to apply it in the appropriate direction. This is often referred to as "axis traction" as you are attempting to apply force in the plane of least resistance. The dominant hand is used to grasp the handles of the forceps and the other hand is placed on the shanks to pull down in a vertical manner, which is called the Pajot maneuver (Hale 2001). This will guide a fetus in the OA position under the pubic symphysis. At times, an instrument called a Bill handle is attached to the handle of the forceps which will accomplish the same axis traction. (See figure 9-6.)

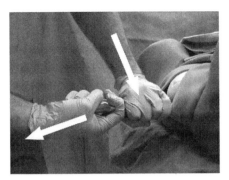

Figure 9-6 Axis traction

The amount of traction applied should be the least possible to accomplish descent of the fetal head. Traction is applied in a steady manner, gradually increasing in intensity as needed, during a contraction with maternal pushing, and then gradually relaxed after the contraction ends.

An episiotomy does not have to be cut just because forceps are placed. If there is significant resistance from the soft tissues, then it can be performed either between pushes, or as the perineum is being distended by the fetal head. If one is performed, care must be taken not to cut the infant, and it is extremely important to support the perineum as the infant delivers to try and avoid extension of the incision into the anal sphincter and rectum.

As the fetal head descends and distends the perineum, the forceps handles are elevated with the dominant hand. The other hand, or an assistant, supports the perineum. (The handles should not be elevated > 45 degrees above a horizontal plane protect against sulcus lacerations.) The blades are then removed by reversing the movements used to apply them, with the right blade first. Make sure to make the same arc motion with removal. After the forceps are removed, delivery of the shoulders and body should proceed in the normal manner.

After the delivery, it is important to examine the vaginal sidewalls for lacerations, as well as the posterior vagina and look for extension of lacerations or an episiotomy into the anal sphincter or rectum.

NOTE: If the fetal head does not descend with appropriate traction, then you can reassess head position. Traction from the OP position is different from the OA position. The most important thing to remember is that, if a fetus does not descend with appropriate traction generated by the arms and shoulders, then there is probably a good reason. It takes practice to understand exactly how much traction to apply, but never make the mistake of applying too much.

Vacuum Delivery

Use of the vacuum device can result in complications just like forceps. After determining that an operative vaginal delivery is indicated, and going through your acronym SLAACKR, consider whether you can use a vacuum. (i.e., gestational age at least 34 weeks, no known bleeding disorders, and no need for rotation) General reasons for choosing a vacuum device over forceps are, more experience with vacuum devices and less need for pain control for placement.

Application and Traction

After counseling the patient and confirming fetal head position, empty the patient's bladder. Then place the vacuum device such that it covers in the midline of the vertex. Make sure that it does not overlap either the anterior or posterior fontanelles, and that there is no vaginal tissue trapped in between the vacuum and the fetal scalp.

When the patient experiences a contraction, have your assistant bring the pressure up to an appropriate level, which should not generally exceed 500-600 mmHg or 0.6 to 0.8 kg/cm^2 (it is important to make sure and review the instructions for the vacuum device that your institution uses so that you will know the appropriate pressure.) After you have done this, apply traction with each push in the appropriate axis (see the forceps section for this description.) It is important to avoid a rocking or jerking motion and instead use gentle and steady traction.

Between pushes release the pressure on the vacuum. This will decrease the risk of cephalohematoma as much as possible.

If the vacuum comes off three times, it is generally wise to abandon the procedure. Also, when this happens, recheck the fetal head position, because, when the fetus is in the OP position, this will often occur.

Sequential Use of Vacuum and Forceps for Delivery

With the increased use of vacuum devices, which are not as successful as forceps in completing delivery, there are times where one instrument is used after the initial one has failed. In a recent study by Gardella et al, they reported on the maternal and neonatal morbidity of over 3,700 combined vacuum/forcep deliveries with an equal number of deliveries by forceps alone and vacuum alone, as well as an additional 11,000 spontaneous vaginal deliveries (Gardella 2001). They found that the risk of intracranial hemorrhage was significantly increased by 3.9-fold when both devices were utilized during delivery. They also reported an increased risk of facial nerve injury, neonatal seizures, and postpartum hemorrhage when both instruments were used compared to

160

only one instrument. Because of this data, extreme care should be taken in both the choice of the first instrument to use, as well as in making a decision to apply a second instrument should the first one fail.

Potential Complications of Operative Vaginal Delivery

There are potential complications involved in the use of both forceps and vacuum devices. It is imperative that you are knowledgeable regarding both maternal and fetal complications so that you can do your best to avoid them, and how to recognize them should they occur. They are as follows:

A. Forceps—

1. Maternal Complications:

a. Cervical lacerations
b. Vaginal sidewall lacerations
c. Third/Fourth degree lacerations (involvement of the anal sphincter/rectum)
d. Vaginal hematoma
e. Postpartum hemorrhage
f. Endometritis (This occurs in 16% of forceps deliveries, Williams 1991.)

2. Fetal Complications:

a. Cephalohematoma
b. Neonatal abducens (6th nerve) injury - 2.4% of forceps deliveries (Gailbraith 1994)
c. Facial marks (These usually resolve within the first few days of life.)
d. Neonatal jaundice
e. Skull fractures

B. Vacuum*—

1. Maternal Complications:

a. Vaginal lacerations: These tend to occur less often than with forceps although if any vaginal tissue is caught between the vacuum device and the fetal head, these can cause significant hemorrhage afterwards. Any operative delivery, especially those that involve an

161

episiotomy, can result in third/fourth degree lacerations although vacuum deliveries are less likely than forceps to cause this. (See Chapter 11.)
   b. Cervical lacerations
   c. Postpartum hemorrhage
   d. Endometritis (This occurs in 8% of vacuum deliveries, Williams 1991.)

2. Fetal Complications:

   a. Scalp lacerations (especially if a twisting movement, or "cookie-cutter" motion is used to attempt to rotate the infant.)
   b. Cephalohematoma—approximately 15% (Johanson 1999)
   c. Subgaleal hematoma—bleeding between cranial periostium and epicranial aponeurosis
   d. Retinal hemorrhages
   e. Neonatal jaundice

* The overall incidence of serious complications with a vacuum extraction is approximately 5% (Robertson 1999).

Long-term Infant Outcomes with Operative Vaginal Delivery

There have been two long-term studies of the cognitive development of children delivered by forceps or vacuum extractor and these found no difference when compared to infants delivered spontaneously (Wesley BD 1993; Ngan HY 1990). The forceps study included nearly 1,200 children delivered via forceps and the vacuum study nearly 300 vacuum deliveries. Another study reported that the risk of intracranial hemorrhage was not increased in over 7,000 operative vaginal deliveries (both vacuum and forceps) when compared with spontaneous vaginal delivery (Garnella 2001). These facts are important to know when counseling patients as they are often nervous when you discuss these interventions with them.

References:

Gailbraith RS. Incidence of neonatal sixth nerve palsy in relation to mode of delivery. Am J Obstet Gynecol, 1994; 170:1158-1159.

Gardella C, Taylor M, Benedetti T, Hitti J, Critchlow C. The effect of sequential use of vacuum and forceps for assisted vaginal delivery on neonatal and maternal outcomes. Am J Obstet Gynecol Oct 2001; 185(4):896-902.

Hale RW, editor Dennen's Forceps Deliveries, 4th edition, American College of Obstetricians and Gynecologists, 2001, Washington, D.C.

Johanson RB, Menon BKV. Vacuum extraction versus forceps for assisted vaginal delivery (Cochrane Review). In: The Cochrane Library, Issue 4, 1999. Oxford: Update Software.

Operative vaginal delivery. American College of OB/GYN Technical Bulletin #17, June 2000.

Ngan HY, Miu P, Ko L, Ma HK. Long-term neurological sequelae following vacuum extractor delivery. Aust N Z J Obstet Gynaecol 1990; 30:111-114.

Robertson PA, Laros RK Jr, Zhao RL. Neonatal and maternal outcome in low-pelvic and midpelvic operative deliveries. Am J Obstet Gynecol 1990; 162:1436-1442.

Wesley BD, Van den Berg BJ, Reece EA. The effect of forceps delivery on cognitive development. Am J Obstet Gynecol 1993; 169:1091-1095.

Williams MC, Knuppel RA, O'Brien WF, Weiss A, Kanarek KS. A randomized comparison of assisted vaginal delivery by obstetric forceps and polyethylene vacuum cup. Obstet Gynecol, 1991; 78:789-794.

Chapter 10

Cesarean Delivery

- Cesarean Delivery
  - Indications for Cesarean Section
  - Preoperative Evaluation
    - Anesthesia
  - Essential Anatomy
  - Surgical Instruments
  - Types of Uterine Incisions
  - Potential Complications
  - Patient Counseling
  - Description of Operation
  - Approach to Intraoperative Hemorrhage
  - Estimation of Blood Loss
  - Emergency Cesarean Section
- Vaginal Birth After Cesarean (VBAC)
  - Brief History
  - Benefits of VBAC
  - Candidates and Contraindications
  - Patient Counseling
    - Success Rates
  - Labor Management
    - Initial Evaluation
    - Induction of Labor
    - Augmentation of Labor
    - Anesthesia during Labor
  - Potential Complications

Cesarean Delivery

Cesarean deliveries are now a routine part of any obstetric practice. The current cesarean rate in the United States is approximately 31% (CDC 2006). Of these operations, the majority are repeat cesarean sections. Once a patient has had a cesarean, for any reason, she may choose to have a repeat cesarean delivery with subsequent pregnancies. While attempting to have a **V**aginal **B**irth **A**fter **C**esarean section (**VBAC**) is a reasonable option for many women, they must be given the option of a repeat cesarean delivery as there are risks involved in a VBAC. This topic is discussed in detail later in this chapter.

Indications for cesarean section. As with nearly everything in obstetrics, there are both maternal and fetal indications for performing a cesarean delivery. Currently, over 85% of cesarean sections performed in the United States are done for one of the following four reasons:

1. Prior cesarean delivery
2. Labor dystocia (Arrest of dilation/Arrest of descent)
3. Fetal distress
4. Breech presentation

(Williams 2001)

Chapter 4 and Chapter 5 contain extensive discussions of exactly when a cesarean delivery is indicated for labor dystocia, as well as what level of fetal distress that may require an immediate cesarean section.

Other, less common indications for cesarean delivery can be categorized as either maternal or fetal. Some of these include the following:

Maternal:
1. Placenta previa or vasa previa
2. Placental abruption
3. CNS lesions that make labor contraindicated
4. Active genital HSV infection during labor
5. HIV infection with a detectable viral load* (>1,000 copies)

Fetal:
1. Transverse fetal lie
2. Breech presentation
3. Umbilical cord prolapse

4. Significant hydrocephalus that makes vaginal delivery impossible
5. Fetal macrosomia **
6. Other fetal conditions that preclude vaginal delivery
7. Triplet pregnancy or higher-order multiple gestations
8. Fetal bleeding disorder

> * This recommendation depends on the patient's antepartum treatment as well as their viral load at the time of delivery (Chen 2001; Minkoff 2003).
>
> ** Presumed fetal macrosomia is rarely an indication for a primary cesarean section without labor. This is because ultrasound estimation of fetal weight is not very accurate at term. ACOG does, however, recommend offering a prophylactic cesarean section if the estimated fetal weight is > 5,000 grams in a non-diabetic patient or > 4,500 grams in a patient with diabetes in an effort to prevent shoulder dystocia (ACOG 2000).

Preoperative evaluation. Prior to beginning a cesarean section, the following steps should be taken:

1. Anesthesia evaluation for determining type of anesthesia required. (This will most often be some form of conduction anesthesia. See Chapter 8.)
2. Baseline laboratory testing to include a measurement of hemoglobin, hematocrit, platelets and an antibody screen.
3. Order antibiotic prophylaxis (usually either ampicillin, an extended-spectrum penicillin or cephalosporin)

Anesthesia. Most commonly, either a spinal or epidural anesthesia is used to perform a cesarean section. In emergent cases, or when a spinal or epidural is contraindicated (such as patients with thrombocytopenia or a coagulopathy), it may be necessary to administer a general anesthesia. This should be undertaken with caution as the risks of a general anesthesia in pregnancy are significantly higher than with conduction anesthesia.

Essential anatomy. Most cesarean sections will be straightforward in terms of anatomy, but a thorough knowledge of female pelvic anatomy is essential for when complications occur. You must know every layer of tissue that you incise and understand the potential problems that can occur at each step of the operation. Always remember that if there are abdominal adhesions or you are having difficulty repairing the uterine incision, *restore normal anatomy first*. This will prevent accidental damage of other structures and ensure an appropriate repair. Both written descriptions as well as diagrams are provided to help you identify important structures during the operation.

A. **Abdominal wall.** When beginning the operation, you will make a sharp incision in the skin with a scalpel. After getting through the skin, you will encounter the following layers in this order:

1. Subcutaneous tissue
   a. Camper's fascia (fatty tissue)
   b. Scarpa's fascia (thick, fibrous tissue)

2. Fascia (musculoaponeurotic layer)
   a. Rectus sheath (formed by the aponeuroses of the external and internal oblique and transversalis muscles)

3. Transversalis fascia
4. Peritoneum

B. **Blood vessels.** In general, during an uncomplicated cesarean delivery, you should not encounter or damage any significant blood vessels. However, some large vessels that you may see and should be aware of include the following:

Abdominal wall vessels. The femoral artery supplies branches to the superficial layers of the abdominal wall, and the external iliac artery gives rise to the inferior epigastric artery. Specifically, some important vessels are the following:

a. ***Branches of Femoral Artery***

   1) Superficial epigastric artery: This vessel is lateral to the rectus muscle and runs over the external oblique muscle.
   2) Superficial circumflex artery: Runs laterally, inferior to the iliac ligament up toward the iliac crest.
   3) Superficial external pudendal artery: This vessel runs in a medial direction just above the inguinal ligament.

b. ***Branches of External Iliac Artery***

   1) Inferior epigastric artery: This vessel runs superiorly on the posterior and lateral portion of the rectus abdominal muscles. It is not incised with a transverse incision, but if a muscle-cutting incision (such as a Maylard incision*) is used, these must be identified and ligated prior to transecting the rectus muscles.

167

* (Note: This type of incision is rarely used in a cesarean as a Pfannenstiel incision should generally not be converted to a Maylard.)

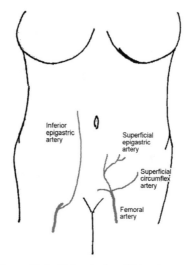

Figure 10-1 Abdominal wall blood vessels

Intra-abdominal:

    a.   Uterine arteries: These arteries are on the lateral sides of the uterus in the broad ligament. They are most commonly injured when a low transverse uterine incision extends laterally.

C. **Uterus**. The uterus is a muscular organ that receives blood from the uterine arteries and the many collateral vessels.

D. **Ureters/Bladder**. The bladder is located anterior to the uterus, and a bladder flap is made prior to the uterine incision in order to avoid injury. The ureters lie lateral to the cervix and may be damaged if there is lateral extension of the uterine incision and they are incorporated in clamps or sutures placed in this area to control bleeding (figure 10-2). Making sure your initial uterine incision is not too lateral and good technique with delivery of the fetus will decrease the risk of the incision extending laterally.

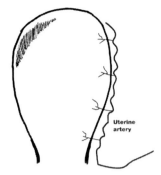

Figure 10-2 Location of uterine arteries with respect to the uterus

Surgical instruments. When in the OR, both as the surgeon and as an assistant, you must be able to ask for the instrument you need in a way that the scrub tech can provide it to you in a timely manner. To do this, you need to know the names of the basic instruments and what they are used for as well as what they look like because sometimes you will be handed a different instrument than what you requested. What follows here is a list of the basic surgical instruments used during a cesarean section. Photos of these instruments, their function and when they are used is described in the cesarean section talk-through in Appendix C.

Scalpel—(usually a No. 10 blade for both abdominal and uterine incisions)

Bovie—(Setting is commonly 40 cut / 40 coagulation)

Suction—(usually a Yankauer-type suction device)

Pickups—(Debakey or smooth pickups, Russian pickups, Rat-tooth pickups)

Clamps—(Allis clamp, Kelly clamp, Hemostat, Pennington, Ring forceps)

Retractors—(Large, medium, small Rich retractors, bladder blade)

Scissors—(Metzenbaum, Mayo)

Laparotomy tapes

Types of Uterine incisions. The most common type of uterine incision made is a low transverse uterine incision. Remember that the incision on the abdomen does not necessary match the type of incision on the uterus. (This is a point that often confuses patients, medical students, and interns alike.) What type of uterine incision is used may depend on the gestational age of the patient, fetal lie, location of the placenta, and the presence of

169

uterine myomas or adhesions. Because the type of uterine incision made has implications for future pregnancies, it is important to clearly note in the operative report which type is made. Four common types of uterine incisions will be described here. They are:

1. Low transverse
2. Low vertical
3. Classical
4. T-shaped

Low transverse incision. This is the most common uterine incision made during a cesarean section. It is used in term or near-term pregnancies with a developed lower uterine segment. The fetus may be in either a breech or vertex presentation and it may also be used with multiple gestations.

Subsequent pregnancies: These patients can labor with subsequent pregnancies. (See discussion of VBAC in this chapter.) The risk of uterine rupture in future pregnancies is 0.2%-1.5% (ACOG 1999).

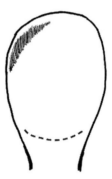

Figure 10-3a Low transverse uterine incision

Low vertical incision. This incision, while vertical like a classical incision, does not extend into the contractile portion of the uterus. It may be performed when one of the following situations is present:

1. Preterm fetus with an undeveloped lower uterine section
2. Anterior placenta previa
3. Scheduled cesarean hysterectomy
4. Back down, transverse lie
5. Transverse lie with oligohydramnios
6. Myomas occupying the lower uterine segment.

This type of incision is associated with increased blood loss and infection rates compared to a low transverse incision (Boyle 1996). A low vertical incision is repaired in layers, in the same manner as a classical incision. While an incision may begin as a low vertical incision, it may extend spontaneously during delivery or be extended with bandage scissors if it is found not to be adequate for delivery. If this occurs, it must be clearly documented in the patient's record and the patient should not labor with her next pregnancy.

Subsequent pregnancies: These patients may be allowed to labor although this is somewhat controversial. (See discussion of VBAC in this chapter.) The risk of uterine rupture in future pregnancies is 1%-7% (ACOG 1999).

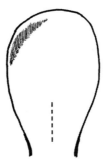

Figure 10-3b Low vertical uterine incision

Classical incision. A classical incision extends vertically into the fundal region of the uterus. The incision is started as low as possible, but above the bladder, and then carried superiorly toward the fundus until it is large enough to allow for atraumatic delivery of the fetus. It is performed in the following situations:

1. Lower uterine segment cannot be entered because of adhesions or fibroids
2. Transverse lie with a large fetus
3. Very small fetus with a poorly developed (or very thick) lower uterine segment
4. Maternal morbid obesity where only the upper uterus can be accessed (Williams 2001).

Subsequent pregnancies: These patients should not be allowed to labor with subsequent pregnancies. The risk of uterine rupture in future pregnancies is 4%-9% (ACOG 2004).

171

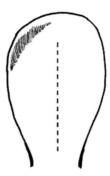

Figure 10-3c Classical uterine incision

T-shaped incision. This incision is almost never made as the initial uterine incision, but rather occurs because a low transverse incision is found not to be adequate to deliver the fetus. At this point, bandage scissors are used to extend the incision upward toward the fundus from the middle of the original incision. (Another variation of this is termed a J-incision in which the original incision is extended upward from one edge with bandage scissors.) The upper portion of the incision is closed with the same technique of a classical incision and the low transverse part as a low transverse incision.

The most common reasons for extending the incision in this manner are malpresentation and breech extraction with fetal head entrapment (Boyle 1996). This extension is associated with surgical complications in 50% of patients, with the most common being excessive blood loss, broad ligament hematomas, cervical lacerations, and uterine artery lacerations (Boyle 1996).

Subsequent pregnancies: These patients should not be allowed to labor with subsequent pregnancies. The risk of uterine rupture in future pregnancies is 4%-9% (ACOG 1999).

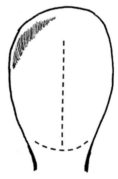

Figure 10-3d T-shaped uterine incision

Potential Complications. Because a cesarean section is a laparotomy and major abdominal surgery, the patient must be counseled prior to the procedure and you must be familiar with the incidence of potential complications that may occur. Some of the more common complications include the following:

> **Hemorrhage/Transfusion.** Hemorrhage, which is defined as an estimated blood loss of greater than 1,000 cc at time of cesarean section, a drop in hematocrit of 10%, or the need for a transfusion, occurs in approximately 6% of cesarean sections. This complication may occur secondary to uterine atony, abnormal placentation (i.e., placenta accreta) or laceration of blood vessels (most commonly the uterine arteries). The risk of transfusion with a cesarean delivery is approximately 1%-2% (Petitte 1985). It is more likely to occur when patients undergo a classical or T-shaped uterine incision.

> **Infection.** Postoperative infections after a cesarean section usually include both wound infections and endometritis. The risk of infection depends on the both the patient's individual risk factors as well as the circumstances surrounding the need for a cesarean section.

> Maternal factors that increase the risk of a postoperative infection include the following:

> > 1. Obesity
> > 2. Diabetes
> > 3. Malignancy
> > 4. Malnutrition

> Additional risk factors for postoperative infection include the following:

> > 1. Prolonged rupture of membranes
> > 2. Chorioamnionitis
> > 3. Manual removal of the placenta
> > 4. Frequent vaginal examinations
> > 5. Emergency cesarean section

> A cesarean delivery is considered a clean-contaminated procedure and has an infection risk of up to 30% in the general population and up to 50% percent in morbidly obese women (Chauhan 2001). It is important to note that the risk of postoperative infection is related to whether or not the patient is in labor or has chorioamnionitis at the time of cesarean section.

Damage to bowel/bladder. These complications are, fortunately, rare with cesarean section, occurring only about 1% of the time (Nielsen 1984). Patients who have had previous abdominal surgery, severe adhesions or scarring from endometriosis or infection, or who require a cesarean hysterectomy are at increased risk of bowel or bladder injury during cesarean section. The risk of bladder injury is decreased by continuous drainage with a foley catheter during the operation, which is why this step should always be taken, even with emergency deliveries.

Thromboembolic disease. Deep venous thrombosis (DVT) with resultant pulmonary embolism (PE) is the leading cause of maternal mortality associated with cesarean section and is more than four times more likely to occur after cesarean section as compared to a vaginal delivery (Simpson 2001). Attempts to prevent this complication include the use of pneumatic compression stockings, early ambulation after surgery, and even prophylactic anticoagulation in high-risk women.

Fascial dehiscence. The risk of fascial dehiscence after cesarean section at approximately 0.3% (Hendrix 2000). The most important risk factor for this complication, which occurs when the fascia comes apart after surgery and may allow protrusion of bowel through the incision, is wound infection. If a fascial dehiscence occurs, then the patient will require surgery to repair the defect. The overall incidence of wound infections after cesarean section has been reported to be approximately 4% (Chaim 2000).

Injury to the baby. The uterus must be entered carefully as it is possible to injure the fetus with the scalpel at this time. The overall incidence of this complication has been reported as between 1.1% and 1.5% (Weiner 2002; Alexander 2006). This risk appears to be the same regardless of the fetal presentation, whether or not the membranes are intact or ruptured. The type of incision may also make a difference, with fetal injury rates of 3.4% reported for a "T" or "J" incision versus only 1.4% for a vertical uterine incision and 1.1% for a low transverse incision (Alexander 2006). If an injury does occur it is important to inform the parents and have the pediatricians and a plastic surgeon evaluate the infant if needed.

Maternal mortality. As with any abdominal surgery, there is a risk of maternal mortality. Even though this risk, especially with an elective cesarean section, is low, it is still present and has been estimated to be approximately 5.8 per 100,000 operations (Sachs 1988).

Retained foreign body. The risk of having a retained sponge or instrument is very low. One analysis of surgical cases over a 16 year period reported that the overall risk was between 1:8,801 and 1:18,760 inpatient operations and this risk was increased if the procedure was an emergency or the patient has an elevated body mass index (Gawande 2003). Care should be taken to ensure that counts of instruments and sponges are correct at the end of the procedure, and that if the procedure was an emergency and there was no count done, that abdominal films are done prior to completing the procedure.

Patient Counseling. The depth of counseling will depend on the urgency of the clinical situation. For scheduled procedures a longer explanation of the risks and benefits listed above should occur and be documented. For emergent cases a brief discussion of the most common potential complications (bleeding/transfusion/infection/damage to bowel or bladder) should occur. Ideally, the discussion regarding cesarean section should occur at the time of admission.

Description of Operation

A. Preparing for Surgery

After the decision has been made to perform a cesarean delivery the patient and spouse should be counseled as to the risks and benefits of the operation and the indications must be clearly explained. When the cesarean is urgent or emergent, the counseling will obviously be more brief. While the American College of Obstetricians and Gynecologists (ACOG) recommends that facilities should have the ability to perform a cesarean section within 30 minutes of the decision being made, the operation will proceed much more rapidly during an emergency, and can safely be delayed longer in non-acute situations (ACOG 1992; Chauhan 1997). Things that should be brought up in counseling include the following:

1. Indication for the cesarean section
2. Potential complications

    a. Hemorrhage
    b. Transfusion of blood products
    c. Damage to bowel, bladder, other abdominal organs
    d. Infection
    e. Hysterectomy
    f. Further surgery if complications occur
    g. Maternal death

A note should be made in the chart detailing the indication for the procedure as well as the fact that the patient was counseled, specifically mentioning the above elements. (See Appendix B for an example.)

Antibiotics should be ordered for the patient to be given in the OR. In general, a single dose of ampicillin, another extended-spectrum penicillin, or a first generation cephalosporin such as cephazolin is given just after the umbilical cord is clamped to decrease the risk of a postoperative infection. If the patient has a well-documented and serious penicillin allergy, then clindamycin or vancomycin may be used for prophylaxis (Mann 2002). If the patient has been laboring and has developed chorioamnionitis prior to a cesarean section, her antibiotics (which will usually consist of ampicillin and gentamycin) should be continued postoperatively, usually with the addition of clindamycin to the regimen, to decrease the risk of postpartum endometritis.

B. In the OR

After the patient is moved to the OR, it is important to document the FHR. In the case of fetal distress, this will help to gauge just how quickly the operation must proceed. After the FHR is documented, anesthesia is administered. In a non-emergent delivery, this usually means a spinal or epidural. This procedure will usually produce a surgical level of anesthesia in 10-20 minutes. In an emergency, general anesthesia may be given or even IV sedation while the operation is started under local anesthesia. (This technique is discussed later.)

When anesthesia has been administered, the FHR monitor is removed (if an FSE is on the fetal scalp, it is removed as well). A foley catheter is inserted, a grounding pad is placed on the thigh, and the abdomen prepped. During this time, the surgeons scrub and gown. After the patient is prepped, the drape is placed by the surgeons and the appropriate suction and bovie attachments are handed off to field to be attached.

C. *Description of Operation*

A final check is performed to ensure that anesthesia is adequate. This is usually done by grasping the skin with an Allis clamp at the level of the intended incision as well as near the umbilicus on both sides of the midline. If significant pain is experienced by the patient, then additional anesthesia is required.

Incision. After adequate anesthesia is obtained, the skin is incised. The two main types of incisions used are the modified Pfannenstiel and the infraumbilical vertical incision.

Modified Pfannenstiel. This is the most common incision for a cesarean section. It is a transverse, slightly curved incision made approximately two fingerbreadths above the superior edge of the pubic bone and extended slightly upward on either side to just past the lateral borders of the rectus muscles (figure 10-4). It has the advantage of being stronger after repair than a vertical incision, and it usually gives a better cosmetic result as it is concealed near the hairline. The procedure for using a modified Pfannenstiel incision is as follows:

After the initial skin incision, the scalpel is used to carry the incision through the subcutaneous tissue down to the underlying fascia. The fascia is then incised in the midline and then, using Mayo scissors, the incision is extended in a transverse fashion on each side. At this point, Kocher clamps are used to grasp the superior edge of the fascia, and it is dissected off the underlying rectus muscles with sharp and blunt dissection. The inferior edges of the fascia are then grasped with Kocher clamps and dissection carried inferiorly to the symphysis. After this, the rectus muscles are separated in the midline and the underlying peritoneum is grasped with two clamps (usually either Kelly or mosquito clamps). Once the surgeon is sure there is no bowel, bladder, or other structures adherent to the peritoneum in that spot, it is incised with Metzenbaum scissors and the abdominal cavity entered.

NOTE: If additional room is needed for the operation, then a Pfannenstiel may be converted to a Cherney incision by sharply dissecting the tendinous insertion of the rectus abdominus muscles from their insertion into the pubic symphysis. The inferior epigastric arteries should be lateral to the insertion and do not need to be ligated. After the operation, the rectus abdominus muscles are then reattached using interrupted permanent sutures.

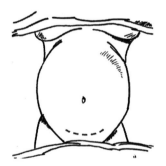

Figure 10-4 Pfannenstiel incision

Vertical incision. Less often, this type of incision is used when rapid entry into the abdominal cavity is needed, such as in the case of fetal distress. It is also the preferred incision in a patient with a coagulopathy, those who refuse transfusion, or who are receiving systemic anticoagulation. It may also be used when the patient has had a previous vertical incision. It is usually started just below the umbilicus and extends inferiorly to approximately 2 cm above the pubic bone (figure 10-5). The advantages of a vertical incision are that it facilitates more rapid access to the uterus, and it is associated with less blood loss and provides better exposure than a modified Pfannenstiel incision. The incision can be extended superior and around the umbilicus if additional exposure is needed. The procedure for a vertical incision is as follows:

A scalpel is used to make an incision in the midline from just below the umbilicus to approximately 2 cm above the pubic symphysis. The subcutaneous tissue is incised down to the sheath of the anterior rectus muscle. The fascia is then incised sharply with the scalpel and then the incision extended superiorly and inferiorly with either a scalpel or Mayo scissors. The rectus muscles are then split in the midline to expose the peritoneum, which is entered above the level of the bladder in the same way as previously described.

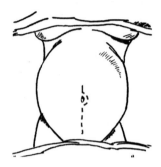

Figure 10-5 Vertical abdominal incision

Creation of bladder flap. After the abdomen has been entered, a bladder blade is inserted to expose the lower uterine segment and the vesicouterine serosa is elevated and incised with Metzenbaum scissors in a curvilinear fashion just superior to the bladder. A clamp is then used to grasp the inferior part of the incision and a bladder flap is made bluntly, always applying pressure against the uterus with care to not injure the bladder anteriorly, or the blood vessels laterally. After this, the bladder blade is replaced between the newly formed bladder flap and uterus.

Uterine incision. Prior to making the uterine incision, it is important to palpate the uterus to determine if it is significantly rotated. Assessing this will help prevent making an incision that is too lateral and should decrease the risk of extension into the uterine arteries. The uterus is then incised approximately 2 cm to 4 cm in a transverse direction (other types of uterine incisions are discussed later in this chapter) in the center of the exposed lower uterine segment. The incision site is then suctioned and palpated after each pass with the scalpel. This is done so that the fetus is not accidentally injured with entry into the uterine cavity. (If you get to the level of the membranes, then you can extend your incision with the membranes intact if desired.) After the uterine cavity is entered, with or without the membranes intact, the incision can be extended either sharply, with bandage scissors, or bluntly, with two fingers inserted into the uterus and traction exerted upward and slightly laterally*. While sharp extension is needed at times with an unlabored lower uterine segment, there is evidence that this may be associated with increased blood loss (Rodriguez 1994; Magann 2002). Because of this, it is recommended that blunt extension be used when possible (Berghella 2005). The key in extending the uterine incision is to ensure you do not extend laterally into the uterine vessels.

It is also important to remember that with ruptured membranes or oligohydramnios, there may be very little fluid between the uterus and baby and in this case you must take extra care not to injure the baby with the scalpel as you make your uterine incision.

* NOTE: It is important that you pull in a mostly vertical/cephalad direction rather than laterally as this should decrease the risk of extension of the incision into the lateral uterine vessels.

Delivery of the infant. The technique for this depends on the presentation of the fetus. The techniques for delivery of vertex and breech fetuses are discussed below.

Vertex presentation. After the uterine incision has been extended, the surgeon's hand is inserted with fingers extended into the uterus inferior to the fetal head. *(Note: If the patient has been pushing prior to the operation, then an assistant may need to push the fetal head up some by inserting a hand into the vagina.) A moderate amount of fundal pressure is applied with either the surgeon's other hand or from an assistant and the fetal head is gently brought through the uterine incision. At this point, the nares and mouth are bulb suctioned and the rest of the fetus delivered. The umbilical cord is clamped x 2 and cut and the infant handed off the field to the pediatricians.

Breech presentation. The operator's hand is inserted in the same fashion as a vertex presentation. The fetal buttocks is then elevated through the uterine incision, again with the assistance of a moderate amount of fundal pressure. The legs are delivered one at a time by splinting the fetal thigh with the fingers parallel to the femur and then sweeping the leg away from the midline. (Note: If the fetus is in a footling breech position, then the feet are grasped and these are then delivered through the incision to the level of the fetal back.) After this, the lower body of the fetus is rotated to a sacrum anterior position if it is not already there and wrapped in a sterile blue towel and gently delivered to the level of the scapula. The fetus is then rotated so that one shoulder is superior, and that arm is then delivered by first splinting the arm with the fingers parallel to the humerus, and then sweeping it downward. The fetus is then rotated to the other side, and the procedure repeated. After this, a Mauriceau-Smellie-Veit maneuver is performed where the index and middle finger of one hand are placed on the fetal maxilla in order to flex the head and complete the delivery.

* (The maneuvers to deliver the breech during a cesarean section are the same as with a breech vaginal delivery which is described and illustrated in Chapter 14.)

Transverse presentation. When a fetus is in a transverse position, then some thought must be given prior to what type of uterine incision will be made prior to beginning the operation. In general, a back-down transverse lie is an indication for a vertical uterine incision as it can be very difficult or impossible to grasp the fetal feet through a low transverse incision with this presentation. If a transverse lie is present, than an intraoperative abdominal version may be attempted in order to allow for a low transverse uterine incision to be made. This is performed in a similar manner to an external cephalic version. (See Chapter 2.) If this is not successful or the operator does not wish to attempt the maneuver, however, it is usually better to initially make a low vertical incision rather than be forced to convert a low transverse incision to a T or J-shaped incision.

Delivery of the placenta. After the infant has been delivered, the umbilical cord is doubly clamped and ligated and the infant is given to the waiting pediatrician. At this time the placenta is delivered, either by manual extraction, or spontaneously with gentle traction on the cord. A prospective randomized study reported that the incidence of postoperative endometritis is significantly higher when the placenta is manually removed, so if it will deliver with simple traction on the cord, this is preferred (Atkinson 1996). In addition, blood loss is also significantly less when cord traction and oxytocin are used when compared to manual removal (McCurdy 1992).

Repair of the uterus. After the placenta is removed, the uterus is exteriorized onto the abdomen and a laparotomy sponge can be used to clear all clots and debris from inside the uterus if desired. It is easier to hold the uterus in this position with a moist laparotomy tape draped over the fundus.

While you can repair a uterus without exteriorizing it, this step gives you better visualization and can allow you to notice uterine atony more quickly. If there is an extension of the uterine incision laterally, then you must exteriorize the uterus to determine how far the extension goes. While this step may increase maternal discomfort slightly, it does not increase the risk of infection (Wilkenson 2000). Another recent study showed that surgical time was decreased with exteriorization of the uterus but there was a slight increase in pain 6 hours postoperatively (Coutinho 2008). There will be some cases where the uterus cannot be exteriorized secondary to adhesions or fibroids, which is why you must know your anatomy in order not to injure the uterine vessels or ureters during your repair.

After the placenta is removed, clamps (which may be ring forceps, Pennington clamps, or Allis clamps) are placed at the lateral edges of the uterine incision, and also at any point where there is significant bleeding along the incision. The incision is then closed with one or two layers of a locked, continuous 0 or #1 absorbable suture, most commonly either polyglactin (vicryl) or chromic. Additional interrupted sutures (usually figure-of-eights) are thrown as necessary for hemostasis. After the uterus is repaired and good hemostasis is noted, the uterus, fallopian tubes, and ovaries are inspected and then replaced into the abdomen.

A recent study involving over 2,100 women by Bujold et al. has reported that the risk of subsequent uterine rupture is increased nearly fourfold when a single-layer closure is performed when compared with a double-layer closure. Because of this study, and the fact that the operating time is minimally increased by this step, a double-layer closure is generally recommended by many (Berghella 2005).

If a vertical incision is used on the uterus, then the repair is performed in several layers with the same types of sutures to reapproximate the incision. This will usually require two or three layers and is made easier if the assistant can compress the uterus with each throw to keep the two edges close together and prevent the suture from tearing through. After the muscular part of the uterus is together, the serosa is repaired in a running fashion with a smaller suture, such as a 3-0 vicryl.

Closure of the abdomen. With the uterus back in the abdomen, the incision is again visualized to ensure hemostasis. The gutters are irrigated and cleared of all clots and debris. Prior to closing the fascia, the scrub nurse should notify you that the sponge and instrument count is correct. If the count is incorrect, you must find the missing item, or if there was no count done because the procedure was an emergency, then you should call for radiology to come up and perform portable films of the abdomen. You should have these results before proceeding with closure of the abdomen.

Some providers will close the bladder flap with a running suture of 2-0 or 3-0 vicryl or chromic. While some feel that this step will decrease bladder adhesions for future surgeries, there is not convincing evidence either way at this time. This step should not be done if the patient has a significant coagulopathy or is in DIC as there is a risk of creating a space for a bladder hematoma to form.

In general, the peritoneum is not closed or reapproximated. While some physicians do prefer to close the peritoneum with a running suture of 2-0 or 3-0 vicryl or chromic suture, there is mounting evidence that this is not necessary and may even increase the risk of complications. These include studies that have demonstrated no difference in the incidence of postoperative fever, wound infection, endometritis, ileus, wound dehiscence, incisional hernia, postoperative pain, or adhesions at the time of subsequent surgery when this is not done (Hull 1991; Tulandi 1988; Chanrachakul 2002). Two additional reviews of the topic also state that at present, there is "no evidence to justify the time taken and cost of peritoneal closure" (Bamigboye 2005; Berghella 2005).

If there is significant diastasis of the rectus abdominal muscles, some surgeons will place a few interrupted sutures of 2-0 chromic or vicryl to reapproximate them in the midline. These throws are not tied tightly as they are for reapproximation and not hemostasis.

The fascia is then closed with a running suture of either a permanent or delayed absorbable type.

Many surgeons prefer to use vicryl for primary cesarean sections and either a delayed-absorbable monofilament suture such as PDS (polydiaxanone) or a permanent monofilament suture like polypropylene for repeat operations, vertical incisions, or other patients at increased risk for fascial dehiscence. After this, the subcutaneous tissue is

181

irrigated with sterile water and any bleeding is stopped using the bovie (electrocautery). The skin is then closed with either a subcuticular suture or staples.

Results from a randomized trial of over 970 patients demonstrated no difference in the risk of wound complications in patients with >/= 2cm of subcutaneous fat when no closure of the subcutaneous tissue was compared with placement of a drain or suture closure of the subcutaneous layer (Magann 2002).

Completing the operation. After the skin is closed, the drapes are removed, the grounding pad taken off, and a vaginal exam performed to clear all clots from the uterus and vagina while the other hand massages the uterine fundus. This allows the operator to assess uterine tone. The patient is then transferred to a bed and taken to the recovery room.

A thorough "talk through" of a cesarean section is included in Appendix C, which explains in detail every step performed and instrument used during a cesarean section. After reading the above description of the operation, it will allow you to run through the procedure in your mind, focusing on what the next step is and what instruments you need to request.

Approach to Intraoperative Hemorrhage. This complication may occur secondary to uterine atony, abnormal placental implantation (i.e., placenta accreta), or laceration of blood vessels (most commonly the uterine arteries). Postpartum hemorrhage occurs in approximately 6% of cesarean deliveries. The risk of hemorrhage is higher with a classical or T-shaped uterine incision as compared to the more common low-transverse incision.

Etiology. The approach to stopping hemorrhage depends on the etiology of the hemorrhage. In general, bleeding will initially occur as a result of either uterine atony or extension of the uterine incision into other vessels, such as the uterine arteries.*

* Another consideration for hemorrhage is the onset of DIC, which may occur after a substantial blood loss has already occurred. If this is the case, then transfusion of blood products will be required to allow the patient to form clots in order to stop the bleeding.

Estimation of blood loss (EBL). Deciding how much blood has been lost during a cesarean section is a very difficult thing to do, especially when there is a significant amount of amniotic fluid. In general, average blood loss at the time of a cesarean section is around 1,000 cc. It is, however, possible to get a slightly better estimate when you consider the following rules of thumb:

-   Make sure and tell the anesthesiologist when you are irrigating, so this fluid does not get counted in the EBL.

- Look at how much blood is in the suction, and then try and subtract out for amniotic fluid. (This will be an estimate.)
- Count the laparotomy tapes and estimate the blood loss based on how much you see on each one:

	% Sponge Covered	Amount of Blood
Standard 18 x 18 Surgical Lap Sponge*	50%	25 mL
	75%	50 mL
	100%	75 mL
	100% + dripping	100 mL

(*Dildy 2004)

Lacerations. Bleeding from lacerations will generally be seen from the uterine incision or laterally if it extends into the uterine vessels.

Uterine incision. If the bleeding is coming from the uterine incision, then you can place Pennington clamps on the edges where the vessels are bleeding the most while you prepare to close the uterine incision. This will decrease your blood loss and allow you better visualization for the repair.

Uterine arteries. If the bleeding appears arterial in nature and your incision extended laterally into the uterine artery, then you will need to perform an O'Leary stitch in order to stop the bleeding. To do this, you will first palpate the vessel inferior to where the bleeding is coming from, then use a 0-vicryl suture and, going anterior to posterior insert the needle into the broad ligament approximately 1cm lateral to the vessel and then bring it through medially to where it exits in the uterine tissue (figure 10-6). This is usually done with a single pass and not a figure of eight because the ureter runs about 2 cm lateral to the uterine artery and you must take care not to injure it.

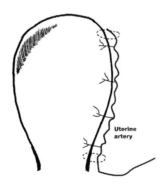

Figure 10-6 Uterine artery ligation and high uterine artery ligation

Uterine atony This is the most common cause for bleeding at the time of a cesarean section. When this occurs, you should first administer medications in the same manner that you would if you had a postpartum hemorrhage after a vaginal delivery. (See Chapter 14: Postpartum Hemorrhage.) If medications fail to improve the uterine tone and bleeding, then you may have to move on to the surgical methods listed below.

Surgical treatment of hemorrhage due to uterine atony is meant to first decrease the pulse pressure of the blood flow to the uterus and second to mechanically compress the uterus and stop bleeding. A general order in which interventions are taken are as follows:

1. Bilateral O'Leary stitches. These are performed as described above, but the sutures are thrown at the level of the internal cervical os. Remember this is a mass ligature and you do not need to dissect into the broad ligament to define the space you will be putting the stitch. This technique is effective in stopping hemorrhage in approximately 75% of cases. It must be done bilaterally and care taken to avoid the ureters. (Figure 10-6)
2. Bilateral Ovarian artery ligation. A single suture of 0-vicryl is thrown at the anastamosis of the ovarian and uterine vessels near the utero-ovarian ligament. (Figure 10-6)
3. Hypogastric artery ligation. You will see many textbooks describe a technique where you can enter the retroperitoneum and divide the anterior division of the hypogastric artery. In practice, however, this has not been shown to be effective in most cases of postpartum hemorrhage.
4. B-Lynch suture. This intervention is an attempt to mechanically compress the uterus. While the original technique describes this being done with the uterine incision intact, it can still be accomplished after the uterine incision is closed.

   A 0-chromic suture is used and inserted below the uterine incision at one of the lateral edges, then exits just above the incision. It is taken over the top of the uterus and then a horizontal suture is thrown on the posterior uterus. The suture is then brought back over the top of the uterus on the opposite side and inserted above the uterine incision on the opposite side the stitch was started and exits below the incision. The assistant then compresses the uterus while the surgeon ties down the suture which will keep the uterus in this position. Please see figure 10-7 for an example of what this will look like.

   This technique is relatively easy to perform, and has been reported to be effective in over 80% of cases (Doumouchtsis 2007).

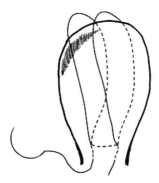

Figure 10-7 B-lynch suture

5. Hysterectomy. If all other treatments (medications and sutures) have failed and the patient continues to bleed and becomes hemodynamically unstable, then you may have to proceed with a hysterectomy as a lifesaving option. The technique for a cesarean hysterectomy is very similar to when the patient is not pregnant. Differences include the fact that the lateral vessels are engorged and more difficult to clamp well and a supracervical hysterectomy is often done because, especially if the patient was in advanced labor, it may be difficult to identify the entire cervix and avoid the ureters.

Blood products may also be required during a postpartum hemorrhage in order to stabilize the patient. The specific blood products and recommendations for giving them can be found in Chapter 14 in the section on Postpartum Hemorrhage.

Emergency Cesarean Section

Definition. A true emergency cesarean section is one that must be performed within minutes secondary to a potential life-threatening situation for either the mother, the fetus, or both. When a true emergency exists, the baby can be delivered in under a minute from the time you make your incision. The delay that usually exists, therefore, is in making the decision and then transitioning the patient to the operating room and obtaining adequate anesthesia.

Potential Indications. An emergency cesarean section may be performed for either maternal indications, fetal indications, or a combination. Some possible situations where an emergency cesarean section may be indicated include:

Fetal: -Prolonged fetal bradycardia
       -Umbilical cord prolapse

Maternal: -Amniotic fluid embolism
                -Myocardial infarction

Combined: -Uterine rupture
                -Hemorrhage (Placental abruption/vasa previa/placenta previa)
                -Trauma

Prevention. The best way to avoid an emergency cesarean section is to monitor any non-reassuring fetal heart rate tracings closely so that you may intervene in such a manner as to prevent the situation from becoming a true emergency. While this will help you avoid an emergency cesarean in many cases it will not help in those that do not have any specific warning signs, such as an amniotic fluid embolism or trauma.

Treatment. A well-rehearsed plan will help you to perform a rapid and safe emergency cesarean section.

Initial actions. Take a quick second and begin by considering your options.

1. Determine the level of fetal/maternal distress. If there is mild to moderate distress, then you may attempt conservative maneuvers (maternal position changes, administration of O2, or terbutaline) as appropriate. If there is severe distress present, or the mild/moderate distress worsens or does not respond to conservative maneuvers, then prompt intervention is required.
2. Call for Assistance. When you have determined that an emergency cesarean delivery is indicated, alert the following personnel:

    -   Chief Resident or Staff
    -   Anesthesia support
    -   Nursing staff
    -   Scrub tech
    -   Pediatricians

3. Counsel patient and family. Briefly counsel the patient and family on the need and indications for an emergent delivery while continuing to make preparations for moving the patient to the operating room.
4. Unhook all monitors and the bed. This step is often overlooked and results in a delay as the cables become entwined on something and are pulled out of the wall as you exit the room.
5. Prep and scrub. As the patient is coming out of the room, run down ahead to the OR and make sure your gloves are out, and if they are not, then get them out. Tell the nurse to place a foley and perform a very rapid prep (splashing the

abdomen versus a quick scrub as time permits). After making sure the patient is in the OR and on the operating table, quickly scrub for the procedure.

6. Recheck the fetal heart rate before prepping the patient. There are times where the fetal heart rate will have recovered and then you can make the decision of whether or not to proceed with the cesarean section or if you can wait. If it has recovered, then at least you can proceed in a more controlled manner and are more likely to be able to use conduction anesthesia rather than a general anesthesia.

Anesthesia. The anesthesiologist should be one of the first people to arrive when an emergency cesarean section needs to be performed. Unless the patient has an extremely dense epidural, it is unlikely that time will permit you the 10-15 minutes needed to obtain an adequate level for the procedure. A decision to proceed with a general anesthesia should not be taken lightly as the risk of complications is significantly higher in pregnant women than with conduction anesthesia. The risk of maternal death from general anesthesia is 16.7 times greater than with regional anesthesia and the incidence of failed intubation is tenfold higher in pregnant women than in the nonpregnant population (Hawkins 1997; Barnardo 2000).

If, for whatever reason, there is a significant delay in obtaining an adequate level or administering a general anesthesia and there is severe fetal distress, the cesarean section can be started under local anesthesia. This is done by filling the largest syringe available with local anesthetic and injecting into the subcutaneous tissue, making the incision, then continuing to alternate injecting and cutting until the peritoneum is entered. (A total of 200-300 mL of 0.5% lidocaine with epinephrine may be required.) This is, fortunately, a very rare occurrence, and the patient is usually asleep before the second incision is made. Maximum doses of local anesthetic are listed in table 10-1.

Table 10-1. Maximum doses of local anesthetic

Marcaine	2 mg/kg
Lidocaine	4.5 mg/kg
Lidocaine w/epinephrine	7 mg/kg

Operation. While the operation is the same as a routine cesarean section after the baby is delivered, the abdominal incision technique and entry into the abdomen are modified slightly.

Foley catheter placement. Make sure the OR nurse has placed a foley catheter, even if this is being done while you make your incision. This will help to decrease the risk of bladder injury.

Choice of abdominal incision. After obtaining adequate anesthesia, make your abdominal incision. Your choices are either a Pfannenstiel or a vertical incision. The classic teaching is that a vertical incision is faster and associated with less blood loss. If the patient has had no previous abdominal surgery, however, it is usually just as quick to perform a transverse (Pfannenstiel) incision for most surgeons.

Initial incision. Make the initial incision deeper than normal, with the goal being to cut through all of the subcutaneous tissue and make your fascial incision with one, or at most two, passes with the scalpel.

Fascia. Once the fascia has been incised in the midline, you may perform a fascial "rip" where you simply place your fingers under the fascia on either side of midline and then spread laterally. If this is too difficult, you may use pickups and Mayo scissors to incise the fascia as you normally do, just very quickly. In general, you will skip the step of placing Kocher clamps on the fascia and separating the underlying rectus muscles.

* (NOTE: When you dictate this part of the procedure, you should state that "the fascial incision was extended bluntly" rather than "a fascial rip technique was used.")

Entry into the abdomen. Bluntly separate the rectus abdominus muscles in the midline and then spread the peritoneum laterally with your fingers as superiorly as possible to minimize the risk of bladder injury and enter the peritoneal cavity. If there are significant adhesions, you may or may not have time to dissect them away prior to entry of the peritoneum.

Bladder flap. Creating a bladder flap, if done very quickly, will only take a few seconds. This step may be skipped if the maternal or fetal situation is extremely emergent.

Uterine incision. You will make the same type of uterine incision as during a routine cesarean section, i.e., a low-transverse incision at term, and a classical incision for a significantly preterm fetus or back-down transverse presentation. (*Take a deep breath when you get to the uterus and remember NOT to cut the baby!) After you have entered the uterine cavity, spread the incision with your fingers bluntly or with bandage scissors if necessary, and deliver the baby.

After delivery. After the baby is delivered, make sure and collect a segment of the cord for gases, then remove the placenta and inspect the following structures very carefully:

1. Uterus. Look for evidence of extension of the uterine incision as well as at the posterior side of the uterus to ensure the posterior wall is intact and was not injured or perforated during the delivery.

2. Bladder. This is especially important if you did not have time to create a bladder flap. Make sure you can clearly see where the bladder begins so that you do not accidentally injure it during the uterine repair. Sometimes you will have to create a small bladder flap after the delivery to allow you to repair the uterine incision.
3. Intestines. Look to make sure there is no bowel in your field. If you see anything that resembles stool, it is a wise idea to run the bowel to look for evidence of injury.

After you have evaluated the above structures, you can proceed with your repair of the uterine incision. At this time, you should do the following:

1. Antibiotics. Make sure the anesthesiologist either has or is administering antibiotics, usually a cephalosporin, as the risk of infection is higher in patients undergoing an emergency procedure.
2. Call for x-ray Because you will almost never get a count of instruments prior to starting an emergency cesarean section, when you are closing the uterine incision, call to have x-ray come up. They will need to do a portable film of the abdomen and pelvis prior to closure of the fascia or at least before closing the skin. (Staples can potentially interfere with the interpretation of the film.) Make sure that you send someone with the film so that they can have the radiologist read it quickly and explain to them that you are attempting to rule out any retained instruments/sponges and that the patient is under anesthesia on the operating table, and that they cannot leave until the film is clear. A study by Gawande et al. reported that risk factors for retained instruments or sponges included an emergency procedure and an increased BMI (Gawande 2003).

Post-operatively. After the procedure, review the indications as well as how the operation went with the family. Make sure that your written and dictated operative notes are accurate and note that the x-ray was negative for any retained instruments and sponges. Be very clear on the type of uterine incision that was made and any implications it has for future pregnancies. Also, try and dictate the operative report as soon as possible after the procedure. When writing postoperative orders, take into consideration the following:

1. Antibiotics. Continue antibiotics for 24-48 hours postoperatively, usually a cephalosporin, or, if the patient had chorioamnionitis prior to the procedure, expand the coverage to triples (ampicillin/gentamicin/clindamycin).
2. Feeding. If you had to run the patient's bowel, then plan to advance the diet more slowly and monitor closely for evidence of a post-operative ileus.

Postpartum. When seeing the patient postpartum, be vigilant for evidence of infection, both endometritis and wound infections, and have a low threshold to treat the patient or change antibiotics as needed.

Vaginal Birth After Cesarean (VBAC)

Brief History. Whereas women who had cesarean sections were told in the past that every subsequent delivery had to be by cesarean delivery, this began to change in the 1970's. As OB care for both the mother and infant improved, the VBAC rate, which was only 3% in 1981, increased significantly, with 27% of women with a previous cesarean delivery attempting VBAC in 1995 (Curtin 1997). However, because of the increasingly publicized cases of patients with uterine rupture and more study into which patients are good candidates for VBAC, the rate of patients attempting vaginal birth has decreased to only 12% (ACOG 2004).

Benefits of VBAC. Women who have a successful vaginal delivery after a cesarean section have less blood loss, fewer transfusions, fewer infections, a shorter recovery time and hospital stay, and usually no increased perinatal morbidity when compared to women who undergo cesarean delivery (ACOG 1999). Some women also feel that their previous cesarean section was a sign they "failed" in their task of having a normal delivery. The risk of postpartum infection and complications is also much lower in these patients as well although their counterparts who undergo a repeat cesarean section are not at risk for significant vaginal and anal sphincter lacerations that may occur during a vaginal delivery. (See Chapter 11.)

From a purely economic perspective, the prevention of a single major adverse neonatal outcome by performing a repeat cesarean section rather than attempting a VBAC requires 1,591 cesarean deliveries at a cost of 2.4 million dollars by some estimates (Grobman WA 2000).

Candidates. The American College of OB/GYN (ACOG) recommends that the following criteria be met before a patient is allowed to attempt a VBAC:

- History of only 1 or *2 previous cesarean deliveries (*only if patient has had a vaginal delivery)
- Clinically adequate pelvis
- No history of uterine rupture or other uterine scars or surgery (i.e., myomectomy with entry into the uterine cavity)
- Physician available during active labor to perform emergent cesarean if indicated
- Anesthesia support and facilities for emergency cesarean

Other patients for whom VBAC is controversial, but is still considered acceptable in some institutions include the following:

-   Unknown uterine scar type
-   Twin gestation
-   Postterm pregnancy
-   Suspected macrosomia
-   History of a low-vertical uterine incision

When you encounter patients such as these who desire VBAC, it is important to consult with their attending physician as different staff will have different comfort levels with these patients.

Contraindications. Because of the serious complications, such as uterine rupture, that can occur while attempting a VBAC, patients with any of the following conditions should be delivered by repeat cesarean section:

-   Prior classical uterine incision
-   History of a T-shaped uterine incision (See types of uterine incisions.)
-   History of uterine surgery with entrance into the uterine cavity (i.e., during myomectomy)
-   Medical or obstetric complications (maternal or fetal) the make vaginal delivery contraindicated.
-   Lack of facilities, physicians, and/or anesthesia support to perform an emergent cesarean section for fetal distress.

Patient counseling for VBAC. Because there are risks associated with attempting a VBAC that can result in fetal distress, emergent surgery, and even hysterectomy, a specific counseling note should be placed on the patient's chart when they are admitted in labor. The counseling note should include the following items:

-   The patient has been offered the option of a repeat cesarean section and she desires to attempt a VBAC.
-   Risks of VBAC and uterine rupture have been discussed as well as the potential complications of a cesarean section (which were listed earlier in this chapter).
-   It is also important to note in the chart that the risk of postpartum endometritis after a cesarean section during labor is slightly higher than with a primary cesarean section and that this was explained to the patient.

A sample form of this counseling is located in Appendix B.

While the list of possible complications sounds horrible, remember that the incidence of any of these events happening is still very small. It is usually reassuring to the patient if you explain that they are rare occurrences and can comment on the general percentages mentioned previously.

> **Success rates.** Depending on the reference cited, overall VBAC success rates are reported to be between 60%-80%. Patients who had their first cesarean for an indication such as fetal distress or malpresentation (i.e., breech or transverse lie) are more likely to be successful in their VBAC attempt than those patients who had a cesarean for arrest of descent (ACOG 2004). Factors that decrease the chances of a successful VBAC include labor augmentation or induction, maternal obesity, and birthweight > 4,000 grams.

Labor management. Because even those patients with a low transverse incision have up to a 1.5% chance of uterine rupture, their care in labor is slightly different than a patient who has never undergone a cesarean.

- Initial evaluation. Once labor has started, the patient should be evaluated promptly, with most authorities recommending the use of continuous electronic fetal monitoring (ACOG 2004). These patients also require prompt attention and evaluation if any signs or symptoms of uterine rupture occur. (See Chapter 14—Uterine rupture.)
- Labor induction. Induction of labor in VBAC patients can be done using several different methods. Most often, mechanical cervical dilators or Pitocin are chosen. It is important to note that misoprostol should NOT be used for induction or augmentation of labor in patients with a previous cesarean section or other scar on their uterus as this significantly increases their risk of experiencing a uterine rupture (ACOG 1999a; ACOG 1999b; ACOG 2002). Recent studies even suggest that no prostaglandins should be used to induce labor in patients with a previous cesarean section (ACOG 2002; Lyndon-Rochelle 2001).
- Labor augmentation. In general, it appears that augmentation of labor using pitocin is safe in patients attempting VBAC. While there are reports that high doses of Pitocin may increase the risk of uterine rupture, there are other studies that have shown no association between the uterine activity patterns of patients with uterine rupture and other VBAC patients who had successful vaginal deliveries (Grubb 1996; Phelan 1998). If Pitocin is used, it should be used cautiously with continuous fetal monitoring.
- Anesthesia. Patients attempting VBAC should be allowed to have an epidural for pain control if desired. An epidural will not mask signs and symptoms of uterine rupture, and the first sign usually present with this complication is fetal distress and not maternal discomfort.

Potential Complications of VBAC

Uterine rupture. The most serious complication that can occur during a VBAC attempt is uterine rupture. It is important to note for documentation purposes that a uterine rupture is different from a uterine dehiscence. Uterine rupture implies a complete opening in the uterus with at least part of the fetus being outside of the uterus, while dehiscence means there is at least a layer of serosa intact and the fetus remains in the uterine cavity. While many studies group these together, each should be documented accurately in the chart should they occur.

The risk of uterine rupture depends on the type of uterine incision that was made previously as rupture of an unscarred uterus is extremely rare. Approximate risks of uterine rupture for different incisions are:

Low-transverse incision	0.2%-1.5%
Low-vertical incision	1%-7%
Classical uterine incision	4%-9%
T-shaped incision	4%-9%

If a patient has had a previous uterine rupture, then the risk of uterine rupture in subsequent pregnancies is reported to be between 6% and 32% depending on whether the initial rupture involved the lower uterine segment or the upper portion of the uterus respectively (Ritchie 1971; Reyes-Ceja 1969). It is also important to take into account when the patient's previous cesarean section was performed.

A study by Shipp et al. of over 2,400 women undergoing VBAC trials found that the risk of uterine rupture was three times higher in women whose VBAC trial was within 18 months of a prior cesarean section (Shipp 2002). While the overall risk for these women was still low, at 2.25%, this is still higher than would be expected for a previous low-transverse uterine incision and should be taken into consideration.

The clinical presentation of uterine rupture, as well as the management, can be found in Chapter 14: Common Obstetric Complications and Emergencies.

Repeat Cesarean Section. Even though the overall success rate for women attempting VBAC is excellent, there will still be some 20%-40% of patients who will require a repeat cesarean section for delivery for a variety of indications. In these patients, the risk of postoperative infection is higher than in women who undergo an elective cesarean section without labor.

References:

Alexander JM, Levno KJ, Hauth J, Landon MB, Thom E, et al. Fetal injury associated with cesarean delivery. Obstet Gynecol 2006; 108(4):885-890.

Barnardo PD, Jenkins JG. Failed tracheal intubation in obstetrics: a 6-year review in the UK region. Anaesthesia 2000; 55:690-694.

Beall M, Eglinton GS, Clark SL, Phelan JP. Vaginal delivery after cesarean section in women with unknown types of uterine scar. J Reprod Med 1984; 29(1):31-35.

Atkinson MW, Own J, Wren A, Hauth JC. The effect of manual removal of the placenta on post-cesarean endometritis. Obstet Gynecol 1996; 87:99.

Bamigboye AA, Hofmeyr GJ. Closure versus non-closure of the peritoneum at caesarean section. Cochrane Database Syst Rev 2005;1.

Berghella V, Baxter JK, Chauhan SP. Evidence-based surgery for cesarean delivery. Am J Obstet Gynecol 2005; 193:1607-1617.

Births: Preliminary data for 2006. CDC: National Vital Statistics Report, Dec 5, 2007.

Boyle JG, Gabbe SG. T and J vertical extensions in low transverse cesarean births. Obstet Gynecol. Feb 1996; 87(2).

Bujold E, Bujold C, Hamilton EF, Harel F, Gauthier RJ. The impact of a single-layer or double-layer closure on uterine rupture. Am J Obstet Gynecol, June 2002; 186(6):1326-1330.

Cesarean delivery and postpartum hysterectomy. In: *Williams Obstetrics* 21st ed, 2001. McGraw-Hill, New York.

Chanrachakul B, Hamontri S, Herabutya Y. A randomized comparison of postcesarean pain between closure and nonclosure of peritoneum. Eur J Obstet Gynecol and Reprod Biology, Feb 2002; 101(1):31-35.

Chauhan SP, Roach H, Naef RW, Magann EF, Morrison JC, Martin JN. Cesarean for suspected fetal distress: Does the decision-incision time make a difference? J Reprod Med, 1997; 42: 347.

Chauhan SP, Magann EF, Carroll CS, Barrilleaux PS, Scardo JA, Martin JN Jr. Mode of delivery for the morbidity for the morbidly obese with prior cesarean delivery: vaginal versus repeat cesarean section. Am J Obstet Gynecol. 2001 Aug; 185(2):349-354.

Chen KT, Sell RL, Tuomala RE. Cost-effectiveness of elective cesarean delivery in human immunodeficiency virus-infected women. Obstet Gynecol 2001; 97(2):161-168.

Chiam W, Bashiri A, Bar-David J, Shoham-Vardi I, Mazor M. Prevalence and clinical significance of postpartum endometritis and wound infection. Infect Dis Obstet Gynecol 2000; 8:77.

Coutinho IS, Ramos de Amorim MM, Katz L, Bandeira de Ferraz AA. Uterine exteriorization compared with in situ repair at cesarean delivery. Obstet Gynecol 2008; 111:639-647.

Cunningham GF, Gant NF et al. eds, Cesarean delivery and postpartum hysterectomy, in Williams Obstetrics 21st ed, McGraw-Hill, New York: 540.

Curtin SC. Rates of cesarean birth after vaginal birth after previous cesarean. National Center for Health Statistics, Monthly vital statistics report, 1997; vol 45, no. 11 (suppl 3).

Dildy GA, Paine AR, George NC, Velasco C. Estimating blood loss: Can teaching significantly improve visual estimation? Obstet Gynecol 2004 Sept, 104:3; 601-606.

Doumouchtsis SK, Papageorghiou AT, Arulkumaran S. Systematic review of conservative management of postpartum hemorrhage: what to do when medical treatment fails. Obstet Gynecol Surv. 2007 Aug;62(8):540-547.

Fetal Macrosomia. ACOG Practice Bulletin #22, Nov 2000.

Gawande AA, Studdert DM, Orav EF, Brennan TA, Zinner MJ. Risk factors for retained instruments and sponges after surgery. NEJM 2003 Jan; 348(3):229-235.

Grobman WA, Peaceman AM, Socol ML. Cost-effectiveness of elective cesarean delivery after one prior low transverse cesarean. Obstet Gynecol May 2000; 95(5):745-751.

Grubb DK, Kjos SL, Paul RH. Latent labor with an unknown uterine scar. Obstet Gynecol 1996; 88:351-355.

Guidelines for Perinatal Care. ACOG Publications, Washington, DC, 1992.

Lyndon-Rochelle M, Holt VL, Easterling TR, Martin DP. Risk of uterine rupture during labor among women with a prior cesarean delivery. NEJM 2001; 345:3.

Hawkins JL, Koonin LM, Palmer SK, Gibbs CP. Anesthesia related deaths during obstetric delivery in the United States 1979-1990. Anesthesiology 1997; 86:277.

Hendrix SL, Schimp V, Martin J, Singh A, Kruger M, McNeeley SG. The legendary superior strength of the Pfannensteil incision: a myth? Am J Obstet Gynecol 2000 Jun; 182(6):1446-1451.

Hull DB, Varner MW. A randomized study of closure of peritoneum at cesarean delivery. Obstet Gynecol 1991; 77:818-820.

Induction of labor with misoprostol. ACOG Committee Opinion #228, 1999a.

Induction of labor for vaginal birth after cesarean delivery. ACOG committee opinion #271, 2002.

Magann EF. Subcutaneous stitch closure versus subcutaneous drain to prevent wound disruption after cesarean delivery: a randomized clinical trial. Am J Obstet Gynecol, June 2002; 186(6):1119-1123.

Magann EF, Chauhan SP, Bufkin L, Field K, Roberts WE, Martin JN, Intra-operative haemorrhage by blunt versus sharp expansion of the uterine incision at caesarean delivery: a randomized clinical trial. BJOG 2002; 109:448-452.

Mann JW. Preoperative evaluation and preparation of women for gynecologic surgery. Up To Date version 11.1, December 2002.

McCurdy CM Jr, Magann EF, McCurdy CJ, Saltzman AJ. The effect of placental management at cesarean delivery on operative blood loss. Am J Obstet Gynecol 1992; 167:1363.

Minkoff H. Human immunodeficiency virus infection in pregnancy. Obstet Gynecol 2003; 101(4):797-810.

Nielsen TF, Hokegard KH. Cesarean section and intraoperative surgical complications. Acta Obstet Gynecol Scand 1984; 63:103.

Phelan JP, Korst LM, Settles DK. Uterine activity patterns in uterine rupture: a case-control study. Obstet Gynecol 1998; 92(3):394-397.

Petitte DB. Maternal mortality and morbidity in cesarean section. Clin Obstet Gynecol 1985; 28:763.

Reyes-Ceja L, Cabrera R, Insfran E, Herrera-Lasso F. Pregnancy following previous uterine rupture. Study of 19 patients. Obstet Gynecol 1969; 34:387-389.

Ritchie EH. Pregnancy after rupture of the pregnant uterus. A report of 36 pregnancies and a study of cases reported since 1932. J Obstet Gynaecol Br Commonw, 1971; 78:642-648.

Rodruguez AI, Porter KB, O'Brien WF. Blunt versus sharp expansion of the uterine incision in a low-segment transverse cesarean section. Am J Obstet Gynecol 1994; 171:1022-1025.

Sachs BP, Yeh J, Acker D, et al. Cesarean section-related maternal mortality in Massachusetts, 1954-1985. Obstet Gynecol 1988; 71:385.

Shipp TD, Zelop CM, Repke JT, Cohen A, Lieberman E. Interdelivery interval and risk of symptomatic uterine rupture. Obstet Gynecol Feb 2001; 97(2):175-177.

Simpson EL, Lawrenson RA, Nightingale AL, Farmer RD. Venous thromboembolism in pregnancy and the puerperium: incidence and additional risk factors from a London perinatal database. British J Obstet Gynaecol 2001; 108:56.

Tulandi T, Hum HS, Gelfand MM. Closure of laparotomy incision with or without peritoneal suturing and second-look lapartomy. Am J Obstet Gynecol 1988; 158:536-537.

Vaginal birth after previous cesarean delivery. ACOG Practice Bulletin #5, July 1999b.

Vaginal birth after previous cesarean delivery. ACOG Practice Bulletin #54, July 2004.

Wiener JJ, Westwood J. Fetal lacerations at caesarean section. J Obstet Gynaecol. 2002 Jan;22(1):23-24.

Wilkinson C, Enkin MW. Uterine exteriorization versus intraperitoneal repair at caesarean section. Cochrane Database Syst Rev 2000:CD000085.

Chapter 11

Lacerations and Episiotomies

- Types of Lacerations
  - Cervical
  - Vaginal/Perineal
    - 1st/2nd/3rd/4th Degree Lacerations
  - Periurethral
- Episiotomy
  - Indications
  - Anatomy
  - Types of Episiotomies
  - Complications
- Repair of Lacerations/Episiotomies
  - Anesthesia
  - Suture Choice
  - Repair Techniques
- Complications
  - Hemorrhage
  - Infection
  - Hematoma
  - Repair Breakdown
  - Anal Incontinence
  - Rectovaginal Fistula
  - Antibiotic Prohylaxis

Introduction

Lacerations are a common occurrence during spontaneous vaginal deliveries and especially after operative vaginal deliveries. After delivery it is important to fully inspect the cervix, vagina, and perineum and identify what lacerations, if any, are present and then repair them appropriately. Knowing how to perform an episiotomy, which is an incision in the perineum during delivery, is an important skill to have, but must be used with care as it inevitably increases the risk of more extensive lacerations.

Types of Lacerations

Cervical lacerations. After delivery of the placenta, one hand should be placed into the posterior vagina and the cervix completely visualized. This is often made easier by grasping the anterior and/or posterior lip of the cervix with a ring forceps. (Make sure you have adequate lighting when examining for lacerations and request additional lighting if needed.) If you notice profuse bleeding from the vagina, and you have good uterine tone, look closely for a cervical laceration. While one study noted cervical lacerations in as many as 50% of vaginal deliveries, most of these are less than 0.5 cm in length and do not require any treatment after delivery (Fahmy 1991). One obstetric text even notes that "cervical lacerations of up to 2 cm must be regarded as inevitable in childbirth" (Williams 2001).

If you identify a cervical laceration that is greater than 2 cm or one that is actively bleeding, then it is important to repair this immediately. In order to do this, first call for an assistant to provide retraction and right angle retractors if needed, then grasp the cervix on either side of the laceration with ring forceps. Your assistant can retract so that you can identify the apex of the laceration and you then place your suture (usually either 2-0 chromic or 2-0 polyglactin (vicryl), just above the apex, which should control most of the bleeding and make visualization easier. You may either run this suture, which is often easier as you can use it for traction, or perform interrupted sutures. Be sure to only repair the laceration and not suture the cervix closed and check to ensure the os is patent after your repair.

Vaginal/Perineal lacerations. Lacerations of the vagina and perineum are common during vaginal delivery. There are many factors that place a patient at risk for more significant lacerations such as nulliparity, episiotomy, operative vaginal delivery, macrosomia, precipitous delivery, prolonged 2nd stage, and individual anatomy. While some dexterous residents will repair lacerations before delivery of the placenta, these repairs can become dislodged after delivery of the placenta if you need to manually explore the uterus secondary to atony or retained membranes. Also, performing a repair a second time on tissue that has had sutures tear through is not nearly as easy as the initial repair. For these reasons, it is recommended that repairs not be started until after the placenta has delivered.*

* (An exception to this is if you have a specific vessel or area that is bleeding profusely. In this case, an interrupted suture to prevent continued hemorrhage is advised rather than waiting for the placenta to deliver.)

Lacerations are classified as being either 1st, 2nd, 3rd, or 4th degree. It is important to know these as you must accurately document what occurred in the medical record, as well as understand how to repair them. Missing a third or fourth degree laceration and failing to repair it properly can result in anal incontinence and the formation of a rectovaginal fistula.

1st degree— Involves the vaginal fourchette, perineal skin, or vaginal mucous membrane
2nd degree— Involves skin *plus* the fascia and muscles of the perineal body*
3rd degree— Involves the skin, fascia/muscles of perineal body *plus* at least some portion of the anal sphincter.
4th degree— Laceration extends into the rectal mucosa

(*Note: By definition, any episiotomy is at least a 2nd degree laceration as it incises the fascia/muscles of the perineal body.)

While 1st and 2nd degree lacerations are usually repaired by junior residents with little trouble, when you have a 3rd or 4th degree laceration, it is important to have a senior resident or staff present for help in identifying anatomy and providing adequate exposure. Repair techniques are discussed later in this chapter.

Periurethral lacerations. Sometimes after delivery, there will be bleeding from the anterior portion of the vagina near the urethral opening. Most of the time this will stop with direct pressure, but if it does require sutures for hemostasis, then it is prudent to place a red robin or foley catheter into the urethra. This will allow you to avoid the urethra while you throw either interrupted or figure of eight sutures for hemostasis. Afterward, you can leave a foley catheter in place if there was an extensive repair, or if you remove the catheter, warn the patient that it will be painful to urinate for the next few days, and monitor them for urinary retention in the postpartum period.

Episiotomy

An episiotomy is an incision in the perineum made in an attempt to enlarge the vaginal opening during delivery. While there was a time in obstetric practice when episiotomies were cut with nearly all deliveries, this is no longer the case. Arguments that a clean cut is easier to repair than a jagged tear, that it protects the woman against pelvic relaxation, or it prevents fetal injury at delivery have not been borne out in studies. It is also well-established that performing a midline episiotomy significantly increases the risk of a 3rd/4th degree laceration (Klein 1992). Because of these findings, the incidence of episiotomy during delivery has decreased significantly in recent years. Currently, episiotomies are still performed in around 40% of deliveries in the United States (Weeks 2001).

Indications. Indications for an episiotomy all involve the need for a larger vaginal opening for delivery. Some commonly cited reasons for making an episiotomy include:

- Shoulder dystocia
- Macrosomic fetus
- Breech vaginal delivery
- Operative vaginal delivery (Forceps or Vacuum)
- Occiput posterior presentation

It is important to note that these are not absolute indications, and the fact that third- and fourth-degree lacerations are much more likely after an episiotomy must be taken into account when making the decision to perform an episiotomy. For example, whereas in the past it was recommended that an episiotomy be cut with every operative vaginal delivery, studies have demonstrated that this increases the risk of third and fourth-degree lacerations and may not be necessary in all cases (Coombs 1990; Helwig 1993). In these situations, clinical judgment must be used with regards to when to perform an episiotomy.

Another thing to consider is the medical-legal matter of informed consent with this procedure because of the potential for long-term morbidity that can result from a significant extension of an episiotomy. Prior to performing an episiotomy, preferably at the time of admission, you should talk with the patient about the possibility of her requiring an episiotomy as well as the potential complications. These complications are discussed later in this chapter.

While there is adequate clinical evidence to argue against performing routine episiotomies, the bottom line when it comes to making an episiotomy is that the benefit of widening the vaginal opening must be weighed against the potential complications and the clinical situation.

Anatomy. With a midline episiotomy, the incision will involve the vaginal mucosa, the perineal body, and the inferior portion of the bulbocavernosis muscle in the perineum (figure 11-1). If the episiotomy extends during delivery, it can disrupt the anal sphincter and rectal mucosa. A mediolateral episiotomy will transect the junction of the bulbocavernosis and transverse perineal muscles. It is important to understand the anatomy well as these structures must be identified during the repair.

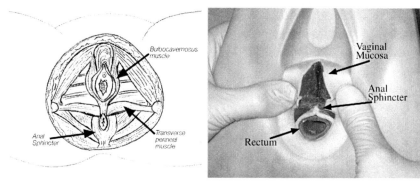

Figure 11-1 Illustration of anatomy of the perineum and muscles

Figure 11-1a Photo of anatomy of perineum

Types of Episiotomies. An episiotomy should always be noted in the delivery record, as well as any extensions that occurred. You must also be specific on the type of episiotomy. The most common types of episiotomies are a midline episiotomy and a mediolateral episiotomy although a modified mediolateral episiotomy is also sometimes used.

Midline episiotomy

The midline episiotomy (MLE) is used almost exclusively in the United States, whereas a mediolateral episiotomy is commonly employed in other parts of the world. When a midline episiotomy is cut, the fingers of the non-dominant hand are placed between the baby and the perineum and scissors are then used to make an incision directly inferior into the perineum into the perineal body. Care is taken to not incise the anal sphincter at the time the incision is made.

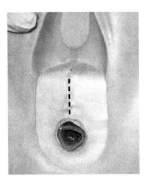

Figure 11-2a Midline episiotomy (MLE)

Mediolateral episiotomy

A mediolateral episiotomy is made the same way as a MLE in terms of how the hands are positioned, but the scissors are angled at approximately a 45-degree angle in an attempt direct any extension that may occur with delivery around the anal sphincter.

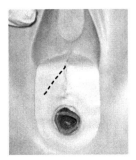

Figure 11-2b Mediolateral episiotomy

Modified mediolateral episiotomy

A modification of the midline episiotomy that is sometimes used is called a modified mediolateral episiotomy. In doing this, the incision is initially directly inferiorly, just like an MLE, for approximately 2cm, and then directed laterally at a 45-degree angle. This prevents the incision from severing the junction of the bulbocavernosis and transverse perineal muscles while still directing the incision, and hopefully any extension, lateral to the anal sphincter.

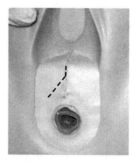

Figure 11-2c Modified mediolateral episiotomy

Complications of episiotomies

Hemorrhage. Patients who undergo an episiotomy generally lose more blood than those who deliver over an intact perineum. The increased blood loss has been estimated to be between 300 mL and 600 mL (Thacker 1983; Rockner 1989). A better study, that used the actual change in hematocrit to define a postpartum hemorrhage, demonstrated that both midline and mediolateral episiotomies are associated with an increased risk of postpartum hemorrhage (Coombs 1991).

Hematoma. If an episiotomy is not properly repaired, and all of the dead space appropriately closed, it is possible for a hematoma to develop. If this becomes infected, then it may result in a rectovaginal fistula. This same complication may occur with spontaneous lacerations as well.

Infection. When an infection or episiotomy breakdown occurs, it will usually happen in the first 7 days after delivery (Sanz 2001). The incidence of episiotomy infection has been reported to be between 0.35% to 10% (Myers-Helfgott 1999). Treatment for an infection includes antibiotics and debridement and this is discussed later in this chapter.

Third/Fourth degree lacerations. The incidence of third/fourth degree lacerations is increased when an episiotomy is performed. This risk is higher with a midline episiotomy when compared with a mediolateral episiotomy although the risk is increased with both.*

(*Note: There have been studies that demonstrate that mediolateral episiotomies can be protective against third and fourth degree lacerations in primiparous women. However, one study of over 43,000 patients demonstrated that it would require 48 episiotomies to prevent one severe tear (Anthony 1994). When the other complications of an episiotomy, such as hemorrhage and infection, are taken into account, it cannot be recommended that a mediolateral episiotomy be made routinely for this indication.)

Repair of Lacerations/Episiotomies

Repairing lacerations caused by delivery can be a time-consuming procedure. It may take longer to do a proper repair of a fourth degree laceration than to complete an uncomplicated cesarean section. It is extremely important to correctly identify all lacerations that are present in order to prevent complications, such as postpartum hemorrhage immediately after delivery, and the potential long-term complications of a rectovaginal fistula or anal incontinence from unidentified injuries or improper repairs. Before doing these types of repairs on your own you should review all pertinent anatomy and perform several with an experienced senior physician.

It is imperative that you actively seek someone out to help you with this and not assume a resident or staff will sit down and teach you these skills as a recent study reported that nearly 60% of residents in the United States did not receive any didactic teaching on either episiotomy repair techniques or pelvic floor anatomy during their residency (McLennan 2002). It is a good knowledge of anatomy as well as the ability to recognize and adequately repair lacerations that will prevent future debilitating complications.

Anesthesia for Repairs. The amount of anesthesia required will depend on the extent of suturing that must be done. In general, a working epidural is almost always adequate for any repair. It may need to be rebolused by the anesthesiologist after delivery if an extensive repair is required. If the patient does not have an epidural, then injecting local anesthetic into the tissue you will suture usually works well. If this is not adequate, then intravenous medications can help. The maximum doses for some common local anesthetics are listed below:

Marcaine 2 mg/kg
Lidocaine 4.5 mg/kg
Lidocaine w/epinephrine 7 mg/kg

(See Chapter 8: Obstetric Analgesia/Anesthesia for additional information on options for anesthesia for laceration repairs.)

Suture Choice. The type of suture used depends on physician preference, the tissues that are to be repaired, and whether or not there is evidence of infection (i.e., Group B streptococcus or chorioamnionitis) at the time of the repair. Recommended sutures for specific sites and tissue can be found in table 11-1.

The reason for the use of different sutures when there is either a positive culture for GBS or evidence of chorioamnionitis during delivery is that the monofilament sutures, such as Monocryl (poliglecaprone) or PDS (polydioxanone), are less likely to harbor bacteria than are the braided sutures (polyglactin, Vicryl) (Sanz 2001).

A recent analysis of the medical literature comparing synthetic sutures, such as polyglactin, versus catgut, or chromic, sutures for perineal repairs found that the synthetic sutures were associated with less pain in the immediate postpartum period as well as a decreased risk of repair dehiscence (Kettle 2000). There were, however, no long-term differences in residual perineal pain or dysparunia.

Table 11-1. Suture choices for episiotomy repair

Recommended Suture

	Negative GBS and No Chorioamnionitis	*+ GBS or + Chorioamnionitis*
Vaginal mucosa	3-0 Vicryl or 3-0 Monocryl	3-0 Monocryl
Perirectal fascia	3-0 Vicryl or 3-0 Monocryl	3-0 Monocryl
Anal sphincter	2-0 Vicryl or 2-0 Monocryl	2-0 Monocryl or 2-0 PDS
Anal mucosa	3-0 Vicryl or 4-0 Monocryl	4-0 Moncryl

Vicryl = polyglactin
Monocryl = poliglecaprone
PDS = polydioxanone

Repair Techniques

1st Degree laceration. First degree lacerations may or may not need to be repaired. Examine them closely and apply pressure for several minutes if there is only a small amount of bleeding present. If hemostasis cannot be achieved this way, then interrupted sutures of 3-0 vicryl or chromic can be used. Also, if there is a wide space created by the superficial laceration, it may be reapproximated using interrupted sutures. Always remember the surgeon's creed: "The enemy of good is better." (which simply means that additional sutures when there is no bleeding can result in additional bleeding or a hematoma.)

2nd Degree laceration. Second degree lacerations must always be repaired. If the vaginal portion of the laceration is deep, then it is prudent to place one finger into the rectum and ensure there are no small "button-hole" defects in the rectum that communicate with the floor of the laceration. If these are present, you actually have a 4th degree laceration and, if you do not repair it properly, you may have a fistula form between the rectum and vagina and the repair will breakdown. Also, after placing a finger in the rectum it is wise to change gloves to prevent bringing fecal matter into the repair.

In order to repair this laceration, start by placing a suture at the vaginal apex. This is done using either 2-0 or 3-0 vicryl (polyglactin), monocryl (poliglecaprone), or chromic suture as previously discussed. Continue your repair toward the hymen in a running and locked manner for hemostasis.

Once you reach the hymenal ring you can continue the repair in one of two ways:

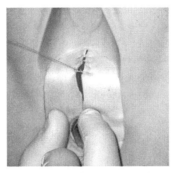

Figure 11-3 Initial repair of vaginal portion of episiotomy

A.

1) Once at the hymenal ring, turn the needle so that it is parallel with the vagina and go from the hymen area out towards yourself on the perineum.

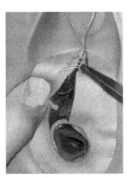

Figure 11-4 Transition from vaginal to perineum with episiotomy repair

2) Close the incised muscles/fascia of the perineum with the same suture in a running fashion

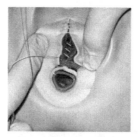

Figure 11-5 Closure of deep portion of muscular tissue

3) Ensure the suture comes through the posterior apex of the incision in the subcutaneous tissue.

4) Run the suture to close the subcutaneous tissue back to the hymenal ring.

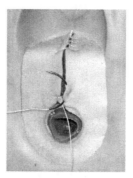

Figure 11-6 Closure of superficial perineum tissue

5) Turn the needle to be parallel with the vagina and place the suture from outside the hymenal ring to inside the vagina

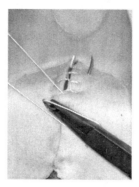

Figure 11-7 Transition back to vaginal tissue to tie final suture

6) Take a small amount of vaginal tissue lateral to your suture and tie.

B.

1) Tie the vaginal suture at the hymenal ring.
2) Close the incised muscles/fascia of the perineum with interrupted sutures (using the same type suture as in the vagina)
3) Close the subcutaneous tissue by starting at the inferior apex and then tie near the hymenal ring.

At the end of either of these repairs, place a finger into the rectum to ensure there are no sutures penetrating the rectum or any hematomas present. If there is a suture that has gone into the rectum, it must be removed in order to prevent a potential fistula from forming.

3rd Degree laceration. When you confirm you have a 3rd degree laceration, place a finger into the rectum to check for a 4th degree extension. Change gloves, then identify both ends of the anal sphincter. These can often retract laterally, and you may need to use Allis clamps to grasp them (figure 11-8). After you have identified the sphincter, the ends are reapproximated using three or four either interrupted or figure-of-eight sutures, usually 2-0 Vicryl, Monocryl, or PDS. After the anal sphincter is reapproximated, the repair is the same as for a 2nd degree. Figure 11-8a shows the initial suture placed in the anal sphincter.

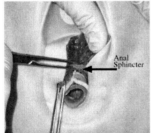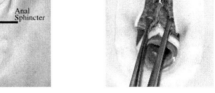

Figure 11-8 Grasping anal sphincter   Figure 11-8a Repair of anal sphincter

Another technique that has been taught is to actually overlap the torn distal ends of the anal sphincter during the repair. The theory is that this will provide a better repair and improved function. To date, however, there is little evidence that this is superior to the reapproximation method (Fernando 2002; Fitzpatrick 2000).

4th Degree lacerations. When you discover a 4th degree laceration, you should ask for a senior resident/staff for assistance, and then ensure you have the following:

- Adequate anesthesia: Usually an epidural is required for this type of repair. Otherwise, IV sedation in addition to local anesthetic is often required, but this will often require the assistance of an anesthesiologist. (See Chapter 8: OB Anesthesia for information on potential medications that can be used.) It is also advisable to inject bupivacaine 0.25% with epinephrine into the perineum around the repair for postoperative pain relief.

- Adequate visualization: If you cannot adequately visualize the apex of the laceration in the rectum, then you may need to transfer the patient to the operating room for better lighting and positioning. (The OR table is equipped for stirrups which will improve visualization considerably.) Additional retractors and an assistant will also make the repair easier. Some retractors that may be helpful include the Breisky-Navratil vaginal retractor, right angle retractors, and long Deaver retractors.

During the repair, make sure that you keep track of the patient's vital signs, urine output, and blood loss. It is easy to concentrate on the repair and not notice continued bleeding until the patient has sustained a significant hemorrhage.

When starting the repair, identify the apex of the rectal injury. (If you must put a sponge into the vagina to keep your view of the field, try and use a laparotomy tape and leave the blue tag on the outside so you do not forget it at the end of the repair.)

Reapproximate the edges of the rectal mucosa and muscularis with a continuous suture of either 3-0 polyglactin (Vicryl) or 4-0 poliglecaprone (Monocryl) on an SH needle. After this, perform your repair of the anal sphincter as previously described and shown in figure 11-8. When closing the remaining vaginal portion of the laceration, be sure to close the deep tissue overlying the rectum and do not leave any dead space where a hematoma could form. The rest of the repair is the same as for a second degree laceration. After the repair is complete, make sure all sponges are removed from the vagina and perform a gentle rectal exam to ensure you have not significantly constricted the lumen or left any significant gaps in the repair. Make sure that you write appropriate postpartum orders, to include stool softeners, the application of an ice pack to the perineum for the next 24-48 hours, and sitz baths BID. There is also some literature to support the use of prophylactic antibiotics (usually a cephalosporin, such as cephalexin) in these patients for the first few days after delivery to prevent infection or breakdown of the repair. (See Appendix B: Sample Notes & Orders.)

Complications of Lacerations/Episiotomies

Both lacerations that occur spontaneously and those that result from an episiotomy can cause a number of complications. It is important to not only recognize the acute problems, such as postpartum hemorrhage, but also to be aware and monitor for those that are delayed for several days or weeks, such as infection, hematomas, and fistulas. Some of the more common complications include the following:

Hemorrhage. All types of lacerations are associated with postpartum hemorrhage, but midline and mediolateral episiotomies are significant risk factors for this as well. One study, which used a decrease in hematocrit to determine if significant blood loss occurred, reported that mediolateral episiotomies in particular were associated with postpartum hemorrhage (Coombs 1991). When evaluating a patient for a postpartum hemorrhage and the uterus is firm, you must consider and inspect for cervical and vaginal lacerations.

Infection. When you consider the amount of trauma that can occur with a vaginal delivery, the normal bacteria in the vagina, and the lochia that flows through the vagina after delivery, it is remarkable that infections of episiotomies are relatively uncommon. When these do occur, it may be a superficial wound infection, or a deeper abscess which can form from a hematoma. Risk factors associated with infection include infected lochia, fecal contamination, and poor hygiene of the incision site. The incidence of an infection of an episiotomy has been reported between 0.35% and 10% (Myers-Helfgott 1999).

In general, whenever a patient who had lacerations repaired after delivery complains of increasing pain and/or fevers, the area should be inspected and examined. This most commonly occurs on postpartum day three or four. Erythema, a tender, fluctuant mass, or purulent drainage may be present. If a superficial infection is present, then it should be treated with antibiotics. If an abscess or infected hematoma is present, it must be incised, drained, and the area surgically debrided and then antibiotics administered.

Hematoma. If the soft tissue dead space of a deep laceration is not properly obliterated, then bleeding may continue into this potential space. A hematoma can form which has the potential to cause significant discomfort as well as become a nidus for infection. When present, these can often be felt on gentle digital examination of both the rectum and vagina. The incidence of hematomas after delivery has been reported to be between 1:300 and 1:1,000 deliveries (Gilstrap 2001). If the hematoma continues to expand, it can even dissect into the retroperitoneum, which should be considered when a patient has a falling hematocrit and an expanding hematoma.

When the hematoma is small to moderate size, not expanding, and the patient is hemodynamically stable, it may be conservatively managed. The patient is given oral pain medication and may use a heating pad for comfort. If it is expanding or the patient is unstable, then it should be evacuated and, after identifying and correcting any bleeding with hemostatic sutures, a vaginal packing is placed for up to 24 hours and then reexamined to ensure they have not reaccumulated. It is important to note that nearly half of women with hematomas that require surgical treatment will require a transfusion (Zahn 1990).

Repair breakdown. Fortunately, this is an uncommon occurrence, seen in only around 4 % of cases (Sanz 2001). When it does occur, it is usually associated with a concurrent infection over 75% of the time (Ramin 1992). While in the past, repair of the breakdown was performed after waiting at least 3-4 months, it has been demonstrated that, with appropriate preoperative care, to include IV antibiotics, bowel preparation, and aggressive cleansing of the wound, that early repair of an episiotomy breakdown (usually within one week) is associated with good outcomes (Hankins 1990; Ramin 1992).

Anal incontinence. In general, this only occurs when there has been damage to the anal sphincter, i.e., with third and fourth-degree lacerations. When a third-degree laceration occurs, the incidence of long-term anal incontinence has been reported as high as 40% (Poen 1998). The risk of sustaining a third or fourth-degree laceration is increased in patients that are primiparous, have an instrumental vaginal delivery, a macrosomic infant, or an episiotomy.

Rectovaginal fistula. This is a rare complication, but can occur when an infected hematoma erodes through the rectovaginal septum, or when an unrecognized injury into the rectum occurs and is not repaired. This latter injury allows for fecal contamination of the incision, which then progresses to become a fistula. This unrecognized "buttonhole" lesion of the rectum has been reported to occur in approximately 0.1% of deliveries (Graber 1957).

Antibiotic prophylaxis. While there has been considerable discussion regarding the need for antibiotics when a patient experiences a 3rd or 4th degree laceration, this has previously been left up to the discretion and preference of the patient's physician. A recent randomized study, however, suggests that patients who have a 3rd or 4th degree laceration should receive a single dose of a 2nd generation cephalosporin after delivery as this will decrease the incidence of perineal wound complications from 24% to 8% (Duggal 2008).

References:

Anthony S, Buitendijk S, Zondervan K, et al. Episiotomies and the occurrence of severe perineal lacerations. Br J Obstet Gynaecol, 1994; 101:1064-1067.

Coombs CA, Murphy E, Laros R. Factors associated with postpartum hemorrhage with vaginal birth. Obstet Gynecol, 1991; 77:69-76.

Duggal N, Mercado C, Daniels K, Bujor A, Caughey AB, El-Sayed YY. Antibiotic prophylaxis for prevention of postpartum perineal wound complications. Obstet Gynecol. 2008 June; 111(6):1268-1273.

Fahmy K, el-Gazar A, Sammour M, Nosair M, Salem A. Postpartum colposcopy of the cervix: Injury and healing. In J Gynaecol Obstet 1991; 34:133-137.

Fernando RJ, Sultan AH, Radley S, Jones PW, Johanson RB. Management of obstetric anal sphincter injury: a systematic review & national practice survey. BMC Health Serv Res. 2002 May 13;2(1):9.

Fitzpatrick M, Behan M, O'Connell PR, O'Herlihy C. A randomized clinical trial comparing primary overlap with approximation repair of third-degree obstetric tears. Am J Obstet Gynecol. 2000 Nov;183(5):1220-4.

Gilstrap LC, Van Dorsten PV, Cunningham FG. Puerperal hematomas and genital tract lacerations. In: Operative Obstetrics, 2nd ed. New York, McGraw-Hill, 2001.

Graber E, O'Rourke J. Rectal injuries during vaginal delivery. Am J Obstet Gynecol, 1957; 73:301.

Hankins G, Hauth J, Gilstrap L, et al. Early repair of episiotomy dehiscence. Obstet Gynecol, 1990; 75(1):48-51.

Helwig J, Thorp J, Bowes W. Does midline episiotomy increase the risk of third and fourth degree lacerations in operative vaginal deliveries? Obstet Gynecol, 1993; 82:276-279.

Kettle C, Johanson RB. Absorbable synthetic versus catgut suture material for perineal repair. Cochrane Database Syst Rev. 2000;(2):CD000006.

Klein M. Does episiotomy prevent perineal trauma and pelvic floor relaxation? Online J Curr Clin Trials, 1992 Jul 1; Doc No 10.

McLennan MT, Melick CF, Clancy SL, Artal R. Episiotomy and perineal repair: An evaluation of resident education and experience. J Reprod Med 2002; 47:1025-1030.

Myers-Helfgott MG, Helfgott AW. Routine use of episiotomies in modern obstetrics. Obstet and Gynecol Clin, June 1999; 26(2): 305-325.

Obstetrical Hemorrhage, in *Williams Obstetrics*, 21st edition, Eds Cunningham GF, Gant NF. 2001 Appleton & Lange, New York.

Poen AC, Felt-Bersma RJ, Strijers RL, Dekker GA, Cuesta MA, Meuwissen SH. Third-degree obstetric perineal tear: Long-term clinical and functional results after primary repair. Br J Surg, 1998; 85:1433-1438.

Ramin S, Ramus R, Little B, et al. Early repair of episiotomy dehiscence associated with infection. Am J Obstet Gynecol, 1992; 167:1104-1107.

Rockner G, Walhbberg V, Olund A. Episiotomy and perineal trauma during childbirth. J Adv Nurs 1989; 14:264.

Sanz LE. Managing episiotomies and their complications. Contemporary OB/GYN, May 2001; vol 46(5).

Thacker SB,Banta HD. Benefits and risks of episiotomy: An interpretative review of the English language literature, 1860-1980. Obstet Gynecol Surv 1983; 38(6):322-338.

Weeks JD, Kozak LJ. Trends in the use of episiotomy in the United States: 1980-1998. Birth 2001; 28:152-160.

Zahn CM, Yeomans ER. Postpartum hemorrhage: Placenta accreta, uterine inversion and puerperal hematomas. Clin Obstet Gynecol, 1990; 33:422-431.

Chapter 12

Neonatal Resuscitation

In most deliveries, after the baby is born, they will cry and breathe spontaneously. In some deliveries, however, the baby will come out blue, apneic, and significantly depressed. Although you are not expected to be an expert in pediatrics, it is incumbent upon you to know when and how to resuscitate a newborn baby as it may take several minutes for the pediatricians to arrive.

APGAR Scores

APGAR scores are routinely assigned at one and five minutes of life, and also at ten minutes if significant resuscitation of the infant is required. APGAR scores take into account several variables which are listed in table 12-1. While many parents may focus on APGAR scores, they are a subjective evaluation of the infant and are meant to guide you in your resuscitation of the baby, not to predict long-term outcomes. (The exception to this is that very low APGAR scores, especially <3 at 5 minutes, may be associated with peripartum insults [Thorp 1999].) Remember that you never wait for a 1 minute APGAR to begin resuscitation.

Table 12-1. APGAR scores

SCORE	0	1	2
Activity (Tone)	LIMP	SOME FLEXION	ACTIVE FLEXION
Pulse (BPM)	ABSENT	< 100 BPM	> 100 BPM
Grimace (Reflex Irritability)	NONE	GRIMACE	WITHDRAWL TO STIMULUS
Appearance (SkinColor)	BLUE	BODY PINK, EXTREMITIES BLUE	COMPLETELY PINK
Respirations	ABSENT	WEAK CRY	STRONG CRY

Neonatal Resuscitation

Apnea. When a baby is born and not breathing, this is called apnea. There are two different types of apnea, primary and secondary. Primary apnea is the initial response of a baby to asphyxia, or oxygen deprivation. It will often resolve without intervention and will always respond to stimulation alone. Secondary apnea occurs after several minutes of asphyxia and will not resolve spontaneously. Secondary apnea also does not respond to just stimulation, but requires respiratory intervention, such as positive-pressure ventilation. The most important thing to remember when an apneic infant is born is that you cannot differentiate between primary and secondary apnea based on the fetal heart rate tracing preceding birth or the physical exam, so you must begin resuscitation efforts immediately. Always assume that apnea is secondary apnea.

Preparing for a delivery. As with nearly everything in obstetrics, it is important to try and anticipate when a baby may require resuscitation. If there is a concerning fetal heart rate tracing prior to delivery, an operative delivery is performed, narcotics have been given to the mother within two hours of delivery, or the fetus is preterm, then pediatricians should be called prior to the delivery. A list of other potential situations where you should be concerned about a depressed infant being delivered can be found in table 12-2. Another situation, which may or may not result in a depressed infant, and where pediatricians should be called prior to delivery, is when an operative delivery of any type is going to be performed.

Table 12-2. Antepartum factors that can be associated with delivery of a depressed neonate.

- Emergency cesarean section
- Premature labor
- Precipitous labor
- General anesthesia
- Maternal narcotic administration within 2 hours of delivery
- Abruptio placenta
- Placenta previa
- Chorioamnionitis
- Meconium stained amniotic fluid
- Operative vaginal delivery

It is also important to have the proper equipment available for resuscitating a newborn and to know where this is kept. A list of the standard equipment required is listed in table 12-3.

Table 12-3. Infant resuscitation equipment

Suction equipment
- Bulb suction
- DeLee suction
- 8F feeding tube and 20 mL syringe
- Meconium aspirator

Bag and Mask
- Infant resuscitation bag with a pressure-release valve
- Face masks (newborn and premature sizes with cushioned rims)
- Oral airways
- Oxygen supply with tubing and flow meter

Intubation equipment
- Laryngoscope with blades (size 0 and 1)
- Check batteries in laryngoscope
- Endotracheal tubes, sizes 2.5, 3.0, 3.5, 4.0 mm
- Stylet

It is also necessary to check the equipment prior to delivery. Besides ensuring you have the proper equipment, check the following:

1. Turn on the oxygen and make sure you have good flow.
2. Check that you can get a good seal with the mask by placing it on your hand, and ensure the pressure-release valve works when you squeeze the bag.
3. Open the laryngoscope and check the light. (You will use a size 0 blade for preterm infants and size 1 blade for term infants.)
4. Make sure you have the proper size endotracheal tube (ET) for the size of baby you expect. ET sizes for different weights and gestational ages as recommended by the American Academy of Pediatrics are listed in table 12-4.

Table 12-4. Endotracheal tube sizes

Endotracheal tube size	Gestational Age	Fetal Weight
2.5 mm	< 28 weeks	< 1,000 gms
3.0 mm	28-34 weeks	1,000-2,000 gms
3.5 mm	34-38 weeks	2,000-3,000 gms
4.0 mm	>38 weeks	>3,000 gms

Algorithm for Delivery and Evaluation. When an infant is born, note the tone of the infant and whether or not the infant is attempting to breathe. If the infant is apneic or has poor tone, quickly clamp and cut the cord and take the infant over to the warmer. If the pediatricians are not in the room for the delivery, make sure at this time that you instruct one of the nurses or assistants to contact the pediatricians and have them come immediately. Most institutions have a "code" button in the delivery room that will alert the pediatric resuscitation team. Make sure you know where this is if your hospital has one.

Start by placing the infant on the radiant warmer with the head toward you. Quickly dry and clean the infant with a warm towel, which will provide gentle stimulation. Suction the mouth first, then nares and then evaluate for respirations and position the infant with the neck slightly extended to open the airway. (Please note that this is not the exaggerated "sniffing" position that adult resuscitation may require as that position can close off the infant's airway.) If meconium is present and the infant is not vigorous then it is important to not dry and stimulate the infant before you remove the meconium with an endotracheal tube under direct visualization, which is achieved with a laryngoscope.

After the airway has been cleared, proceed with the evaluation and resuscitation in the following order: Respiratory effort, Heart rate, Color.

- **Respiratory effort.** After the airway has been cleared, evaluate the infant for spontaneous respirations. If apnea is present, always presume secondary apnea and start positive pressure ventilation (PPV) with 100% O2. After this step, check the infant's heart rate with a stethoscope or by palpating the umbilical stump.

  When PPV is required, the initial breaths should be between 30-40 cm H_2O and then subsequent breaths should be 15-20 cm H_2O for normal lungs after this.

- **Heart rate.** If the infant is breathing spontaneously, then check the fetal heart rate. If the heart rate is less than 100 bpm, start PPV, even if the infant has normal respirations. If the heart rate is normal, then evaluate the infant's color (next step). If the infant requires PPV, then after 30 seconds, reevaluate the infant's heart rate. If the heart rate is greater than 100 bpm, you can discontinue the PPV and go to the next step of evaluating the infant's color. If the heart rate is less than 60 bpm and not increasing, then ensure PPV is effective, consider intubation, and begin chest compressions. If the heart rate is > 60 bpm then continue PPV and recheck the heart rate in another 30 seconds. (See figure 12-1)
- **Color.** Evaluate the infant's color. Check for central cyanosis, which means the infant will appear blue over the abdomen and truncal area as opposed to acrocyanosis, which means that cyanosis is only present in the extremities. If central cyanosis is present, and there are spontaneous respirations and a heart rate of over 100 bpm, then administer free-flow oxygen by face mask. As the infant's color improves, you can gradually remove the oxygen.

(A flow diagram of this algorithm is shown in figure 12-1.)

Algorithm for Medications. If the infant requires chest compressions and the heart rate remains under 60 bpm after at least 30 seconds of both chest compressions and PPV, then medications should be administered. The common medications given during a resuscitation are listed in table 12-5. The first medication always given in this situation is epinephrine, which can be administered either intravenously or through the endotracheal tube. An algorithm for medication administration is shown in figures 12-2a and 12-2b. Usually, by the time medications are required, the pediatric team will have arrived. But, just in case, it is good to know the indications and initial medications needed during a resuscitation.

Table 12-5. Medications used in neonatal resuscitation

Medication	Concentration And Preparation	Dosage	Route of administration	Rate of administration
Epinephrine	1:10,000	0.1-0.3 mL/kg ___ 0.3-1.0 mL/kg	IV ___ ET	Give rapidly ___ Dilute w/1–2 mL of normal saline if given in ET
Volume expanders	Type O, Rh - blood 5% Albumin Normal Saline Lactated Ringers	10 mL/kg	IV	Give over 5-10 minutes
Naloxone	0.4 mg/mL	0.1 mg/kg	IV ET SQ IM	Give rapidly ___ Slower onset of action if given SQ/IM

ET = endotracheal tube
IM = intramuscular
IV = intravenous
SQ = subcutaneous

Umbilical Artery Blood Acid-base Analysis

Whenever an infant is born and has an APGAR score of less than 7, it is prudent to obtain an arterial blood sample from the cord for analysis. This information provides a much more objective measure of the infant's acid-base status at the time of delivery as compared to APGAR scores (ACOG 1994). The goal is to determine the degree of acidosis, if any, that is present, and what type of acidosis, i.e., respiratory, metabolic, or mixed, it is. This is important because if the acidosis is respiratory, it is probably secondary to an acute event whereas a metabolic acidosis reflects a more chronic process.

Basic Physiology. The pH of fetal blood is directly correlated with concentration of base, or bicarbonate, and inversely related to the concentration of carbonic acid (H_2CO_3) that is present (ACOG 1995). This is shown in the Henderson-Hasselbach equation:

$$pH = pK + log \frac{HCO_3 \, (base)}{H_2CO_3 \, (acid)}$$

The carbonic acid dissociates to a hydrogen ion (H+) and bicarbonate (HCO3).

As long as there is adequate placental perfusion, oxygen is supplied to the fetus and carbon dioxide ($CO2$) and acid metabolites are removed by the placenta and the fetus is able to maintain its normal acid-base balance. When, for whatever reason, this process is interrupted, fetal acidemia may occur. This is first seen with the accumulation of $CO2$.

Acidemia is classified as respiratory, metabolic, or mixed depending on the levels of PCO_2 and bicarbonate (HCO_3-) present. Table 12-6 demonstrates these different combinations.

Table 12-6. Fetal acidemia

Type of Acidemia	PCO_2 (mm Hg)	HCO_3-(meq/L)
Respiratory	Elevated	Normal
Metabolic	Normal	Low
Mixed	Elevated	Low

Respiratory acidosis, which is associated with an accumulation of $CO2$ with a normal level of HCO3, is most commonly caused by an abrupt decrease in either uteroplacental or umbilical perfusion. The presence of respiratory acidosis is not predictive of long-term injury. Some potential causes for this are listed below:

- Maternal hypoxia from narcotic administration
- Hypotension from the administration of regional anesthesia
- Uterine hyperstimulation
- Magnesium sulfate toxicity
- Umbilical cord compression
- Placental abruption

A metabolic acidemia may occur in the presence of either a chronic or prolonged metabolic imbalance. In this situation, the PCO_2 is relatively normal and the bicarbonate (HCO_3) level is decreased. Some potential causes of a metabolic acidemia include chronic uteroplacental insufficiency, intrauterine growth restriction, and maternal acidemia from diabetes, preeclampsia, or chronic hypertension (Thorp 1999).

The presence of a metabolic acidosis results in both a decreased amount of buffer base and an excess of acid. This results in a base deficit, which is also measured on a standard blood gas analysis.

When respiratory acidemia occurs for a prolonged period of time, it may result in a mixed acidosis, which is characterized by both elevated PCO_2 and a decreased bicarbonate (HCO_3) levels. When either a severe metabolic or mixed acidemia is present, there is a much higher risk of fetal problems.

Technique. The cord is clamped immediately after the infant is delivered, and a 10-20 cm length of cord is obtained and set aside on the delivery table. If it is necessary to obtain an arterial blood sample then a small 1-2 mL heparin-flushed syringe is used to aspirate one of the umbilical cord arteries. If you cannot obtain an adequate sample, then you can aspirate from an artery on the chorionic surface of the placenta (the arteries should be visible as they cross over the veins). After this, obtain a similar sample from the umbilical vein. The samples are then sent to the laboratory for acid-base assessment. It is worthwhile trying to obtain both arterial and venous samples as it is not uncommon for a specimen to clot.

While some people have recommended sending blood-gases with every delivery, this is probably not a cost-effective or necessary procedure. Since you cannot always predict which infants will have low APGAR scores based on antepartum monitoring, following the procedure in table 12-7 will ensure you can send a sample if needed by clamping the cord at every delivery until the 5-minute APGAR is assigned.

Table 12-7. Protocol for umbilical cord gas collection during delivery.

1) Double clamp a segment of the umbilical cord after the infant is delivered in all deliveries.*
2) If either APGAR score is less than 7, then obtain a sample of blood from an umbilical artery and the umbilical vein (if possible).
3) If the specimen cannot be obtained from the cord, you may draw it from the chorionic side of the placenta.
4) If the 5-minute APGAR score is 7 or greater, and the infant is stable, then you can discard the segment of umbilical cord.

Notes:

* You must clamp the cord immediately after delivery, as a delay of only 20-30 seconds can alter the results (ACOG 1995).

* The sample is stable at room temperature for 30-60 minutes (Strickland 1984).

Normal Values. The normal values from over 3,500 infants after vaginal delivery, as well as the accepted normal ranges are listed in tables 12-8 and 12-9. Note that the normal pH for the umbilical vein is higher than for the umbilical artery. This is because the umbilical artery samples blood directly from the fetus and is a better measure of fetal acid-base status, whereas the umbilical vein is more representative of maternal status.

Umbilical cord gases may be affected by multiparity, the altitude at which the patient lives, and smoking, with all of these patients having slightly elevated pH values (Thorp 1999). These differences are, however, rarely significant.

Table 12-8. Normal mean blood gas values

Arterial blood	Value (+/- SD)
pH	7.27 (+/-0.069)
PCO_2 (mm Hg)	50.3 (+/-11.1)
HCO_3-(meq/L)	22.0 (+/-3.6)
Base excess (meq/L)	-2.7 (+/-2.8)
Venous blood	
pH	7.34 (+/-0.063)
PCO_2 (mm Hg)	40.7 (+/-7.9)
HCO_3-(meq/L)	21.4 (+/-2.5)
Base excess (meq/L)	-2.4 (+/-2)

(Riley RJ, Johnson JWC. Collecting and analyzing cord blood gases. Clin Obstet Gynecol 1993; 36:13-23.)

Table 12-9. Normal range for blood gas values

	ARTERY	*VEIN*
pH	7.15-7.38	7.20-7.41
PCO2	35-70	33-50
Bicarbonate (HCO_3-)	17-28	15-26
Base excess	-2.0 to -9.0	-1.0 to -8.0

Source: Thorp JA, Rushing SR. Antepartum and intrapartum fetal assessment. Obstet Gynecol Clinics 1999 Dec 26(4):695-709.

Interpretation of values. After obtaining the values from the samples (assuming you were able to obtain both arterial and venous samples), compare the pH values to ensure they are labeled correctly. (The pH should be higher in the venous sample.) After doing this, determine if the pH is in the normal range and what categories the PCO2 and HCO3 fall into (normal, elevated, or low). If the pH is low, then look at table 12-6 to determine what type of acidemia, if any, is present.*

If a metabolic or mixed acidemia is present, the base deficit should also be noted. The risk of significant newborn complications increases with the amount of the base deficit, with infants with values greater than 16 mmol/L having a fourfold higher incidence than those with a level between 12 and 16 mmol/L (Low 1997).

The umbilical PO2 is not predictive of fetal outcome as normal newborns may be hypoxic according to this value until extrauterine respirations are well-established.

* While there is much disagreement about what pH cutoff should constitute fetal acidemia, many experts suggest a cutoff of < 7.10 for defining acidemia at birth. It should be noted that the risk of perinatal morbidity or mortality does not increase unless the pH is less than 7.00 (Fee 1990; Freeman 1988).

As a final note, there is much confusion over certain terms used to describe the depressed neonate, and the word asphyxia is often misused. It is extremely important for medicolegal reasons to be precise in your notes. The American College of OB/GYN gives the following definitions which will help you:

- Hypoxemia: Decreased oxygen content in the blood
- Hypoxia: Decreased level of oxygen in the tissue
- Acidemia: Increased concentration of hydrogen ions in the blood
- Acidosis: Increased concentration of hydrogen ions in the tissue
- Asphyxia: Hypoxia with evidence of a metabolic acidosis

References:

Fee SC, Malee K, Deddisch R, et al. Severe acidosis and subsequent neurologic status. Am J Obstet Gynecol 1990; 162:802.

Freeman JM, Nelson KB. Intrapartum asphyxia and cerebral palsy. Pediatrics 1988; 82:240-249.

Low, JA. Intrapartum fetal asphyxia: Definition, diagnosis, and classification. Am J Obstet Gynecol 1997; 176:957-959.

Riley RJ, Johnson JWC. Collecting and analyzing cord blood gases. Clin Obstet Gynecol 1993; 36:13-23.

Strickland DM, Gilstrap LC III, Hauth JC, Widmer K. Umbilical cord pH and PCO2: effect of interval from delivery to determination. Am J Obstet Gynecol, 1984; 148:191-193.

Textbook of Neonatal Resuscitation, American Heart Association and American Academy of Pediatrics, Bloom RS, Croply C. eds, Copyright 1994.

Thorp JA, Rushing SR. Antepartum and intrapartum fetal assessment. Obstet Gynecol Clinics 1999 Dec; 26(4):695-709.

Umbilical artery blood acid-base analysis, ACOG Technical Bulletin #216, November, 1995.

Utility of umbilical cord blood acid-base assessment, ACOG Committee Opinion #138, April, 1994.

Figure 12-1. Flow diagram for neonatal resuscitation

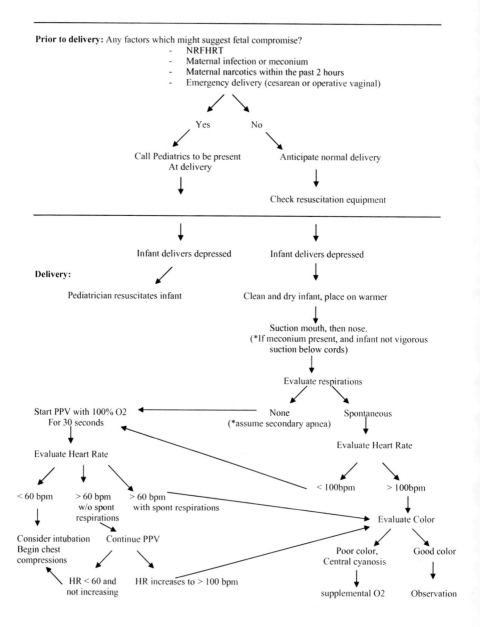

Prior to delivery: Any factors which might suggest fetal compromise?
- NRFHRT
- Maternal infection or meconium
- Maternal narcotics within the past 2 hours
- Emergency delivery (cesarean or operative vaginal)

Yes No

Call Pediatrics to be present At delivery Anticipate normal delivery

Check resuscitation equipment

Infant delivers depressed Infant delivers depressed

Delivery:

Pediatrician resuscitates infant Clean and dry infant, place on warmer

Suction mouth, then nose.
(*If meconium present, and infant not vigorous suction below cords)

Evaluate respirations

Start PPV with 100% O2 For 30 seconds None (*assume secondary apnea) Spontaneous

Evaluate Heart Rate

Evaluate Heart Rate

< 60 bpm > 60 bpm w/o spont respirations > 60 bpm with spont respirations

< 100bpm > 100bpm

Consider intubation Begin chest compressions Continue PPV

Evaluate Color

Poor color, Central cyanosis Good color

HR < 60 and not increasing HR increases to > 100 bpm

supplemental O2 Observation

Figure 12-2a-b. Algorithms for medication use in neonatal resuscitation

Figure 12-2a.

Infant with respiratory depression and a history of recent maternal narcotic administration

↓

Administer Naloxone

Figure 12-2b.

If either of the following are present:

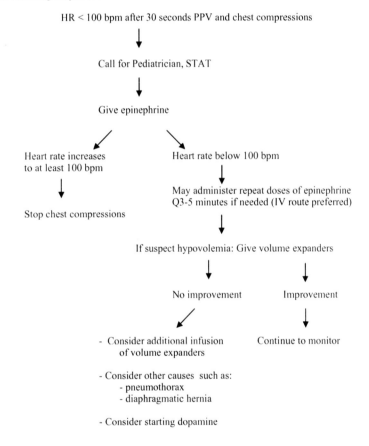

HR < 100 bpm after 30 seconds PPV and chest compressions

↓

Call for Pediatrician, STAT

↓

Give epinephrine

Heart rate increases to at least 100 bpm

Heart rate below 100 bpm

↓

Stop chest compressions

May administer repeat doses of epinephrine Q3-5 minutes if needed (IV route preferred)

↓

If suspect hypovolemia: Give volume expanders

↓

No improvement   Improvement

- Consider additional infusion of volume expanders

Continue to monitor

- Consider other causes such as:
  - pneumothorax
  - diaphragmatic hernia

- Consider starting dopamine

227

Chapter 13

Postpartum Care

- Routine Care after SVD
  - Rounds
  - Physical Exam
  - Episiotomy/Laceration Care
  - Pain Medication
- Routine Care after an Operative Vaginal Delivery
- Routine Care after Cesarean Section
  - Rounds
  - Physical Exam
  - Incision Care
  - Pain Medication
  - Foley Catheter Management
  - Return of Bowel Function
- Breastfeeding
  - Contraindications
  - Common Problems
- Common Infections/Complications
  - Postpartum Fever
  - Endometritis
  - Mastitis
  - Preeclampsia
  - Postpartum Blues
  - Urinary Retention
  - Wound/Episiotomy Infections
  - Postpartum Hemorrhage
- Discharge issues

- Discharge Criteria
  - Timing of Discharge
- Immunizations
- Rhogam
- Contraception
- Resuming Coitus

Routine Care after SVD

Rounds. After a vaginal delivery, even those assisted with forceps or vacuum devices, the infant and mother are monitored for several hours to ensure both are stable. They are then transferred to the postpartum service for the remainder of their stay. This may be on a separate floor or in the same room depending on the institution. For mothers who are doing well, you will see them at least once a day on rounds to check on their recovery and issues. Important questions to ask are as follows:

1. How is the patient feeling?

    - Remember that most mothers will be somewhat tired after having been through labor.

2. How much bleeding (lochia) is the patient having?

    - In general, they should not be passing large clots, and they should not be soaking more than one pad per hour. If they are, then it is important to investigate this further by checking vital signs, fundal height and tone, complete blood count (CBC), and for vaginal lacerations that are bleeding. If the patient is dizzy or lightheaded (i.e., orthostatic symptoms) then you must find the etiology quickly and should order a stat CBC. See Chapter 14 for more details on postpartum hemorrhage.

3. Any fevers or chills?

    - If the patient has fevers or cheers, then a further investigation is required to determine the etiology.

4. Is the patient able to void spontaneously?

    - While it is not uncommon for a patient to have difficulty urinating after delivery, especially after an operative vaginal delivery or when they received an epidural during labor. It is important to monitor for urinary retention as an overdistended bladder that is neglected or unnoticed for a long period of time may result in damage to bladder innervation. This complication is discussed later in this chapter.

5. How is the patient's pain?

    -   Uterine cramping. This complaint, which is usually more intense with breastfeeding, is very common. It is best treated with analgesics such as ibuprofen. In cases where this is not adequate, a mild narcotic, such as Percocet (which is a combination of acetaminophen and oxycodone) can be given. During the physical exam, you must make sure the patient's complaint of uterine cramping is not actually a manifestation of endometritis, which will demonstrate significant uterine tenderness with palpation.
    -   Perineal pain. Patients who had significant lacerations may have dysuria and pain in the perineal region. This is again treated best with ibuprofen and/or acetaminophen, but mild narcotics may be required. Any complaint of a significant increase in pain should be investigated with a gentle physical exam to look for evidence of infection or hematomas.
    -   Headache. This is a common complaint after delivery. It may simply be due to a lack of sleep, but it is important to look for other causes that could be more serious.

6. Is the baby breastfeeding?

    -   Difficulty with breastfeeding is one of the more frustrating things a new mother may encounter. This is also discussed later in this chapter.

7. How is the baby feeding?

    -   While you are not the pediatrician, you will almost certainly be rounding before them. If the baby is having difficulty feeding, this should be placed in your note so they can be aware of this.

    *   Note: A sample postpartum note is contained in Appendix B: Sample Notes and Orders

Physical Exam. The physical exam should generally include a brief exam of the heart and lungs, and the head and neck if there are specific complaints such as headache or sinus congestion. The breasts should be examined if there have been any fevers or if the patient complains of tenderness or pain.

The abdominal exam after a vaginal delivery focuses on palpation of the uterus and ensuring that it is firm and appropriately contracted, which will prevent excessive bleeding. The fundal height is usually described in relation to the umbilicus in terms of centimeters. If the fundus is 2 cm below the umbilicus, it is referred to as U-2 in the progress note. Alternatively, if it is 1 centimeter above the umbilicus, it is at U+1. If it is at the umbilicus, the fundus is at "U." This exam, while usually very easy, can be very difficult in obese patients. If the fundus is at U + 2 or higher, then there is some concern for retained clots in the uterus although this is not a specific finding for this problem. More commonly, the fundal height is increased by a full bladder. In the absence of significant bleeding, simply checking the fundal height again after the patient has urinated usually results in an exam that falls in the normal range.

It is also important to evaluate the uterus for tenderness. In general, the uterus may be mildly tender, especially with contractions during breastfeeding, but it should not be significant. If it is, then you must consider the possibility of endometritis, which is described later in this chapter.

The perineum is inspected if there was a significant laceration or repair, or if the patient has significant pain in that area. Care and evaluation of the perineum is discussed in the next section.

The extremities should be evaluated for edema, which is almost always a normal finding when bilateral, especially in the lower extremities. Concerning findings are unilateral edema accompanied by significant pain or a palpable cord on examination. Remember that pregnancy and the postpartum period are marked by a hypercoaguable state and you must keep deep venous thrombosis in your differential diagnosis. If the patient has hypertension and worsening edema, then you should also consider the possibility of postpartum preeclampsia.

As with everything on labor and delivery, if you have a question about a physical exam finding, ask someone above you or a colleague to evaluate the patient.

Episiotomy/Laceration care. If either an episiotomy was made or a laceration requiring sutures occurred, then the patient should be asked about increasing pain or discomfort in that area each day. An ice pack should be applied just after delivery and continued for several hours to help reduce swelling. The area should also be visually inspected to monitor for early signs of infection. If the patient has fevers, chills, or increasing discomfort in the area, then a gentle digital exam is needed to make sure no hematomas are present. A rare, but potentially fatal infection, necrotizing fasciitis, can occur which requires immediate surgical debridement.

Pain medication. Most women will not require any pain medication other than ibuprofen after an uncomplicated vaginal delivery. Women who have significant lacerations and repairs may require mild narcotics, such as oxycodone. (See medication database.)

Routine Care after an Operative Vaginal Delivery

Care after an operative vaginal delivery is the same as after a spontaneous vaginal delivery with the following small differences:

1. Inspect the perineum, especially since operative vaginal deliveries are more likely to have had an episiotomy or more extensive lacerations.
2. Look at the infant. With a vacuum delivery, inspect the fetal scalp (and take off the hat if the child has one on during rounds) and look for evidence of hematomas. For forceps delivery, make sure and note any facial marks and if they have diminished as they will usually begin to fade in the days after delivery.
3. Be aware of the potential for urinary retention and ask if they are having any difficulty with urination.

Routine Care after Cesarean Section

Rounds. After a cesarean section, the mother and infant are taken to a recovery room where they are monitored for several hours. As long as she remains stable, the mother is transferred to the postpartum service at this time. The questions you will ask a postoperative patient are the same as after a vaginal delivery with the following additions:

1. Are you having any nausea or vomiting?
2. Are you dizzy or lightheaded?
3. Have you been able to ambulate?
4. Have you had any drainage from your incision?

After a cesarean section, which is major abdominal surgery, you are more concerned about postoperative bleeding and return of bowel function compared to a patient who had a SVD. Because of this, you need to note any symptoms that could be related to hypovolemia from bleeding, such as dizziness or lightheadedness, especially with ambulation as some patients may feel fine lying down, then become very symptomatic when they attempt to ambulate. The vital signs are also important for this and you need to note tachycardia and hypotension. Urine output, which should be at least 0.5 cc/kg/hour, is a good way to monitor the patient's hemodynamic status. (If the patient's kidneys are not seeing enough blood, they won't make as much urine.) Record the amount of urine output overnight and then put the number in cc's/hour in your note as well. This is most important for the first 12-24 hours after surgery as the foley catheter is usually removed then.

Physical exam. The physical exam after a cesarean delivery is essentially the same as after a vaginal delivery, with the addition of an incision to evaluate.

Incision care. After cesarean section, the incision is covered with a sterile dressing. This dressing is generally left in place until the next morning, or approximately 12 hours. For vertical skin incisions, the dressing is often left on for 24 hours after the operation although both of these times are subject to a wide range of provider preference.

When evaluating an incision, the bandage is removed and the incision visualized. Sometimes this is difficult in obese patients as the incision is under the pannus. (If this is the case, then placing a clean sanitary pad over the incision between the incision and pannus can help to keep the incision dry.) Regardless of whether sutures or skin staples were used, make sure the incision is intact, look for areas of erythema, and note any drainage coming from the incision. If erythema is present, you can mark the extent of it with a pen to compare at the next exam. A small amount of serosanguinous drainage is common, and a piece of 4 x 4 gauze can be placed over this and checked later. Frank bleeding, a significant increase in drainage, or purulent discharge will need to be evaluated immediately. If any of these are present, have the senior resident or staff see the incision. (Wound infections and treatment are discussed in detail in Chapter 10.)

Pain medication. After a cesarean section, many patients receive a long-acting narcotic in their epidural, which will usually provide adequate analgesia for the next 12-24 hours. If they do not, then patient-controlled anesthesia (PCA), which is a pump that administers a small dose of a narcotic when the patient pushes a button, can be used for the initial postoperative period. Another option is simply using IV narcotics on an as-needed, or prn, basis. A nonsteroidal medication such as ketorolac can be given as well if there was not excessive bleeding during the cesarean section.

When the patient is able to tolerate PO, a nonsteroidal medication, such as ibuprofen, is given on a schedule, i.e., 800 mg PO every 8 hours. A mild narcotic, usually medications such as either Percocet or Darvocet (see medication database), is given every 4-6 hours as needed to control breakthrough pain.

Foley catheter management. The foley catheter is usually removed on postoperative day one. It is an important tool for monitoring hemodynamic status as mentioned previously. If the patient is not making adequate urine, or they had excessive bleeding and require a transfusion, then the foley should remain in place until they are stable.

After the catheter is removed, it is important to write an order that the patient is due to void (DTV) in 4-6 hours in order to prevent her bladder from becoming overdistended. If the patient is not able to void by that time, then the foley catheter can be replaced and removed again the next day. If the patient has continued urinary retention, they will need further evaluation. (This complication is discussed in detail later in this chapter.)

Return of bowel function. In the past, patients were not given anything by mouth after a cesarean section until they had flatus due to the belief that this would prevent a postoperative ileus. This notion has been challenged with several studies in recent years which have shown that early feeding for both gynecologic abdominal surgery and cesarean sections are associated with decreased time in the hospital and no significant increase in the incidence of postoperative ileus (Soriano 1996; Fanning 2001; Patolia 2001; Kramer 1996).

Breastfeeding

Breastmilk is the ideal food for new infants and decreases the risk of infection, including diarrhea, otitis media, urinary tract infections, and many other common infant infections. There are even studies that show it may be protective against sudden infant death syndrome and the development of insulin-dependent diabetes (American Academy of Pediatrics 1997). In 2005, as many as 72% of new mothers were at least starting with breastfeeding (ACOG 2007). Although breastfeeding has so many proven benefits, it can be frustrating at first, and it is important to recognize and intervene early when problems occur to ensure that as many women as possible can continue to breastfeed. Unfortunately, not all women can breastfeed. Contraindications to breastfeeding are listed below.

Contraindications to breastfeeding

- HIV infection is a contraindication to breastfeeding in developed countries as the infection may be transmitted to the infant
- Active HSV infection of the nipple
- Maternal medications that make breastfeeding contraindicated

(Most antibiotics and medications do not pose a problem with breastfeeding. There is a category in the medication database included with this curriculum that comments on the safety of each with breastfeeding. If you are using another medication, then a helpful reference is the book *Drugs in Pregnancy and Lactation* which is listed in the references and is currently in its 8th edition.)

- Active, untreated tuberculosis
- Patients with an infant with galactosemia
- Patients undergoing treatment for breast cancer
- Patients taking illicit drugs or who abuse alcohol
    (ACOG 2007)

Common problems with breastfeeding

It is important to know how to manage common complications in order to allow for the mother to continue to breastfeed. With appropriate and prompt care, most problems can be overcome.

Sore nipples/fissures. These complications usually result from incorrect positioning of the infant and poor latching-on rather than prolonged nursing (Berens, 2001). If the nipple appears infected, then treatment with an antibiotic to cover Staphylococcus aureus should be started. (See Medication Database) In addition, the use of over the counter topical creams, such as those containing lanolin, may also be helpful.

Mastitis. This infection occurs in between 1%-2% of lactating women and is most common in the first and fifth weeks postpartum (ACOG 2000). Some risk factors include missed feedings, nipple fissures, and untreated breast engorgement.

Clinically, the patient will usually complain of the rapid onset of fevers, unilateral breast pain, and myalgias. The most common responsible organism is Staphylococcus aureus, which accounts for approximately 40% of cases (Matheson 1988). A narrow-spectrum antibiotic, such as Dicloxacillin or a cephalosporin, is the first line therapy and should be given for 10-14 days. (If the patient is allergic to penicillins and cephalosporins, then erythromycin can be given.) See the medication database for more information on these antibiotics.

The patient should continue to breastfeed, as the milk is not harmful and both penicillins and cephalosporins are safe in breastfeeding. If this is too uncomfortable for the patient, then the infected breast should be expressed by hand if possible.

Mastitis should be treated early and aggressively, because delaying treatment increases the risk of developing a breast abscess.

Breast abscess. Between 5%-11% of women with mastitis will go on to develop a breast abscess (Berens 2001). The symptoms are essentially the same as mastitis, but a fluctuant mass is present. It is diagnosed by either a palpable mass or failure to respond to antibiotic treatment for a presumed mastitis within 48-72 hours.

The most common treatment of a breast abscess is surgical incision and drainage, with continued antibiotic treatment. If multiple abscesses are present, all must be drained and meticulous hemostasis obtained to prevent hematomas from forming. After surgery, breastmilk from the affected breast is generally disposed of for the first 24 hours. Breastfeeding after surgery from the infected breast can be restarted after this time as long as there is not drainage from the incision onto the nipple.

Another therapy that has been utilized for breast abscesses involves the drainage of the abscess by needle aspiration guided by ultrasound (Karstrup 1993). Check with your staff and residents as to what is most commonly done at your institution.

Galactocele. These are caused by plugged milk ducts and create a tender, palpable lump in the breast. They are not accompanied by evidence of infection such as fevers, chills, or erythema. Some risk factors for these include missing a feeding, overabundant mild supply, and poor latch-on (Berens 2001). Treatment is symptomatic and includes increasing the frequency of feeding, massaging the area during feeding, and applying a moist, warm compress to the area. These should generally resolve within 72 hours. If signs of infection become evident, then patients should be evaluated for mastitis or an abscess.

Bloody nipple discharge. This can be a normal finding during the third trimester because of increased vascularity of the breast, or during the postpartum period from nipple trauma. It is not harmful to the infant, and should resolve spontaneously within approximately 7 days. If the bloody discharge lasts longer than this, or appears to be coming from a single duct, then further evaluation, including a breast exam, cytologic evaluation of the discharge, and possibly mammography or ultrasound, should be pursued as this can be the presentation of a malignant tumor.

Breast mass. When a breast mass is found postpartum, and it is not felt to be due to a galactocele or breast abscess, then further workup is required. Fortunately, the incidence of breast cancer in breastfeeding mothers is only 1:3,000 to 1:10,000 patients and there is no difference in survival rates when compared to nonpregnant women (Berens 2001). The same diagnostic workup, including breast exam, fine needle aspiration, mammography, and ultrasound as required are all acceptable and safe in breastfeeding patients.

Contraception issues. When breastfeeding is used exclusively, lactational amenorrhea is a very effective form of contraception. This method is also beneficial in that it does not affect the milk supply. Barrier methods such as condoms also do not affect the milk supply, but they are less effective. Progesterone-only contraceptives may be started as soon as the patient is discharged from the hospital and do not affect the milk supply. Depot medroxyprogesterone acetate can be given prior to hospital discharge, especially in patients who may not follow up for a postpartum visit, but is normally given at 4-6 weeks postpartum. Combination birth control pills (OCPs), which contain estrogen, are not generally started until 6 weeks after delivery because of the concern about the risk of venous thromboembolic events (VTE) in the immediate postpartum period.

Common postpartum infections/complications

Postpartum Fever. If a patient develops a fever in the postpartum period, they should be examined closely for a source. One useful memory aid to help to remember what to look for is:

Wind: Atelectasis (This is more common after a cesarean delivery, especially if the patient has not been ambulatory.) Sinus/Upper respiratory tract infections
Water: Urinary tract infection
Walking: Thrombophlebitis
Wound: Infection of the incision or episiotomy
Wonder drug: Medication-induced fevers
Womb: Endometritis
Woman: Mastitis

A thorough review of systems and a physical exam should be performed. If a source is not obvious, such as endometritis, then a urinalysis and culture, and a complete blood count with differential should be sent and acetaminophen administered. If the fever continues to increase or the patient's condition worsens, then two sets of blood cultures and a chest x-ray should be done as well.

When a source is found, the infection should be treated with the appropriate antibiotics and the patient should not be discharged until they have been afebrile for at least 24 hours.

Endometritis. This is much more common in patients who undergo a cesarean delivery. It generally presents with fevers and chills in combination with significant uterine tenderness on abdominal exam. Please refer to Chapter 14 for a complete discussion of the diagnosis and treatment of this infection.

Mastitis. This complication was discussed previously in this chapter.

Preeclampsia. While the treatment and cure for preeclampsia is delivery, it is possible for patients to develop preeclampsia in the postpartum period. Early postpartum preeclampsia develops within 48 hours of delivery, and late-onset postpartum preeclampsia is generally defined as having on onset between 48 hours and 4 weeks after delivery. This complication is also discussed in detail in Chapter 14.

Postpartum blues. Mild depressive symptoms, referred to as the postpartum blues occur in up to 50% of women after delivery, usually within the first week after delivery (Kendell 1987). Common symptoms include anxiety, difficulty concentrating, labile mood swings, insomnia, and weepiness.

The most important characteristic of postpartum blues is that symptoms only last for a few hours or days and the patient, while labile, does not completely lose touch with reality. Treatment is initially just supportive and you should reassure the patient that this is most likely simply a transient phase. Make sure the patient does not have any suicidal ideations and that she is able to care for the infant prior to discharge, and arrange early followup and provide phone numbers where she can contact her provider if she continues to experience problems. If the symptoms persist then a psychiatrist should be consulted and the diagnosis of postpartum depression considered.

Urinary retention. It is not uncommon for women to have difficulty voiding after either vaginal delivery or a cesarean section. It is important to diagnose this as prolonged urinary retention and overdistention of the bladder can result in permanent damage and voiding problems.

Urinary retention is usually diagnosed when a patient has been unable to void for 4-6 hours after a foley catheter has been removed and when an enlarged bladder, which feels like a cystic mass in the lower abdomen on exam, is palpated.

A differential of the causes of urinary retention after delivery that must be considered includes the following:

- Effects of medication/anesthesia
- Vaginal hematoma causing obstruction
- Urethral obstruction by sutures from laceration repair

A physical exam can usually rule out a hematoma or suture as the etiology of urinary retention.

Treatment of urinary retention initially consists of a physical exam and then placing a foley catheter to provide drainage of the bladder. If the catheter is placed in the afternoon, it is often left in place overnight and removed the next morning. After the catheter is removed, immediately after the first time the patient urinates, a post-void residual is checked by an in-and-out catheterization. If the residual is less than 200 cc, then the foley does not need to be replaced. If it is greater than this, the foley is either replaced or post-void residuals continue to be checked, ensuring the patient does not go more than four hours between voids. If the residuals do not decrease and are consistently greater than 200 cc, then a foley catheter may be replaced to rest the bladder and voiding trials conducted again the next day.

If the patient is still unable to void appropriately when she meets all other discharge criteria, then she must either be taught how to self-catheterize herself or have a foley catheter inserted with a leg bag attached to go home with. Close follow-up and bladder trials are important to monitor for return of normal function.

Fortunately, it is uncommon for urinary retention to persist more than a couple of days after delivery. One study of over 8,000 deliveries found the incidence of persistent urinary retention, which was defined as present if the patient was still unable to void spontaneously on the third postpartum day, to be only 0.05% (Groutz 2001). Risk factors for this included VBAC, a prolonged second stage of labor, epidural analgesia, and delayed diagnosis and intervention.

Wound/episiotomy infections. When the normal bacterial content of the vagina and the continued normal lochia that occurs after delivery are taken into account, the incidence of episiotomy infections is surprisingly low.

While an episiotomy infection often presents with increased pain, erythema, fevers, and chills, an abdominal wound infection can present with an increased amount of drainage in addition to erythema, fever and chills.

Please see the following for a complete discussion of these problems:

- Chapter 10: Wound infections after cesarean section.
- Chapter 11: Episiotomy infections

Postpartum hemorrhage. While this usually occurs at the time of delivery, it may occur while the patient is on the postpartum ward. This complication is addressed in detail in the next chapter.

Discharge issues

Discharge criteria. Prior to discharge, all patients must be able to do the following:

- Ambulate
- Spontaneously void (or if not, then they must have a catheter, or learn how to self-catheterize themselves as described previously in this chapter.)
- Tolerate a regular diet
- Be hemodynamically stable
- Have no evidence of serious infection that requires inpatient treatment
- Adequate follow-up for both the patient and the child is arranged
- All immunizations/Rhogam given as indicated
- Contraception has been discussed with patient

Timing of discharge. The time from delivery to discharge differs between vaginal deliveries and cesarean deliveries, but the same criteria as listed above must be met for the patient to leave the hospital.

- Vaginal delivery. If there are no complications, then patients are usually not kept any longer than 48 hours. In some cases, patients may leave as early as 24 hours after delivery, if they desire.
- Cesarean delivery. Patients may be discharged when they meet the discharge criteria above. This will occur in most patients by 72 hours, but there are times where they will have slow return of bowel function and need to stay another day.

Immunizations. Patients who are rubella non-immune should be vaccinated prior to discharge. You can reassure the parents that breastfeeding is not a contraindication to the immunization and does not place the infant at risk of contracting the disease (APGO 1999).

Rhogam. If the mother is Rh-negative and the infant is Rh-positive, then prior to discharge, the patient should receive the standard dose of 300 mcg of anti-D immune globulin (Rhogam) in order to prevent isoimmunization and complications with subsequent pregnancies.

Contraception. While this may be the last thing on a new mother's mind, it is important to discuss prior to discharge. If the patient is breastfeeding on demand, then ovulation is usually suppressed, but in the nonlactating mother, ovulation usually occurs between three and 10 weeks after delivery. In general, the following options are available for women who are not using lactational amenorrhea for contraception:

- Barrier methods
- Progestin-only oral contraceptive pills may be given to patients at the time of discharge, or at anytime postpartum. (Ovulation generally does not return before three weeks postpartum even in nonlactating women.)
- Intrauterine device (may be placed at 6 weeks postpartum)
- Combination oral contraceptive pills (OCPs) may be started at 6 weeks postpartum
- Depot medroxyprogesterone acetate is generally given prior to discharge from the hospital or at approximately 6 weeks postpartum*

* Note: An additional benefit of the depot medroxyprogesterone over OCPs is that adolescents are much less likely to discontinue this form of birth control as compared to OCPs. In one study, 72% of women under the age of 18 discontinued OCPs within a year compared to 44% using depot medroxyprogesterone (Templeman 2000).

Resuming coitus. While there is not a specific time period that must lapse before coitus is resumed, this is an area where common sense should be used. Women with significant vaginal lacerations will require more time for healing than women without lacerations. It is also important to inform breastfeeding patients that, because they will produce less estrogen, they may experience vaginal dryness. In general, after two or three weeks postpartum, coitus can be resumed depending on the patient's desire and level of comfort. For patients who had a cesarean section, they should generally wait for 4-6 weeks to resume coitus to permit adequate healing of their incision.

References:

American Academy of Pediatrics, Work Group on Breastfeeding and the use of human milk. Pediatrics, 1997; 100:1035-1039.

Association of Professors of Gynecology and Obstetrics, Immunization for Women's Health. APGO Educational Series on Women's Health Issues, Washington, DC, 1999.

Berens PD. Prenatal, intrapartum, and postpartum support of the lactating mother. Pediatric Clin of North America. April 2001; 48(2):356-375.

Breastfeeding: Maternal and Infant Aspects. ACOG Educational Bulletin # 361, Feb 2007.

Briggs GG, Freeman RK, Yaffe SJ (eds) *Drugs in Pregnancy and Lactation* 6th edition, Williams & Wilkins, Baltimore, MD, 2001.

Resnick R. "The Puerperium" in *Maternal-Fetal Medicine*, 4th ed.Creasy RK, Resnick R. eds. W.B. Saunders, Philadelphia, PA, 1999:pg 102.

Fanning J, Andrews S. Early postoperative feeding after major gynecologic surgery: Evidence-based scientific medicine. Am J Obstet Gynecol, July 2001; 185(1): 1-4.

Groutz A. Persistent postpartum urinary retention in contemporary obstetric practice. Definition, prevalence and clinical implications. J Reprod Med, Jan 2001; 46(1):44-48.

Karstrup S, Solvig J, Nolsoe CP, Nilsson P, Khattar S, Loren I, et al. Acute puerperal breast abscesses: Ultrasound-guided drainage. Radiology, 1993; 188:807-809.

Kendell RE, Chalmers JC, Platz C. Epidemiology of puerperal psychoses. Br J Psychiatry, 1987; 150:662-673.

Kramer R, Van Someren J, Qualls C, Curet L. Postoperateve management of cesarean section patients: The effect of immediate feeding on the incidence of ileus. Obstet Gynecol, 1996; 88:29-32.

Matheson I, Aursnes I, Horgan M, Aabo O, Melby K. Bacteriological findings and clinical symptoms in relation to clinical outcome in puerperal mastitis. Acta Obstet Gynecol Scand, 1988; 67:723-726.

Patolia DS, Hilliard RLM, Toy EC, Baker B. Early feeding after cesarean: Randomized trial. Obstet Gynecol, July 2001; 98(1):113-116.

Soriano D, Dulitzki M, Keidar N, Barkai G, Mashiach S, Seidman DS. Early oral feeding after cesarean delivery. Obstet Gynecol, June 1996; 87(6): 1006-1008.

Templeman CL, Cook V, Goldsmith LJ, Powell J, Hertweck P. Postpartum contraceptive use among adolescent mothers. Obstet Gynecol, May 2000; 95(5):770-776.

CHAPTER 14

Common Obstetric Complications and Emergencies

- Chorioamnionitis
- Endometritis
- Hemorrhage
    - Antepartum
    - Postpartum
    - Use of Blood Products
- Magnesium Toxicity
- Malpresentation
    - Breech Vaginal Delivery
    - Transverse Lie
- Oligohydramnios
- Preeclampsia
- Eclampsia
- Preterm Labor
- Preterm Premature Rupture of Membranes (PPROM)
- Shoulder Dystocia
- Umbilical Cord Prolapse
- Uterine Inversion
- Uterine Rupture

While the vast majority of deliveries are uncomplicated and you wind up with a healthy child and happy parents, when complications occur, they occur quickly and rapid and correct interventions can be lifesaving for both mother and baby. Always remember that every delivery is an emergency waiting to happen.

What follows in this chapter is by no means a comprehensive discussion of these complications (entire books have been devoted to some of these subjects), but it does cover some of the most common obstetric complications and emergencies as well as how to treat them. References are listed for more detailed reading as desired.

Chorioamnionitis

This refers to an intraamniotic infection that occurs prior to the delivery of the fetus. Treatment of the infection prior to delivery has been demonstrated to decrease both maternal and neonatal morbidity as well as the risk of neonatal sepsis (Gibbs 1988).

Incidence: It is reported to occur in between 0.5% to 10.5% of all deliveries (Newton 2002).

Clinical Picture: A patient should demonstrate a temperature of at least 38°C (100.4°F) and two or more of the following criteria in order to be diagnosed with Chorioamnionitis:

- Maternal tachycardia (>100 bpm)
- Fetal tachycardia (>160 bpm)
- Foul-smelling amniotic fluid
- Uterine tenderness to palpation
- Elevated WBC count (>15,000)

Risk factors:

- Preterm labor
- Meconium-stained amniotic fluid
- Nulliparity
- Internal monitors (FSE or IUPC)
- Prolonged labor
- Frequent vaginal examinations (with ruptured membranes)

Causes: The bacteria that are responsible for chorioamnionitis are usually polymicrobial and represent much of the normal flora of the vagina. Some of the more common bacteria include Gardnerella, Bacteriodes, Mycoplasma, gram-negative anaerobes, and ureaplasma, as well as Group B streptococcus (Sperling 1988).

Complications: Chorioamnionitis increases the risk of neonatal sepsis and morbidity. It also nearly doubles the risk of postpartum hemorrhage and puts the patient at risk for developing a significant bacteremia (Mark 2000).

Treatment: The treatment of Chorioamnionitis is aimed at covering the usual polymicrobial infection. The standard regimen used when this infection is diagnosed is Ampicillin (2 grams IV Q6 hours) plus Gentamycin (1.5 mg/kg IV Q8 hours) until the time of delivery. (Alternative regimens, such as Cefoxitin (2 gm IV Q6 hours) or Ampicillin-Sublactam (3 gm IV Q6 hours) have also been reported for treatment of chorioamnionitis.) The duration of therapy depends on the patient's status as well as the route of delivery.

If the patient progresses to have a vaginal delivery, then antibiotics are usually stopped at that time as the infected tissues have been expelled. If, however, the patient undergoes a cesarean section, they are at significant risk for developing a postpartum endometritis and clindamycin (900 mg IV Q8 hours) should be added to the current antibiotic regimen of ampicillin and gentamycin. In general, the patient should remain afebrile for 24-48 hours on antibiotics before they are discontinued.

Please refer to figure 14-1 for a treatment algorithm for Chorioamnionitis.

Figure 14-1. Treatment of Chorioamnionitis

Chorioamnionitis Diagnosed

Begin Treatment
- Ampicillin 2 grams IV Q6
- Gentamycin 1.5 mg/kg Q8

(If allergic to Penicillin, substitute clindamycin 900 mg IV Q8 for ampicillin.)

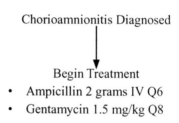

Vaginal Delivery

Cesarean Section

Stop antibiotics

Add clindamycin 900 mg IV Q8

OR
metronidazole 500 mg IV Q12

- Continue antibiotics until at least 24 hrs afebrile

Endometritis

Endometritis refers to a postpartum infection of the endometrium and surrounding tissues.

Incidence: Endometritis occurs rarely after vaginal delivery, in only about 3% of cases, but it may occur in up to 50% of cesarean sections (Chauhan 2001; Gibbs 1985).

Clinical Picture: While the diagnosis of this infection is often clinical, these patients usually present in the first several days postpartum with the following:

- Fever (> 100.4°F or 38°C)
- Uterine tenderness
- Foul-smelling lochia
- Leukocytosis
- Absence of other possible infections (i.e., mastitis, cellulitis, urinary tract etc.)

Risk factors:

- Prolonged rupture of membranes
- Maternal diabetes
- Low socioeconomic status
- Multiple vaginal examinations with ruptured membranes
- Cesarean section
- Chorioamnionitis

Causes: This infection is polymicrobial and includes gram positive, gram negative, anaerobic bacteria and even mycoplasma in many cases.

Treatment: The initial treatment includes the administration of broad spectrum antibiotics, usually Gentamycin (1.5 mg/kg IV Q8 hours)* plus Clindamycin (900 mg IV Q8 hours) until the patient has been afebrile for 24-48 hours. If the patient does not respond to these antibiotics, then Ampicillin (2 gm IV Q6 hours) should be added to cover enterococcus.

Other regiments that have been reported for the treatment of postpartum endometritis include Cefoxitin (2gm IV Q6 hours) or Ampicillin-Sublactam (3 gm IV Q6 hours).

* Note: Gentamycin may also be administered in a Q24 hour dose in the postpartum period. This is generally given as 5 mg/kg IV Q24 hours and multiple studies have demonstrated that this regiment is less expensive, requires less nursing time, and is as safe and effective as the Q8 hour dosing (Del Priore 1996; Mitra 1997).

Hemorrhage

In obstetrics it is common to see significant blood loss on a fairly regular basis and this may occur in both the antepartum and postpartum periods. A life-threatening hemorrhage will occur in approximately 1% of all deliveries, so it is imperative that you be familiar with both potential causes and treatments (Drife 1997; Mantel 1998).

Antepartum Hemorrhage. Third trimester bleeding complicates between 3%-4% of pregnancies (Russo-Stieglietz 2002). The most common causes for this are placental abruption (31%), placenta previa (22%), and cervical dilation from labor or, rarely, neoplasms (Hibbard 1966). In general, bleeding due to cervical change is rarely significant enough to result in fetal or maternal distress, but may alert the physician to the presence of labor. The most important thing to remember about the evaluation of a patient with bleeding during the second or third trimester of pregnancy is NOT to perform a digital examination until you have ruled out a placenta previa as this may precipitate a catastrophic hemorrhage. The evaluation and workup of these patients should proceed as follows:

- Take a thorough maternal history (onset and amount of bleeding, any evidence of rupture of membranes, trauma or motor vehicle accident, history of bleeding problems, medication use such as aspirin or heparin)
- Assess maternal hemodynamic status (Vital signs, CBC, Fibrinogen, PT/PTT)
- Assess fetal status (Fetal heart rate, Continuous monitoring if >24 weeks, monitor for contractions)
- Perform abdominal ultrasound and determine placental location, if there is any possibility of a placenta previa, perform vaginal ultrasound
- If no evidence of a placenta previa, then perform a speculum examination and digital examination to look for cervical source of bleeding (from polyp or dilation)

Placenta previa. A placenta previa is defined as placental tissue either covering the cervical os or being in very close (<2cm) proximity.

Incidence: Placenta previa occurs in between 1:200 and 1:390 pregnancies after 20 weeks (Cunningham 2001; Comeau 1983). It is important to note that 4%-6% of pregnancies will demonstrate evidence of placenta previa on ultrasound between 10-20 weeks gestation, but that 90% of these resolve prior to delivery (Russo-Stieglietz 2002).

Clinical Picture: The classic presentation of a placenta previa is painless vaginal bleeding although as many as 20% of patients may also have uterine contractions at the time of diagnosis. (Cotton 1980; Silver 1984). The bleeding ranges from minimal to massive with maternal shock and fetal distress. The first episode of bleeding generally occurs around 34 weeks gestation, with one third of patients presenting prior to 30 weeks, one-third between 30-36 weeks, and one-third after 36 weeks (McShane 1985). Placenta previa is also associated with fetal malpresentation and preterm premature rupture of membranes. It may also be accompanied by a placenta accreta in 5%-10% of cases, which represents a placenta that has abnormally implanted in the uterine wall and may result in hemorrhage and the need for hysterectomy. Some common nomenclature relating to different degrees of placenta previa are listed in Table 14-1.

Table 14-1. Placenta Previa

Complete previa: Placental tissue covers the entire internal cervical os

Partial previa: Placental tissue only partially covers the internal cervical os

Marginal previa: Placental tissue is within 2 cm of the internal cervical os

Low-lying placenta: The placental edge is 2-3 cm from the internal cervical os

Risk factors:

- Maternal age > 40
- Multiparity
- Previous uterine curettage
- Previous cesarean delivery
- Smoking
- Male fetus
- Multiple gestation

Cause: A previa occurs when the placenta implants in such a manner that it is either in very close proximity or overlying the cervical os. This may be idiopathic or occur as a result of previous uterine scarring from either a curettage or cesarean section.

Diagnosis: The diagnosis is generally made by ultrasound. While an abdominal ultrasound is quite accurate for making the diagnosis, a gentle transvaginal ultrasound examination is safe and effective and nearly 100% accurate. The important thing to remember is, again, do not perform a digital examination until you are sure that a previa is not present as your fingers may disrupt the placental vessels and precipitate a profuse hemorrhage.

Treatment: The initial treatment is aimed at stabilization of the mother and assessing the fetal status. If there is profuse hemorrhage in conjunction with fetal distress in a viable (i.e., >24 week) fetus, then rapid delivery by cesarean section is warranted. If the patient is more than 34 weeks along, then delivery is generally indicated regardless of the amount of bleeding. If the patient is less than 34 weeks and hemodynamically stable with no evidence of fetal distress, then corticosteroids may be administered and careful monitoring undertaken in an attempt to prolong pregnancy.

In terms of route of delivery, when a significant previa is present, a cesarean section is the only acceptable route of delivery to prevent hemorrhage.

Placental abruption. A placental abruption occurs when the placenta prematurely separates from the uterine wall, usually after 20 weeks gestation and before delivery. As the separation occurs, bleeding occurs and is clinically evident in approximately 80% of cases. This problem accounts for approximately one-third of all cases of antepartum hemorrhage.

Incidence: Placental abruption occurs in approximately 1% of all deliveries in the United States, but is severe enough to cause a stillbirth in only 1:830 deliveries (Gillen-Goldstei 2002; Pritchard 1991; Oyelese 2006). It is also important to note that patients who smoke during pregnancy have an increased risk of severe abruption leading to fetal death.

Clinical Picture: Placental abruption usually presents with vaginal bleeding and strong uterine contractions, uterine tenderness, and fetal distress as evidenced by a nonreassuring fetal heart rate tracing. Because a large of amount of blood can be stored behind the placenta, the amount of hemorrhage seen is not an accurate gauge of actual blood loss. Also, in 20% of patients, the bleeding will be concealed.

Risk factors: While there are multiple risk factors associated with placental abruption, there is not usually a single precipitating event that can be determined in most cases. Some risk factors include:

- **Trauma:** Motor vehicle accidents are the most common cause of blunt abdominal trauma in pregnancy followed by falls and physical abuse. Abuse during pregnancy is unfortunately common and is estimated to occur in 10% of pregnancies (Pearlman 2002). Placental abruption has been reported to occur in 1%-5% of minor trauma cases and 20%-50% of major trauma cases (Pearlman 1991).

- **Chronic hypertension/Preeclampsia:** Patients with chronic hypertension have a fivefold increased risk of placental abruption and treatment with medication to lower blood pressure does not decrease this risk (Sibai 1990).
- **Increased maternal age and parity**
- **Cocaine abuse:** Up to 10% of patients who use cocaine in the third trimester will experience a placental abruption (Hoskins 1991).
- **Preterm premature rupture of membranes (PPROM)**
- **Cigarette smoking:** Not only are these patients at increased risk for abruption, but they tend to have more severe abruptions. The risk of abruption increases by 40% for each pack per day they smoke (Kramer 1997).
- **Thrombophilias:** Patients with thrombophilias, which may include protein C or S deficiency, antithrombin III deficiency, and the factor V Leiden mutation as well as several others, are at increased risk of experiencing placental abruption during pregnancy.
- **Previous abruption:** The risk of recurrence of placental abruption is between 5%-15% (Ananth 1996). This risk is affected by cigarette smoking and can be decreased somewhat if the patient will stop smoking.
- **Multiple gestations**

Diagnosis: The diagnosis is primarily made by clinical suspicion and the presence of vaginal bleeding with contractions and uterine tenderness, but there are certain laboratory and imaging studies that should also be performed.

Physical examination: The maternal examination consists of assessing the patient for other causes of vaginal bleeding (which always begins with an ultrasound) to exclude the possibility of a placenta previa, cervical polyps, or labor as the source of bleeding. It is also important to look for evidence of uterine contractions and tenderness to palpation in the absence of a fever. The patient should be evaluated for evidence of hypovolemic shock and vital signs and urine output monitored closely. A large-bore IV should be started if fluid resuscitation is needed or anticipated. The evaluation of the fetus includes looking at the fetal heart rate tracing for evidence of fetal distress.

Laboratory evaluation: Maternal labs should include a CBC, fibrinogen level, and PT/PTT to evaluate both the patient's hemodynamic stability as well as to look for evidence of disseminated intravascular coagulopathy (DIC).* A fibrinogen of < 200

251

mg/dL and/or a platelet count of < 100,000 are both highly suspicious for an abruption. Fortunately, DIC occurs in a small number of abruptions.

*Note: The Kleihauer-Betke test, D-dimer, and CA-125 have been used in an attempt to make the diagnosis of abruption. They are, however, not of any significant value and do not need to be performed (Gillen-Goldstein 2002).

Ultrasound: It is important to rule out a placenta previa by ultrasound. While it is often possible to see a retroplacental hemorrhage on sonogram, its appearance depends on when the ultrasound is done as the blood at first may appear similar to placental tissue and may not become hypoechoic for nearly a week.

Treatment: The treatment of the patient depends both on the gestational age as well as the extent of the abruption. In a preterm fetus (i.e., < 34 weeks gestation), with a mild abruption and no evidence of fetal distress or maternal instability, conservative management, which includes close monitoring and the administration of corticosteroids, may be attempted. Because these patients tend to have significant uterine contractions, tocolysis may be considered in stable cases. This is best done in consultation with a maternal-fetal medicine specialist.

In the term patient, the fetus should be delivered. A vaginal delivery is preferable in the patient who is stable, but a cesarean delivery is required should there be significant fetal distress, life-threatening hemorrhage, or evidence of DIC. In this case, the patient must receive appropriate fluid resuscitation and blood products, which usually includes packed red blood cells (PRBCs), fresh frozen plasma (FFP), and platelets to prevent further compromise.

Postpartum Hemorrhage (PPH). A postpartum hemorrhage (PPH)is defined as either a 10% decrease in hematocrit between admission and the postpartum time period or the need for a blood transfusion (ACOG 2006). The average blood loss at vaginal delivery and cesarean have been reported as 500 mL and 1,000 mL respectively, but the estimated blood loss (EBL) at delivery is often significantly underestimated, often by as much as 50%, so you have to take into account both the estimated blood loss and the patient's clinical picture. Also, remember that the hematocrit does not drop immediately in response to hemorrhage and will not equilibrate until nearly 12 hours later. So, the bottom line is, treat the patient not the labs. While there are definite risk factors associated with PPH, many such as obesity, placenta previa, placental abruption, etc, cannot be prevented. Because of this it is imperative that you recognize risk factors and are prepared should a PPH occur.

Incidence: The incidence of PPH differs based on the type of delivery. PPH occurs after approximately 4% of vaginal deliveries and around 6% of cesarean deliveries and for women who have had a previous PPH, the risk of recurrence is as high as 10% (Hall 1985; Bonnar 2000).

Clinical Picture: Blood loss may be obvious at either vaginal or cesarean delivery. At times, though, it may be masked by amniotic fluid. As blood loss continues, however, the patient will become tachycardic and then hypotensive. She may also complain of shortness of breath, chest pain, or demonstrate an altered level of consciousness.

Risk Factors: There are multiple risk factors for a patient developing a postpartum hemorrhage. Some of these include the following:

- Previous postpartum hemorrhage
- Multiple pregnancy
- Preeclampsia
- Prolonged second or third stage of labor
- Episiotomy
- Obesity
- Placenta abruption/previa
- Chorioamnionitis
- Birthweight > 4000gms
- Coagulopathy

(Adapted from Bukowski 2001)

Causes: While there are multiple possible etiologies for PPH, the most common causes are uterine atony, retained placental tissue, and lacerations. Because of this, your initial treatment will be directed at ruling these out and treating whatever cause is found.

Prevention: Active management of the third stage of labor, which includes early cord clamping, oxytocin after delivery of the baby, and controlled cord traction, will prevent around 60% of PPH (Bukowski 2001). In addition to this, recognizing possible risk factors for PPH will allow you to have the proper personnel and equipment available should it occur.

Additionally, it is important to monitor for the presence of "audible bleeding." This refers to when you are performing a laceration repair after delivery of the placenta and you hear a steady stream of blood dripping off the drapes and into the either the placenta basin or the pocket of the drape. If you do hear this, then evaluate the patient's vital signs and investigate further. Remember that a woman can lose up to 15% of her blood volume without demonstrating any change in her vital signs (Oyelese 2007).

Treatment: The treatment of PPH should include efforts to both stabilize the mother and correct the underlying cause. The initial steps that should be taken are:

- Call for help (staff/anesthesia)
- IV access/fluid bolus (crystalloid)
- O$_2$ by face mask
- Monitors (Ensure you have someone to check BP/pulse.)
- Determine cause—Think of risk factors
- Check uterine tone
- Manually explore uterus for retained products.
- Examine for lacerations

Treatment by etiology*:

Lacerations: If lacerations are present and the etiology for a postpartum hemorrhage, then repairing them as discussed in Chapter 11 will correct the problem.

Retained placenta: When checking for retained products of conception, perform a manual sweep of the uterus. If you are unsure if you have been able to remove everything you can perform a transabdominal sonogram. If retained products are there they will appear as an echogenic mass and significantly thickened endometrial stripe.

Uterine atony: If the uterus is palpated and noted to have poor tone, or if the patient is continuing to bleed and you have ruled out the other causes listed above, then you should proceed in the following manner:

1. Perform uterine massage with one hand on the maternal abdomen and the other in the vagina, compressing the uterus between the two.
2. Administer medications to correct uterine atony. Which one you give first will depend on the patient's medical conditions. The three most common medications for this are the following:

   - Methergine
   - Hemabate
   - Cytotech

(See Table 14-2 for doses and contraindications.)

3. Continue to monitor the patient's vital signs and blood loss and consider either an intrauterine balloon for tamponade or even uterine packing. This may be done with either a Bakri balloon, which is made and marketed specifically for postpartum hemorrhage, or a Sengstaken-Blakemore tube, with the stomach end cut off and inserted into the uterine cavity and then inflated with between 150 mL to 250 mL of saline. If this stops the bleeding, then the device is left in place for approximately 24 hours and the patient monitored.

4. If the patient continues to bleed and is unstable, then you may need to move to the operating room and consider surgical interventions. When you make the decision to go to the operating room, you should notify the following people:

   o Anesthesia
   o Nursing personnel
   o OR scrub tech

   When you have made the decision to go to the OR, make sure and counsel the patient and family about the need for surgical intervention and your plans.

* (A comprehensive discussion of the surgical treatment of postpartum hemorrhage, or hemorrhage during a cesarean section can be found in Chapter 10: Cesarean Section.)

Table 14-2. Medications / Dosage for Postpartum Hemorrahge

MEDICATION	DOSE	CONTRAINDICATIONS
Methylergonovine (Methergine)	0.2 mg IM OR into myometrium Q2-4 hours	Hypertension, preeclampsia, asthma, Raynaud's syndrome
Prostaglandin F-2alpha (Hemabate)	250 mcg IM OR into myometrium Q15 minutes (up to 8 doses)	Asthma, renal disorders, pulmonary hypertension
Misoprostol (Cytotech, PGE-1)	600 mcg-1,000 mcg per rectum x 1 dose	Known hypersensitivity to NSAIDs, active GI bleeding

* See figure 14-2 for a complete treatment algorithm for postpartum hemorrhage.

After managing a patient for a postpartum hemorrhage, it is often helpful to place a foley catheter to monitor urine output. A follow-up CBC is usually drawn 12 hours later as well.

FIGURE 14-2. Treatment algorithm for postpartum hemorrhage (PPH)

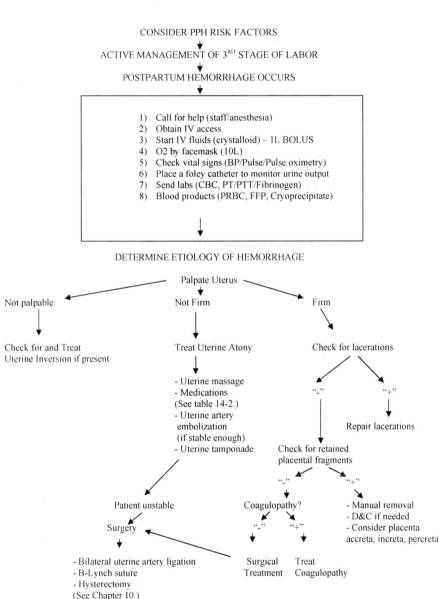

Use of blood products. The use of blood products in patients who experience a significant postpartum hemorrhage can be life-saving. Patients who refuse blood transfusions, such as Jehovah's witnesses, are at increased risk for maternal mortality from postpartum hemorrhage, with one study reporting a 44-fold increase in the risk of death from hemorrhage in this population (Singla 2002). However, because a transfusion

257

involves some risk to the patient in terms of viral infection and transfusion reactions, treatment should be carefully considered and the appropriate products ordered. The most commonly used blood products on labor and delivery include packed red blood cells (PRBC), platelets, fresh-frozen plasma (FFP), and cryoprecipitate.

Packed red blood cells (PRBCs). Most patients who suffer a significant hemorrhage will first receive a transfusion of PRBCs. They are indicated when a patient is hemodynamically unstable due to hemorrhage, especially if the hemoglobin level falls to less than 8 or 9 gm/dL (Strong 1997). While red blood cells are critical to transport oxygen to tissues in the body, care must be taken to monitor the patient for pulmonary edema when multiple transfusions are required. In general, you can expect the patient's hemoglobin and hematocrit to increase by 1 gm/dL and 3% per unit transfused.

Platelets. Platelets should be transfused when there is evidence of hemorrhage as a result of either thrombocytopenia or platelet dysfunction. It may also be given in the face of massive transfusion of PRBC's and abnormal bleeding as a dilutional thrombocytopenia can occur in this situation. While a patient is considered thrombocytopenic if their platelet count falls below 100,000/mm^3, there is generally no problem with surgery (i.e., cesarean section) as long as the level does not fall to below 50,000/mm^3. When a patient has a platelet count of less than 20,000/mm^3, then they should be prophylactically transfused to prevent spontaneous bleeding. A single unit of platelets will increase the patient's platelet count by approximately 7500/mm^3.

Fresh-frozen plasma (FFP). This is extracted from whole blood and contains both significant amounts of fibrinogen as well as multiple clotting factors. This is given when disseminated intravascular coagulation (DIC), vitamin K deficiency, or clotting factor deficiencies related to liver disease (and therefore vitamin K dependent clotting factors) are present. It can be expected to increase the patient's fibrinogen level by 10-15 mg/dL per unit transfused. The goal of treatment with FFP in the presence of DIC or hypofibrinogenemia is a fibrinogen level of at least 100 mg/dL.

It is important to think ahead when you encounter a significant postpartum hemorrhage as it takes at least 30 minutes for this blood product to be thawed and made available in most blood banks.

(Of note, this is the only blood product with clotting factors V, XI, and XII.)

Cryoprecipitate (Cryo). This blood product is a fraction of FFP that is rich in factors VII, XIII and fibrinogen, as well as von Willebrand's factor. Because of the small amount of volume of each unit as compared to FFP (40 mL vs. 250 mL) it is a more efficient way to raise the patient's fibrinogen level. (This may be important in a patient with DIC with pulmonary edema secondary to fluid overload from multiple transfusions of PRBCs where you need to increase the fibrinogen level, but need to give as little additional volume as possible.) One unit of cryoprecipitate will increase the patient's fibrinogen level by 10-15 mg/dL. In general, cryoprecipitate is given specifically for the treatment of von Willebrand's disease, factor VII deficiency, or hypofibrinogenemia.

See table 14-3 for a comparison of all the different blood products.

Table 14-3. Blood products

Blood product	Contains	Indications	Volume (mL)	Effect
Packed red blood cells	Red cells, some plasma	Increase red cell volume	300	Increase Hct 3%/unit Increase Hgb 1 gm/unit
Platelets	Platelets, some plasma, few RBC/WBC	Hemorrhage from thrombocytopenia	50	Increase platelet count by 7,500 mm³/unit
Fresh frozen plasma	Plasma, clotting factors	Treatment of coagulation disorders	250	Increase total fibrinogen 10-15 mg/dL/unit
Cryoprecipitate	Fibrinogen, factors V, VIII, XIII, von Willebrand's factor	Hemophilia A, von Willebrand's disease, hypofibrinogenemia	40	Increase total fibrinogen 10-15 mg/dL/unit

Complications of Blood Transfusions. While the transfusion of blood products is often lifesaving in obstetrics, there are risks involved and these are important to discuss with patients when they are required.

Adverse reactions. Adverse reactions that may occur with the transfusion of blood products generally either involve acute reactions or transmission of infectious agents to the recipient.

Acute hemolytic transfusion reaction. This is most commonly a result of a clerical error resulting in the transfusion of incompatible blood products. It usually presents with a fever, which may be accompanied by nausea, emesis, dypsnea, back pain, and discomfort at the infusion site. It may progress to shock, disseminated intravascular coagulation (DIC), or acute renal failure. The incidence of this type of reaction is, however, only 1:25,000. The risk of a fatal acute hemolytic reaction is much less at 1:600,000. If there is any suspicion of a hemolytic reaction, then the transfusion should be stopped and the blood product returned to the blood bank with a description of the possible reaction. Supportive care of the patient is indicated as well.

Febrile non-hemolytic transfusion reaction. This type of reaction occurs in approximately 1:10,000 transfusions. When this occurs, the patient will generally experience a headache, shaking chills, or a fever within an hour of the transfusion beginning. If this occurs, then the transfusion should be stopped and the blood product sent back to the laboratory for testing. A hemolytic reaction should be ruled out by demonstrating no evidence of hemolysis (i.e., absence of hemoglobinemia, hemoglobinuria, and a negative direct antiglobulin test). Patients should receive acetaminophen for the fever and given supportive care.

Anaphylactic reaction. Anaphylactic reactions, which are characterized by urticaria, angioedema, dypsnea, nausea or abdominal cramping, and even shock, occur approximately 1:150,000 units of blood transfused. When this occurs, you should again, stop the infusion and send the products to the laboratory. Treatment of the patient involves stabilizing the airway and administering antihistamines and epinephrine as needed.

Infections. Although all blood products are screened prior to administration to patients, the possibility of acquiring an infection, usually viral, still exists. Current estimates of these risks can be found in table 14-4.

Table 14-4. **Incidence of viral infection after transfusion (per unit infused)**

INFECTION	RISK
Hepatitis B	1:63,000-1:233,000
Hepatitis C	1:120,000
HIV 1-2	1:676,000
HTLV	1:640,000

* (Modified from Menitove 2000)

Magnesium Toxicity

Magnesium sulfate is used routinely on labor and delivery for both seizure prophylaxis in patients with preeclampsia and in an attempt to stop preterm labor.

Incidence: Serious side effects occur in between 2%-5% of patients treated with magnesium sulfate during pregnancy although this number appears to be higher in multiple gestations (Elliot 1997).

Clinical Picture: In order to detect a patient who is toxic from magnesium sulfate, it is important to know what are normal side effects from the medication. Some common side effects include:

- Nausea/emesis
- Headache
- Dry mouth
- Intense flushing
- Drowsiness
- Blurred vision
- Decreased FHR variability

Clinical signs and symptoms that are indicative of potential magnesium toxicity include the following:

- Absent deep tendon reflexes (DTRs)
- New onset hypotension
- Pulmonary edema
- Respiratory depression

Serum magnesium levels at which different complications may occur include:

- EKG changes 5-10 mEq/L
- Decreased DTRs 10 mEq/L
- Respiratory depression 15 mEq/L
- Cardiovascular collapse >25 mEq/L

Risk factors: Some conditions that may place a patient at increased risk for magnesium toxicity include:

- Multiple gestations
- Renal insufficiency
- Concurrent use of calcium-channel blockers

Treatment: 1 gram (10 mL of 10% solution) of calcium gluconate IV given over 3 minutes will reverse the effects of magnesium sulfate. Additional treatment should include:

- Stop magnesium infusion
- Administer supplemental oxygen and continuously monitor mother with pulseoximetry
  (Intubation if necessary for respiratory failure)
- Administer diuretics (Furosemide 20-40 mg IV) as needed for pulmonary edema

Prevention: In order to prevent a patient from going from therapeutic on magnesium sulfate to the toxic range, they should be closely monitored according to the following protocol:

- Continuous pulse oximetry
- Monitor urine output Q hour (This is important as magnesium is excreted almost exclusively through the kidneys and a decrease in urine output can result in significantly increased serum levels.)
- Check DTR's Q hour
- Monitor IVF given and do not run at higher than a maintenance (usually around 125 cc/hour total) dose
- If the patient demonstrated any evidence of possible magnesium toxicity (as previously discussed) obtain a serum magnesium level STAT

NOTE: If a patient has experienced significant side effects from magnesium sulfate, it is best to use a different tocolytic should the patient require one in the future.

More information on contraindications to magnesium sulfate therapy can be found in the Medication Database.

Malpresentation

Breech Presentation. A breech presentation occurs when either the fetal buttocks or lower extremities are the presenting part or parts rather than the head. While there are different types of breech presentations (for example, a frank breech is where the buttocks is the presenting part and the legs are extended at the knees with the feet up by the fetal head, and a footling breech is where the feet are the presenting parts) the management of them is very similar as vaginal breech deliveries are not recommended.

Incidence: At term, approximately 3%-4% of all fetuses will be in some form of breech presentation (Hikock 1992).

Clinical Picture: A breech presentation is usually first suspected either during Leopold's maneuvers or at the time of cervical examination. Whenever it is suspected, an ultrasound if performed to confirm the fetal position.

Risk factors: There are multiple risk factors for a breech presentation. Most of them are related to either too much or too little room for the fetus to move around in. Some of these include:

- Uterine abnormalities (bicornuate or uterine septum)
- Placenta previa
- Multiparity
- Polyhydramnios
- Fetal anomalies (hydrocephaly)
- Multiple gestation
- Neurologic impairment (anencephaly)
- Large fibroids
- Short umbilical cord
- Prematurity (at 32 weeks, up to 16% of fetuses are breech (Scheer 1976))

Treatment: In general, breech presentations are delivered by cesarean section, especially if they present with ruptured membranes or in labor. Depending on the clinical scenario, an external cephalic version (ECV), which is usually performed around 36 weeks and attempts to turn the fetus to the vertex position through external manipulation, may be offered. If the patient declines this intervention, or the ECV is unsuccessful, then a cesarean section is recommended as this is associated with a significant reduction in perinatal and neonatal death (Hofmeyr 2001).

If a vaginal delivery is imminent, make preparations for a standard vaginal delivery, but add Piper forceps to the delivery tray, call for additional staff and a pediatrician, and make sure the patient has adequate anesthesia if possible.

As the mother pushes, the infant's buttocks will present at the introitus. No assistance should be given to the infant at this point (i.e., avoid the urge to grasp the trunk and pull!). Allow the mother to push and deliver the buttocks and, if the legs are flexed, the lower limbs as well. If the legs are extended, then flex each leg at the knee and move it laterally to deliver each foot. (Figure 14-3a)

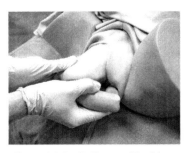

Figure 14-3a Delivery of fetal legs

At this point, wrap the infant's body in a sterile towel and continue to have her push while applying gentle downward traction with your thumbs on the fetal sacrum and fingers in the groin (figure 14-3b). When the infant has delivered to the level of the scapula, the shoulders should be rotated to the anterior-posterior plane and the arms/shoulders delivered individually. If they do not come spontaneously, then placing a finger over the shoulder into the antecubital fossa and sweeping it across the body will allow delivery (figure 14-3c).

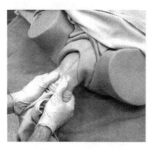 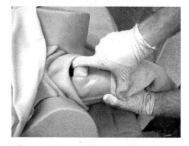

Figure 14-3b Hands on bones and groins   Figure 14-3c Delivery of fetal arms

After the shoulders are delivered, the fetal head is delivered either by the placement of Piper forceps or with a Mauriceau-Smellie-Veit (MSV) maneuver with care to make sure to avoid hyperextension of the infant's cervical spine (figure 14-3d). The MSV maneuver includes hooking fingers over the fetal neck with one hand and placing the fingers of the other hand on the fetal maxilla while an assistant provides suprapubic pressure with all of this done to ensure the fetal head remains flexed during the delivery. An episiotomy may be helpful in this situation to provide more room posteriorly.

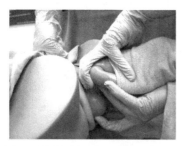 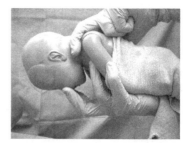

Figure 14-3d Mauriceau-Smellie-Veit   Figure 14-3e Mauriceau-Smellie-Veit
            maneuver   demonstration

Transverse Lie. A transverse lie occurs when the fetal spine is perpendicular to the mother's spine and may be referred to as either a "back-up" or "back-down" transverse lie depending on the orientation. It is often suspected by visual inspection of the maternal abdomen when the uterus appears unusually wide.

Incidence: A transverse lie is an uncommon finding in singleton pregnancies, but it is encountered often in twin gestations with the second twin.

Clinical Picture: This abnormal presentation in singletons is usually first suspected at the time of Leopold's maneuvers or cervical examination although the appearance of the maternal abdomen or an abnormally small fundal height measurement may also raise suspicions.

Risk factors:

- Uterine abnormalities
- Large myomas
- Polyhydramnios
- Placenta previa
- Preterm fetus
- Multiple gestation

Treatment: Similar to a breech presentation, an external cephalic version (ECV) may be offered to these patients who have intact membranes and are not in active labor. (See Chapter 2 for a description of an ECV.) If they present in early labor, an ECV may be attempted at this time as well. If the patient declines or the ECV is not successful, then a cesarean section is performed as the fetus cannot deliver vaginally in this position. (Refer to the section of Chapter 10: Cesarean section that deals with uterine incisions and a transverse fetal lie.) These fetuses are at increased risk of complications if they go into labor or rupture membranes as the risk of umbilical cord prolapse is significantly increased.

Oligohydramnios

This term refers to a significantly decreased amount of amniotic fluid around the fetus. It is not an uncommon occurrence on labor and delivery, and will often lead to further testing or other interventions. The most common definition of oligohydramnios is an amniotic fluid index (AFI—See Chapter 2) of less than 5.

Incidence: Oligohydramnios occurs in between 0.5%-8% of pregnancies depending on the gestational age and actual definition used (Ahanya 2003).

Clinical Picture: Laboring patients who have oligohydramnios are more likely to have fetal heart rate abnormalities requiring cesarean section, which includes variable decelerations from cord compression, than patients with a normal amount of amniotic fluid.

265

In the preterm fetus, long-standing oligohydramnios may result in muscle contractures, lung hypoplasia, and even skeletal deformations. These severe problems, however, are usually seen only when the process begins in the second trimester.

Causes: In the third trimester, the most common causes of oligohydramnios are:

- Rupture of membranes (Term or Preterm)
- Uteroplacental insufficiency (due to preeclampsia or chronic hypertension)
- Idiopathic

Treatment: The treatment of a patient with oligohydramnios depends on the gestational age of the patient.

Preterm (<37 weeks): After ensuring that PPROM has not occurred, these patients should undergo antepartum testing including an NST, AFI, and BPP once or twice weekly to ensure that there is no evidence of fetal compromise. If there is evidence of fetal distress, then further testing or delivery is indicated. The patient is usually delivered once they reach term.

Term: When a term patient is diagnosed with oligohydramnios, they are usually delivered. If the patient is not already in labor, then an induction is started. During labor, you should pay attention to the FHRT and monitor for variable decelerations as an amnioinfusion can be helpful should they occur. Alternatively, if the patient has a low-normal AFI (5-8) then oral hydration with water can increase placental blood flow and the AFI (Hofmeyr 2000).

Preeclampsia

This is an unfortunately common occurrence in obstetrics that is characterized by the development of hypertension, edema, and proteinuria after 20 weeks gestation. It can be either mild or severe and may be complicated by generalized seizures (eclampsia).

Incidence: 5%-10% of pregnancies (Mattar 1999).

Clinical Picture: These patients present after 20 weeks gestation with elevated blood pressures, edema, and proteinuria (at least 300 mg in a 24-hour specimen or $\geq 1+$ urine dipstick). While many patients will have all three components (hypertension, edema, and proteinuria), some will only demonstrate hypertension and proteinuria. While it is rare for patients with preeclampsia not to demonstrate some degree of proteinuria, it is possible and patients with new onset hypertension and edema should be evaluated with additional laboratory testing.

Preeclampsia is generally classified as either mild or severe. This is important in terms of management, especially in the preterm fetus. The features of mild and severe disease are listed below:

Mild

- BP ≥ 140/90 mm Hg (2 readings at least 6 hours apart)*
- Edema (feet, hands, and facial)
- > 300mg protein (24hr urine collection) or dipstick 1+

Severe

- BP ≥ 160/110 mm Hg (2 readings at least 6 hours apart)
- Headache
- Right upper quadrant pain
- Visual disturbances (scotomata)
- Convulsions (eclampsia)
- Pulmonary edema
- Fetal growth restriction
- > 5 grams protein (24hr urine collection)

There is often controversy in exactly how the blood pressure should be taken, i.e., upright versus lying on the left side. The most recent recommendations from ACOG recommend that it may be taken in either the sitting or left lateral recumbent position with the arm at the level of the heart (ACOG 2002a). The blood pressure cuff should be the appropriate size (the bladder of the cuff should encompass at least 80% of the arm), and the patient should not use tobacco or caffeine for at least a half hour prior to the measurements.

* Note: The diagnosis is made more difficult in a patient with chronic hypertension as they will already meet the blood pressure criteria for diagnosis. Also, if a patient has a single elevated blood pressure when you begin their evaluation, you must consider this in the differential and rule it out, especially if they have any severe symptoms.

Laboratory abnormalities with preeclampsia:

	Mild Preeclampsia	*Severe Preeclampsia*
Blood pressure:	≥ 140/90 mm Hg	≥ 160/110 mm Hg
Proteinuria (dipstick)	≥ 1+	≥ 2+
Proteinuria (24 hr)	≥ 300 mg	≥ 5 grams
Uric acid	> 6 mg/dL	
Platelets	Normal	< 100,000 mm^3
AST and ALT	Normal	> 40 IU/L and/or > 40 IU/L
LDH	Normal	> 600 IU/L
Serum creatinine	Normal or slightly elevated (1.0-1.5)	Significantly elevated (>1.5)

Note: An additional screening test that can be used to determine if there is proteinuria present is the urine protein/creatinine ratio. This is most valuable for its negative predictive value as ratio of < 0.19 essentially excludes significant proteinuria (i.e., 300 mg or greater). A description of how to calculate and use this ratio can be found in figure 14-4.

Figure 14-4. Urine protein/creatinine ratio

- **Send a single urine sample (at least 200 cc if possible) for a spot urine protein and spot urine creatinine.***

    * The timing of the specimen, i.e., morning or afternoon, does not matter.

- **Calculate the ratio****

$$\frac{\text{Urine spot protein (mg/dL)}}{\text{Urine spot creatinine (mg/dl)}} = \text{Urine protein/creatinine ratio}$$

    ** Make sure and check the units that your lab reports the results in as you may have to convert them to match.

- **Interpret the results:**

    o A ratio of less than or equal to 0.19 indicates less than 300 mg of protein in a 24-hour period (Negative predictive value 95%-97%; Al 2005; Rodriguez-Thompson 2001).

The correlation between the ratio and significant proteinuria is reportedly poor in the current literature, so any value of 0.20 or greater should be followed with a 24-hr urine protein collection.

Risk factors:

Nulliparity
Family history of preeclampsia
History of preeclampsia
Smoking
Diabetes mellitus
Multiple gestations
Chronic hypertension
Obesity
Low socioeconomic status
Advanced maternal age (> 35 years old)
African-American race

Causes: The cause of this disease is unknown.

Treatment: The only treatment for preeclampsia, mild or severe, is delivery. When the decision to deliver is made, the patient is given magnesium sulfate for seizure prophylaxis. The patient is given a loading dose of 6 grams which is followed by a continuous infusion of 2 grams per hour (Alexander 2006).

After delivery, the disease process resolves. The decision to deliver a patient, however, is dependent on both the severity of the disease as well as the gestational age of the patient. For both mild and severe disease, after delivery, the patient is continued on magnesium sulfate. While the magnesium is usually continued for 24 hours postpartum, recently, there is some evidence that the duration of treatment may be determined by the clinical status of the patient, with patients who demonstrate a brisk diuresis, no severe hypertension, and no severe neurologic symptoms, such as a headache, being able to discontinue the magnesium treatment at 12 hours (Isler 2003). See figure 14-5 for a treatment algorithm to determine if a patient's magnesium sulfate treatment may be discontinued before 24 hours (Ascarelli 1998; Ehrenberg 2006; Fontenot 2005).

Figure 14-5. Discontinuation of postpartum magnesium sulfate prophylaxis for preeclampsia.

Begin/Continue Magnesium Sulfate Seizure Prophylaxis After Delivery

↓

May discontinue at 12 hours if the patient meets the following criteria:

- No persistent headache or visual changes
- No epigastric pain
- No severe hypertension (>160/110)
- At least half of BP's are less than 150/100
- No indication for antihypertensives for at least 2 hours
- Spontaneous diuresis of > 100 mL/hour for at least 2 consecutive hours

↓

Restart magnesium sulfate therapy if any of the following occur:*

- Sustained BP's of >160/110 for at least 2 hours
- Severe headache or visual changes

* If therapy is restarted, it should be continued for a full 24 hours

Mild Disease. The treatment of preeclampsia after 34 weeks gestation may be to deliver the patient, however, conservative management and close monitoring are usually undertaken in cases of mild preeclampsia. If there is any evidence of progression to severe disease, however, then delivery is indicated. It is important to note that preeclampsia is not an indication by itself for cesarean section and that a cesarean should only be performed for obstetric indications.* (See Chapter 10.) Anytime after 37 weeks, delivery may be undertaken, and should be accomplished by 39 weeks. When the decision to deliver is made, the patient should be placed on magnesium sulfate for prophylaxis against seizures according to one of the protocols listed in table 14-6.

Table 14-6. Antiseizure treatment for preeclampsia and eclampsia

PREECLAMSIA

Continuous IV infusion

- 6 gm loading dose diluted in 100 mL of IV fluid over 15-20 minutes
- 2 gm/hr in 100 mL for maintenance infusion
- Continue magnesium during labor and until 24 hours after delivery

Intermittent IM injections

- Give 10 gm of a 50% magnesium sulfate solution with 5 gm into each buttock
- Follow this with 5 gm of a 50% solution of magnesium sulfate IM every 4 hours
- Continue magnesium during labor and until 24 hours after delivery

Severe Disease. When a patient has severe disease and they are at least 34 weeks along, then delivery is indicated. If this occurs prior to 34 weeks, then consideration can be given to conservative management, which includes inpatient monitoring and the administration of corticosteroids. Consultation with a maternal-fetal medicine specialist is recommended in these cases.

* When patients have severe preeclampsia and delivery is indicated, the general rule is to try and have the patient delivered within 24 hours. Because of this, if the patient is preterm, especially less than 34 weeks, and she has an unfavorable cervix, then a cesarean section may be performed.

Eclampsia

Eclampsia is characterized by generalized tonic-clonic seizures which are not attributable to other medical or neurologic problems.

Incidence: Approximately 1:3,250 deliveries in the United States (Ventura 1998). It is the second-most common cause of maternal death in the United States and accounts for 15% of all maternal deaths here in the states and up to 50,000 maternal deaths worldwide every year (Rochat 1988; Duley 1992). After a woman has experienced an eclamptic seizure, she is at increased risk with subsequent pregnancies for several complications. Some of these include the following:

- Mild preeclampsia (13%)
- Severe preeclampsia (9%)
- Eclampsia (2%)
- Placental abruption (2.5%-6.5%)
- Preterm delivery (15%-21%)
- Intrauterine growth restriction (12%-23%)
- Perinatal mortality (4.6%-16.5%)

(Chesley 1976; Sibai 1986; Sibai 1991; Sibai 1992)

Note: These risks may be even higher in patients who experience preeclampsia/eclampsia remote from term, i.e., < 28-30 weeks gestation.

Clinical Picture: The seizures are generally self-limited and rarely last longer than 4 minutes. It is common to have significant fetal heart rate decelerations during a seizure, but these almost always resolve soon after the seizure ends.

Risk factors: Patients with preeclampsia are at risk for developing eclampsia. Actual eclamptic seizures are more common in patients who are nonwhite, nulliparous, less than 20 or greater than 35 years-old, or from lower socioeconomic backgrounds (Norwitz 2002).

Causes: The exact cause of eclampsia is not known, but some theories implicate cerebral vasospasm and hypertensive encephalopathy.

Treatment: The treatment of eclampsia is to stabilize the patient and stop the seizures, which will result in resuscitation of the fetus.

- **Call for assistance:** This should include nursing staff, an anesthesiologist, and additional obstetricians.
- **Protect the airway:** Roll patient to left side, place padded tongue blade in mouth if possible, but do not force this in as you do not want to cause the patient to gag when they regain consciousness.
- **Control seizures:** This begins with the administration of medication to stop the seizures. The most common medication for this is magnesium sulfate. Doses for this include:

   Magnesium sulfate

   - 6 grams in 100 mL crystalloid over 15-20 minutes followed by 2 gm/hr as a continuous infusion
   - Or, if unable to obtain IV access
     10 gm of a 50% magnesium sulfate solution with 5 gm into each buttock

- **Treat severe hypertension (i.e., >160/110):** This is also accomplished with medications including:

   Hydralazine

   - 5 mg IV push then 5-10 mg Q20 minutes as needed

   Labetalol

   - 10-20 mg IV then double every 10 minutes as needed up to 80 mg doses with a total cumulative dose of 220 mg

- **Continue seizure prophylaxis:** The recurrence risk of an eclamptic seizure is approximately 10% if the patient does not receive seizure prophylaxis (Pritchard 1984). Because of this, after the eclamptic seizure has resolved, all patients should receive magnesium sulfate seizure prophylaxis for at least 24 hours. This regimen has been demonstrated to be superior to the use of phenytoin (Duley 2001).
- **Consider delivery:** The definitive treatment of the disease is delivery, but this does not necessarily mean a cesarean section is indicated. In general, induction of labor is reasonable, but factors such as a very unfavorable cervix and the fetal status must be taken into consideration. Some studies suggest that less than one-third of women with either severe preeclampsia or eclampsia <32 weeks gestation with an unfavorable cervix will deliver vaginally (Norwitz 2002). In these women, a cesarean section may be indicated as a long induction, often defined as > 24 hours, is not recommended.
- **Monitor patients for development of complications:** Complications occur in up to 70% of women who experience eclamptic seizures. These may include disseminated intravascular coagulopathy with resulting hemorrhage, acute renal failure, pulmonary edema, intracerebral hemorrhage, cardiac arrest, liver rupture, and transient blindness (Lopez-Llera 1992).

Prognosis: Maternal mortality rates of 0% to nearly 14% have been reported, with perinatal mortality ranging from 9% to 23% although an even higher rate (93%) was reported in one series of eclampsia occurring prior to 28 weeks gestation (Norwitz 2002; Lopez-Llera 1992). The risk of recurrence of eclampsia in subsequent pregnancies is approximately 2%.

Preterm labor

Preterm labor refers to cervical change with regular uterine contractions prior to 37 weeks gestation. It is a leading cause of neonatal morbidity and mortality and accounts for between 60%-80% of deaths among infants without congenital anomalies (Goldenberg 2002). Although this is a very common problem, accounting for 40%-50% of all preterm deliveries, the approaches to its management vary widely although there is some general agreement on the basic treatment (Tucker 1991).

Incidence: The preterm delivery rate in the United States is approximately 11% and spontaneous preterm labor is responsible for more than half of all preterm births (Goldenberg 2002).

Clinical Picture: Patients with preterm labor will often present with abdominal cramping, which they may or may not identify as being a result of uterine contractions. Other possible presenting complaints may include back pain, vaginal spotting or bleeding, pelvic pressure, or increased vaginal discharge. Because the presenting complaints are not always specific, you must maintain a reasonably high index of suspicion.

Risk factors/Causes: There are multiple risk factors for preterm labor. Some of these include:

- **African American race:** African American women have a preterm delivery rate of up to 18% versus 9% for Caucasian women (Goldenberg 2002).
- **Age:** Women who are younger than 17 or older than 35 are at increased risk of preterm delivery.
- **Tobacco use:** Women who smoke during pregnancy have a 20%-30% increase in the risk of preterm delivery (Shiono 1986).
- **Previous preterm delivery:** This increases the risk of subsequent preterm delivery approximately 2.5-fold (Mercer 1999).
- **Multiple gestation:** This accounts for 13% of all births less then 37 weeks gestation and approximately 55% of twin gestations deliver preterm (Robinson 2003; Iams 2003).
- **Infection:** Several different infections, such as Neisseria gonorrhea, Chlamydia trachomatis, Group B streptococci, and Ureaplasma urealyticum, have been associated with preterm delivery.
- **Uterine malformations:** Anomalies such as a unicornuate or bicornuate uterus increase the risk of preterm delivery.
- **Low socioeconomic status:** This has been associated with preterm delivery although there are often other associated risk factors.
- **Periodontal disease:** The risk of preterm delivery has been reported to increase with worsening periodontal disease, with a risk of up to 11% for patients with severe disease (Offenbacher 2001).

Workup and Evaluation: Whenever a patient calls with complaints that may be related to preterm labor, she should be told to come to labor and delivery for evaluation. When she arrives she should be placed on the monitor to both check the fetal heart tracing as well as to watch for contractions. She should be questioned about the following:

- When the symptoms began

- Bleeding
- Rupture of membranes
- History or presence of any risk factors for preterm labor (as above)

After the history has been taken, an examination and tests should be performed and include the following:

- Speculum examination with collection of the following:

  - Vaginal cultures for Gonorrhea, Chlamydia
  - Wet prep for bacterial vaginosis
  - Fetal fibronectin swab
  - Rectovaginal swab for GBS

- Digital examination of the cervix
- Ultrasound examination of the cervical length if the cervix is not dilated
- Send a urine specimen and culture

Treatment: The treatment of preterm labor depends on the presence or absence of contractions as well as the condition of the cervix. If any evidence of infection is found during the initial examination, for example, bacterial vaginosis, vaginal candidiasis, or a urinary tract infection, then these should be treated.

A general treatment algorithm for preterm labor can be found in Figure 14-7. This algorithm combines the Ohio State University Protocol as well as a study by Guinn et al that incorporated the use of subcutaneous terbutaline during the evaluation of preterm labor patients (Iams 2003; Guinn 1997).

The most important interventions for preterm labor that have been shown to decrease perinatal morbidity and mortality are:

1. Transfer of the preterm labor patient to an institution with a neonatal intensive care unit.
2. Administration of glucocorticoids to the mother.
3. Treatment with antibiotics for group B beta-hemolytic streptococcus.

(Iams 2003)

If the patient is found to be in preterm labor, then tocolysis is undertaken, most often with magnesium sulfate or nifedipine and a course of glucocorticoids, either dexamethasone or betamethasone, is started, and antibiotics, usually penicillin G or ampicillin, is started until the results of the GBS culture are available.* A list of common medications as well as dosages and specific indications that may be used for tocolysis can be found in Table 14-6.

Table 14-6. Medications for tocolysis

Medication	Dose	Mechanism of Action	Contraindications	Side Effects
Magnesium Sulfate	4-6 gram IV bolus followed by 2-4gm/hr	Decreases neuromuscular conduction and inhibits uterine contractions	Myasthenia gravis Cardiac conduction abnormalities Renal failure	Diaphoresis, flushing, nausea, vomiting, pulmonary edema
Terbutaline	0.125-0.25mg (intermittent SQ/IV dosing) Q3-4 hours 5-10 mcg/min (continuous IV) 2.5-5.0mg (PO) Q4-6hrs	beta-adrenergic receptor agonist	Cardiac disease Hyperthyroidism	Tachycardia, palpitations, pulmonary edema, tremors
Nifedipine	10-20mg PO Q4-6 hrs	Calcium channel blocker	Magnesium sulfate Congestive heart failure	Hypotension, nausea, flushing, dizziness, headache
Indomethacin	50mg loading dose Followed by 25mg Q6hrs for 48-72 hours	Prostaglandin synthase inhibitor	Bleeding disorders Liver disease Gastric ulcer Asthma, renal dysfunction	Nausea, gastritis esophageal reflux, emesis

*   (The antibiotics should be discontinued if the GBS culture is negative and this is the only reason for the antibiotics being given.)

The reason for beginning tocolysis is that these medications have been shown to be able to prolong pregnancy for between 2-7 days, which allows for a full course of glucocorticoids to be administered to the patient (Berkman 2000). It is important to remember, however, that there is no consensus on exactly when to begin tocolysis and that no evidence based guidelines exist for making this decision (Simhan 2002). The most common medications utilized are magnesium sulfate, beta-adrenergic receptor agonists (ritodrine and terbutaline), calcium channel blockers (nifedipine), and cyclooxygenase or prostaglandin synthase inhibitors such as indomethacin.

The most common first line choices for tocolysis are magnesium sulfate, terbutaline, or nifedipine, with nifedipine becoming the first choice at many institutions. Each of these is given by itself and the contraction pattern is monitored. If there is no significant response, then indomethacin is sometimes added for 48 hours if the patient is at less than 32 weeks gestation. If the patient progresses and enters active labor, then tocolysis is generally discontinued and preparations are made for delivery. If the patient responds to the medication, then it is usually continued for 24-48 hours as long as the uterine contractions do not persist. (These medications, including common doses, indications, contraindications, and maternal and fetal side effects can be found in the medication database.)

The purpose of the glucocorticoids is that they have been shown to promote fetal lung maturity and decrease the risk of severe respiratory distress after delivery.

The important thing to remember about preterm labor is that there is significant variation in how physicians approach and treat these patients. The recommendations in the treatment algorithm are based on the current literature and the fact that preterm delivery before 34-35 weeks is very unlikely (only 1%-3%) in women evaluated for preterm labor who have intact membranes, cervical dilation of less than 3 cm, a cervical length of >30mm, and within 14 days of a negative fetal fibronectin (Iams 2003). What has been presented here is the current evidence about potential interventions and there will definitely be more to follow in the future.

Figure 14-7. Treatment algorithm for preterm labor

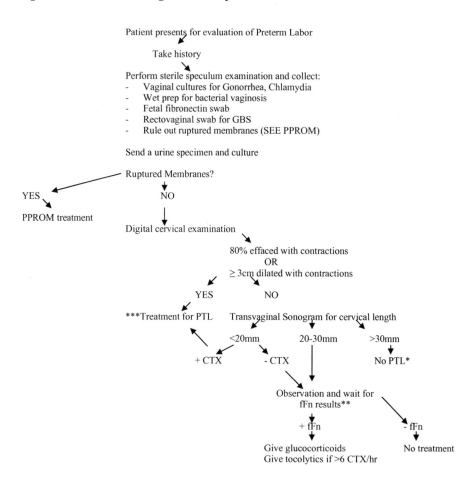

* If the cervical examination and TV sonogram are equivocal (i.e., cervix is dilated 2 cm and/or the cervical length is 20-30 mm) or give conflicting results (i.e. the patient is <3 cm but has demonstrated cervical change from a previous examination but the cervical length is > 30 mm) then the patient should be observed as well and the fFn results used to determine treatment. Also, in the presence of > 4 contractions/hour, a dose of subcutaneous terbutaline may be given to see if this will stop the contractions.

** If the patient's contractions become stronger or she demonstrates cervical change during observation, she is treated for preterm labor.

*** See table 14-6 for a list of medications commonly used for tocolysis

(Adapted from Iams 2003 and Guinn 1997)

Preterm Premature Rupture of Membranes (PPROM)

PPROM is defined as the rupture of the amniotic sac prior to 37 weeks gestation. This is an important complication to recognize as the accurate diagnosis will allow you to treat the mother with antibiotics and possibly corticosteroids to improve the outcome for both the mother and baby.

Incidence: PPROM complicates approximately 3% of all pregnancies and is responsible for nearly one-third of all preterm (<37 weeks) deliveries (Mercer 2003).

Clinical Picture: Patients presenting with PPROM generally present with the same complaints as term patients present with spontaneous rupture of membranes (SROM). They complain of either a large gush of fluid or a continuous leakage of fluid from the vagina. (See Chapter 4: Rule Out Ruptured Membranes.)

Risk factors: There are many risk factors associated with PPROM. Some of these include the following:

- Smoking during pregnancy
- Previous preterm delivery
- Low body mass index (BMI < 19)
- Multiple gestation
- Polyhydramnios
- Sexually transmitted disease during pregnancy
- Cerclage or previous cervical conization
- Amniocentesis*
- Vaginal bleeding during pregnancy
- Pulmonary disease in pregnancy
- Lower socioeconomic status

(Mercer 2003; ACOG 2007)

* Most cases in which PPROM occur after amniocentesis reseal with reaccumulation of the normal amniotic fluid volume. The attributable pregnancy loss from PPROM after amniocentesis is only approximately 0.06% (Eddleman 2006).

Causes: The exact cause of PPROM is not always evident although infection or inflammation is often implicated.

Complications:

Maternal. With PPROM, there is an increased risk of chorioamnionitis and placental abruption (4%-12%) (Ananth 1996; Gonen 1989). Maternal sepsis is, fortunately, a rare event, and occurs in only about 1% of cases.

Fetal. When preterm delivery occurs, the risk of perinatal sepsis is twofold higher if PPROM occurred when compared to preterm labor with intact membranes (Seo 1992). The fetal survival rate depends greatly on both the gestational age at the time of PPROM as well as the presence or absence of infection. A recent meta-analysis of 201 cases demonstrated a 21% survival rate after expectant management when PPROM occurred before viability (Dewan 2001). It is also difficult to say with certainty what the risk of lethal pulmonary hypoplasia (which results from essential anhydramnios during lung development) is with PPROM as the reported risk of this has been reported between 1% and 27% between 16-26 weeks gestation (ACOG 2007).

Recurrence: The risk of recurrence for preterm PROM is quite high, between 16% and 32% (ACOG 2007). Those patients with PPROM who deliver prior to 34 weeks may be candidates for progesterone treatment in subsequent pregnancies, which may decrease the risk of recurrence (deFonseca 2003).

Treatment:* After the diagnosis has been made (See Chapter 4: Rule out Ruptured Membranes), the treatment depends on the gestational age of the fetus. It is important that these patients be monitored closely for evidence of labor, chorioamnionitis, fetal distress, and placental abruption. Usually, the fetal heart rate is continuously monitored and the patient is placed on strict bedrest for the first 24 hours. Corticosteroids are administered if the patient is less than 34 weeks, and antibiotics are given as well, which have been shown to both increase the latency period from PPROM to delivery, as well as reduce major infant morbidity, to include death, RDS, early sepsis, and significant intraventricular hemorrhage (IVH) or necrotizing enterocolitis (NEC) (Mercer 1997).

(Of note, there has been controversy about administration of corticosteroids with PPROM, with the NIH Consensus Development Panel recommending steroids for PPROM patient before 32 weeks gestation. Two subsequent meta-analyses, however, have suggested that steroids for fetal lung maturity are still beneficial (i.e., reduce the risk of Respiratory Distress Syndrome, NEC, and IVH) without increasing the risk of infection up to 34 weeks gestation and the most recent ACOG guidelines support this as well. (Roberts 2006; Harding 2001; ACOG 2008). Because of this, figure 14-8 contains the recommendation to administer steroids up to 34 weeks with PPROM in the absence of infection.)

If there is evidence of significant fetal distress in the form of a non-reassuring fetal heart rate tracing, then delivery is indicated, regardless of gestational age. After approximately 24 hours, if the patient is stable and the FHRT is reassuring, the fetal status may be followed with a biophysical profile done at least twice weekly and often every other day. If, at any time, there is evidence of chorioamnionitis, fetal distress, or placental abruption, then delivery is also indicated.

In addition to corticosteroids and antibiotics, some physicians consider the use of tocolytics in preterm (<34 weeks) PROM in order to attempt to gain at least 48 hours to complete a course of corticosteroids (ACOG 1998b). There is currently no convincing data that this is either beneficial or harmful to either the mother or fetus although there have been some small studies that suggest it may result in a small increase in pregnancy prolongation (Christensen 1980; Levy 1985; Weiner 1988). While tocolytics may be considered in this case, further study is needed to evaluate whether or not this is efficacious in conjunction with antibiotics and corticosteroids.

In general, delivery is indicated whenever fetal lung maturity is demonstrated (done by testing amniotic fluid either from an amniocentesis or by sampling pooled fluid from the vagina) or the patient reaches 34 weeks. The reason for this is that, after 34 weeks, conservative management is associated with an increased risk of chorioamnionitis and lower umbilical cord pH values at delivery without any significant benefit in terms of reducing perinatal complications associated with premature delivery (Naef 1998).

(*It should be noted that there remains significant controversy and discussion about the optimum treatment for the premature fetus with PPROM, so do not be surprised if you find varying opinions among well-educated physicians.)

Figure 14-8: Treatment Algorithm for PPROM

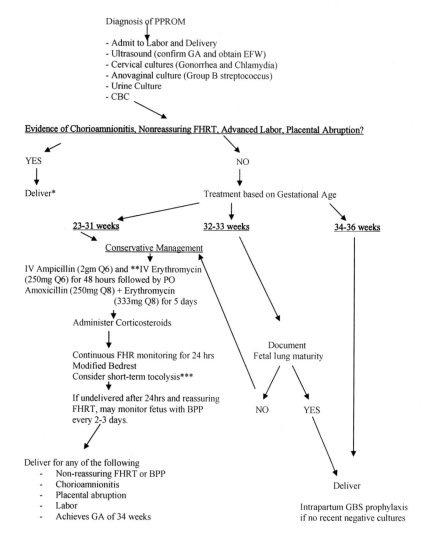

*Treat chorioamnionitis if present and give intrapartum group B streptococcus prophylaxis if no recent negative cultures.
**Some people substitute Azithromycin IV for Erythromycin
***Short-term tocolysis may be considered in patients with early preterm labor who would benefit from a full course of corticosteroids as long as there is no evidence of chorioamnionitis and there is no evidence of fetal distress.

*   Treat chorioamnionitis if present and give intrapartum group B streptococcus prophylaxis if no recent negative cultures.

**   Some people substitute Azithromycin IV for Erythromycin

***   Short-term tocolysis may be considered in patients with early preterm labor who would benefit from a full course of corticosteroids as long as there is no evidence of chorioamnionitis and there is no evidence of fetal distress.

Shoulder Dystocia

This complication occurs when the shoulders fail to deliver either spontaneously or with gentle downward traction after the fetal head has delivered. It is usually caused by the anterior shoulder being wedged behind the pubic symphysis. When this occurs it is imperative to have a well-rehearsed plan of action so that the fetus can be delivered in the most expedient and safest manner possible. It is also important that your assistant and/or nurses are well-prepared for this drill.

Although there are well-known risk factors for a shoulder dystocia, most cases cannot be predicted, so you must be ready for this complication with every delivery. In certain cases, such as when the estimated fetal weight is >5,000 grams in a nondiabetic patient or > 4,500 grams in a diabetic patient, a prophylactic cesarean section may be performed. Elective induction of a patient with presumed macrosomia in an effort to avoid shoulder dystocia is not supported by the literature or ACOG.

Most cases will resolve with only a few maneuvers, but complications, such as a brachial plexus injury, can occur in anywhere from 4%-40% of cases. Fortunately, less than 10% of all brachial plexus injuries result in permanent damage to the child (ACOG 2002b).

Incidence: 0.6%-1.4% of vaginal deliveries of vertex fetuses.

Recurrence risk: 1%-16%

Clinical Picture: After delivery of the head, the shoulders fail to deliver spontaneously or with gentle downward traction. Prior to delivery of the head, it may be noted to retract back significantly after each push (Turtle sign).

Risk factors:

- Prior shoulder dystocia (recurrence risk 1%-16%)
- Diabetes
- Fetal macrosomia (> 4000gms)
- Maternal obesity
- Multiparity
- Postterm gestation
- Previous history of a macrosomic fetus
- Epidural anesthesia
- Induction of labor*
- Operative vaginal delivery

*(While the induction of labor has been associated with shoulder dystocia, there is no compelling evidence that shows either a protracted active phase of labor or the duration of pushing can reliably predict the occurrence of shoulder dystocia [Lurie 1995].)

Treatment: There are many standard maneuvers that are taken when this complication occurs. There is disagreement about exactly what order to do them in, but what follows is a list of possible maneuvers that can be attempted and a detailed description of each. They are listed in the order that they are generally implemented, but there will be some variation between providers.

1. McRobert's maneuver: It is generally agreed that the initial maneuver of choice is McRobert's maneuver which involves hyperflexion and abduction of the patient's legs back to flatten the lumbar lordosis and potentially free the impacted shoulder. After this maneuver is done, attempt again with gentle traction to deliver the anterior shoulder.

2. Suprapubic pressure: This is usually performed at the same time as McRobert's maneuver. An assistant stands up on a stool or high enough to provide downward pressure just above the pubic symphysis in an attempt to dislodge the anterior shoulder. It is important to remember NOT to apply fundal pressure as this has been shown to actually make the situation worse rather than better (Phelan 1997).

3. Generous episiotomy: There is debate as to whether or not this is helpful as the limiting factor is rarely the posterior soft tissue. However, if it is very difficult to perform the rotational maneuvers listed later, then an episiotomy, and even a proctoepisiotomy (which intentionally extends into the rectum) may be made.

4. Modified Woods screw maneuver: This maneuver is meant to turn the shoulders to an oblique position in order to deliver the child. It is performed by placing two fingers behind the posterior shoulder and rotating the child to release the anterior shoulder from behind the symphysis.

5. Rubins maneuvers: The first maneuver involves attempting to disimpact the anterior shoulder by transabdominal manipulation and then placing a hand vaginally behind the anterior shoulder to move it to an oblique angle for delivery.

6. Delivery of the posterior shoulder: A hand is placed into the posterior portion of the vagina and the posterior elbow/wrist grasped and swept across the body to deliver the posterior arm. When this occurs, the anterior shoulder will almost always deliver easily. If this is difficult to perform because there is minimal room posteriorly, a generous episiotomy may be cut to create additional room.

7. Fracture of the clavicle: The fetal clavicle can be fractured by placing two fingers underneath it and pulling outward. It should not be pushed toward

the fetus as angulation in this manner can result in a fetal pneumothorax. This is actually much more difficult than it sounds, but may allow for compression of the fetal shoulder toward the thorax if successful.

8. All-Fours maneuver: This maneuver involves having the patient move from her back to a position on her hands and knees. It may free the anterior shoulder by rotation of the patient's pelvis. It may, however, be a very difficult position to have the patient get into if they have a functioning epidural.

9. Symphysiotomy: In order to perform this maneuver, the patient should be in the lithotomy position. Local anesthetic is injected into the skin and ligament of the symphysis pubis. (This step helps to identify the exact area to be incised and the needle can be left in place as a guide if needed.) A foley catheter or red robin catheter is inserted and the urethra is deviated to the side with a vaginal hand. The ligament of the symphysis is then incised in a downward action beginning at the junction of the upper and middle third of the ligament. The scalpel is then rotated and the remaining upper third of the ligament is incised pushing superiorly. After this, the symphysis can be opened approximately 2.5 cm. In terms of postdelivery management, care should be taken to ensure hemostasis at the incision and the urinary catheter is left in place for five days. The woman should remain on her side with her knees strapped together for three days and then ambulation may be started. (Wykes 2002). It should be noted that major orthopedic disability has been reported in approximately 1%-2% of women after this procedure (Hartfield 1975).

10. Replacement of the fetal head (Zavanelli maneuver): This is a last-ditch effort if all reasonable efforts have failed to deliver the fetal shoulder. In doing this, the cardinal movements of labor are reversed and the fetal head is flexed and replaced into the vagina and upward while the patient is quickly moved to have an emergent cesarean section. The risk of significant fetal morbidity and mortality is increased greatly when this has to be performed.

After the delivery of the fetal shoulders, regardless of what maneuvers are required, you should collect a section of the umbilical cord for cord gases.

After everything is over, it is imperative to sit down with the parents to explain exactly what occurred and what measures you took to deliver their child. Later, when things have calmed down, make sure you counsel them regarding the risk of recurrence should they decide to have another child. It is also extremely important to meet with everyone involved in the delivery and write a detailed note in the chart noting the time of delivery of the head, what maneuvers were performed, what the time of delivery of the impacted

285

shoulder occurred, which shoulder was stuck (left or right), APGAR scores, umbilical cord gases, and whether or not the child was moving its extremities after delivery. In addition, it is wise to dictate the delivery note as a supplement to your written note as soon as you have all of this information.

Umbilical Cord Prolapse

This complication occurs when the umbilical cord falls through the cervix into the vagina ahead of the presenting fetal part after the membranes have ruptured. It is an obstetric emergency that requires prompt intervention as the umbilical vessels are usually compressed resulting in fetal distress and at times fetal demise. Although the prematurity that often accompanies this complication definitely contributes to fetal morbidity, one study reported that the risk of fetal death was 10% (Critchlow 1994).

Incidence: This complication occurs in between 0.14 to 0.62% of all deliveries (Koonings 1990). This number is somewhat misleading, though, as the fetal lie is an important determinant of the actual risk. For example, the risk of cord prolapse is only 0.24% when the fetus is in the vertex position, 3.5% when the fetus is breech, and nearly 10% when the fetus is transverse (Barclay 1989).

Clinical Picture: An acute and severe fetal bradycardia or severe repetitive variable decelerations are almost always seen. These are usually in contrast to a normal and reassuring FHRT prior to the event. When a cervical examination is performed in an attempt to determine the etiology of the fetal distress, the umbilical cord is palpable in the vagina. When this occurs, the diagnosis is clear.

Risk factors:

- Preterm fetus (especially < 1,250 gms) (Yla-Outinen 1985)
- Fetal malpresentation (breech, transverse)
- Second twin (vaginal delivery)
- Multiparity
- Polyhydramnios
- Premature rupture of membranes
- Manual rotation of the fetal head

Causes: The ultimate cause of umbilical cord prolapse is any situation that causes the membranes to rupture and allow the cord to descend ahead of the presenting part. While there are risk factors, which are outlined above, this complication may occur when any of several routine obstetric procedures are performed. Some of these include:

- Artificial rupture of membranes *
- Fetal scalp electrode placement
- Intrauterine pressure catheter placement
- Amnioinfusion

* Note: Because amniotomy may precipitate a cord prolapse, it is imperative that the fetal position be known and the presenting part well-applied to the cervix in an attempt to minimize the risk of this happening.

Treatment: Whenever the umbilical cord is palpated in the vagina, the examiner should not remove their hand, but rather attempt to elevate the presenting part off of the umbilical cord. The patient is taken immediately to the operating room for an emergency cesarean delivery. The initial examiner's hand remains in the vagina until the baby is delivered by cesarean section. If there is any delay in performing the cesarean section you can consider administering terbutaline to decrease uterine contractions, or filling the bladder with 500 mL of fluid to elevate the presenting part off of the cord.

Uterine Inversion

This is a relatively uncommon occurrence, but when it happens immediate intervention is necessary to prevent disastrous hemorrhage. It can be a result of overzealous traction on the umbilical cord after delivery but abnormal placentation is often a key element. The reason that one hand gives suprapubic pressure during the delivery of the placenta is an attempt to prevent this complication by keeping the uterus in its normal position.

Incidence: 1:2,500 deliveries (ACOG 1998)

Clinical Picture: Prolonged 3rd stage of labor
If, with the delivery of the placenta, you see a beefy red mass of tissue that is not obviously placenta, then you have a uterine inversion.

Risk Factors:

- Fetal macrosomia
- Fundal placentation
- Placenta accreta
- Use of oxytocin
- Primiparity
  (Brar et al. 1989)

Treatment:

- Call for help (Staff/Anesthesia)
- Immediately attempt to replace uterus*
- Bolus IV Fluids/IV access (2 large bore IV's)
- Crossmatch blood (at least 2 units to start)
- If unable to replace uterus, give agent to relax uterus.
  - Options:
    - Terbutaline 0.25 mg IV
    - Nitroglycerin 50-100mcg IV (This will result in uterine relaxation within 30 seconds and will last approximately one minute)
    - Halogenated anesthetic agent (anesthesiologist)

- If these attempts are unsuccessful, then the patient must be taken emergently to the operating room where a laparotomy is performed. The round ligaments are used for traction to restore the uterus to its normal position. (This is called the Huntington maneuver.)

- * (Replacing the uterus involves applying gentle manual pressure to the most distal part of the uterus that is seen and pushing it back into the vagina and through the cervix. Once the uterus is back in position, a fist is kept inside the uterus, and uterotonics are given to make sure the uterus contracts.)

Uterine Rupture

Uterine rupture occurs in approximately 1:2,000 deliveries. It can cause significant morbidity and mortality for both the mother and fetus. The amount of fetal and maternal distress and blood loss depends on where the rupture occurs and how large the defect is. If the uterus ruptures laterally, where the uterine vessels are located, then blood loss may be rapid and severe. Also, if the rupture is large, then the fetus may be found floating in the abdomen at the time of emergency cesarean section.

Incidence:

- 1:2,000 of all deliveries
- 1:100 of patients with a previous cesarean section attempting vaginal delivery (See Chapter 10: VBAC.)
- 1:8,000 to 1:15,000 deliveries with an unscarred uterus (Langton 1997)
- In patients with a prior low-vertical, classical, or T-shaped uterine incision or a previous rupture, the risk of subsequent rupture is much higher:

Low-vertical incision = 1%-7%
Classical incision = 4%-9%
T-shaped incision = 4%-9%
Prior rupture = 6%-32% (Ritchie 1971; Reyes-Ceja 1969)

Clinical Picture: While the clinical presentation of a uterine rupture may occur suddenly or develop over a period of time, some common findings often include the following:

- Fetal distress with either a prolonged bradycardia or variable decelerations that progress to late decelerations and bradycardia.
- Loss of pressure on IUPC
- Loss of fetal station (fetal vertex not palpable or much higher than previous exam)
- Sudden onset of focal pain (despite functioning epidural)
- Vaginal bleeding (not required for diagnosis)
- Maternal hypovolemia, hypotension, shock

Risk Factors:

- Previous classical uterine incision
- Prior deep myomectomy (with entry into uterine cavity)
- Midforceps delivery
- Internal podalic version with breech extraction
- Use of misoprostol in patient with previous cesarean section
- Maternal age > 30 years
- Fetal weight > 4,000 grams
- Induction of labor
- No previous vaginal delivery
- Previous cesarean delivery for dystocia (Hamilton 2001)
- Interval of < 18 months between this labor and previous cesarean section (Shipp 2001)

Treatment: A uterine rupture is an obstetrical emergency and requires delivery by cesarean section immediately. Time is of the essence as the fetus is usually in significant distress. Steps that should be taken immediately include the following:

- Call for staff backup/OR scrub technician/Anesthesiologist/Pediatrician.
- Call for blood products (PRBC's/Platelets) and antibiotics on the way to the OR.
- Deliver the fetus by emergency cesarean section.*
- Control bleeding, perform hysterectomy if unable to salvage uterus.

Postpartum:

- Continue antibiotics if the procedure was performed emergently.
- Patients with a previous uterine rupture should not be allowed to labor in subsequent pregnancies.

  * Note: A general anesthesia will often be required in this situation.

References:

Ahanya SN, Ross MG. Oligohydramnios. Up To Date, Version 11.1, Dec 2002.

Al RA, Baykal C, Karacay O, Geyik PO, Altun S, Dolen I. Random urine protein-creatinine ratio to predict proteinuria in new-onset mild hypertension in late pregnancy. Obstet Gynecol 2005; 104:367-371.

Alexander JM, McIntire DD, Leveno KJ, Cunningham GF. Selective magnesium sulfate prophylaxis for the prevention of eclampsia in women with gestational hypertension. Obstet Gynecol 2006; 108(4):826-832.

Ananth CV, Savitz DA, Williams MA. Placental abruption and its association with hypertension and prolonged rupture of membranes: a methodologic review and meta-analysis. Obstet Gynecol 1996; 88:309.

Antenatal corticosteroid therapy for fetal maturation. ACOG Committee Opinion #402, Mar 2008.

Ascarelli MH, Johnson V, May WL, Martin RW, Martin JN. Individually determined postpartum magnesium sulfate therapy with clinical parameters to safely and cost-effectively shorten treatment for preeclampsia. Am J Obstet Gynecol, 1998; 179(4):952-956.

Barclay M. Umbilical cord prolapse and other cord accidents. In: Gynecology and Obstetrics, Sciarra, JJ (ed), JB Lippencott, Philadelphia, PA 1989, page 1.

Berkman ND, Thorp JM Jr, Hartmann KE, Lohr KN, Idicula AE, McPheeters M, et al. Management of preterm labor. Evidence report/technology assessment no. 18. AHRQ publication no. 01-E021. Rockville, MD: U.S. Dept of Health and Human Services, Agency for Healthcare Research and Quality. 2000.

Bonnar J. Massive obstetric haemorrhage. Baillieres Best Pract Res Clin Obstet Gynaecol, 2000; 14:1-18.

Brar HS, Greenspoon JS, Platt LD, Paul RH. Acute puerperal uterine inversion: new approaches to management. J Reprod Med 1989; 34:173-177.

Bukowski R, Hankins, GDV. Managing postpartum hemorrhage. Contemporary OB/GYN 2001 Sept; 46:92-102.

Chauhan SP, Magann EF, Carroll CS, Barrilleaux PS, Scardo JA, Martin JN Jr. Mode of delivery for the morbidity for the morbidly obese with prior cesarean delivery: vaginal versus repeat cesarean section. Am J Obstet Gynecol. 2001 Aug; 185(2):349-354.

Chesley LC, Annitto JE, Cosgrove RA. The remote prognosis of eclamptic women. Am J Obstet Gynecol 1976; 124:446.

Christensen KK, Ingemarsson I, Leideman T, Solum T, Svenningsen N. Effect of ritodrine on labor after premature rupture of the membranes. Obstet Gynecol 1980; 55:187-190.

Combs CA, Murphy EL, Laros RK Jr. Factors associated with postpartum hemorrhage with vaginal birth. Obstet Gynecol 1991; 77:69-76.

Combs CA, Murphy EL, Laros RK Jr. Factors associated with hemorrhage in cesarean deliveries. Obstet Gynecol 1991; 77:77-82.

Comeau J, Shaw L, Marcell CC, Lavery JP. Early placenta previa and delivery outcome. 1983: 61:577.

Cotton DB, Read JA, Paul RH, Quilligan EJ. The conservative aggressive management of placenta previa. Am J Obstet Gynecol 1980; 137:687.

Critchlow CW, Leet TL, Benedetti TJ, Daling JR. Risk factors and infant outcomes associated with umbilical cord prolapse: a population-based case-control study among births in Washington State. Am J Obstet Gynecol 1994; 170:613.

Cunningham FG, Gant NF, Leveno KJ, Hauth JC, Wenstrom KD (eds) Williams Obstetrics 21st ed, NY McGraw-Hill, 2001.

da Fonseca EB, Bittar RE, Carvalho MHB, Sugaib M. Prophylactic administration of progesterone by vaginal suppository to reduce the incidence of spontaneous preterm birth in women at increased risk: A randomized placebo-controlled double blinded study. Am J Obstet Gynecol 2003:188:419-24

Del Priore G, Jackson-Stone M, Shim EK, Garfinkel J, Eichmann MA, Frederiksen MC. A comparison of once-daily and 8-hour gentamicin dosing in the treatment of postpartum endometritis. Obstet Gynecol 1996; 87(6):994-1000.

Delgado-Escueta AV, Wasterlain C, Treiman DM, Porter RJ. Current concepts in neurology: management of status epilepticus. NEJM 1982; 306:1337.

Dewan H, Morris JM. A systematic review of pregnancy outcome following preterm premature rupture of membranes at a previable gestational age. Aust N Z J Obstet Gynaecol 2001; 41:389-394.

Diagnosis and management of preeclampsia and eclampsia. ACOG Practice Bulletin #33, Jan 2002a.

Drife J. Management of primary postpartum haemorrhage. BJOG 1997; 104:275-277.

Duley L. Maternal mortality associated with hypertensive disorders of pregnancy in Africa, Asia, Latin America, and the Carribean. Br J Obstet Gynaecol 1992; 99: 547.

Duley L, Henderson-Smart D. Magnesium sulfate versus phenytoin for eclampsia. The Cochrane Library, Issue 3, 2001.

Eddleman K, Malone F, Sullivan L, Dukes K, Berkowitz R, Kharutli Y, et al. Pregnancy loss rates after midtrimester amniocentesis. Obstet Gynecol 2006; 108:1067-1072.

Ehrenberg HM, Mercer BM. Abbreviated postpartum magnesium sulfate therapy for women with mild preeclampsia: A randomized controlled trial. Obstet Gynecol, 2006; 108;4:833-838.

Elliot JP. Management of complications associated with tocolytic agents. In *Obstetric Intensive Care: a practical manual.* Eds. Foley MR and Strong TH. W.B. Saunders, Philadelphia, PA, 1997.

Fontenot MT, et al. A prospective randomized trial of magnesium sulfate in severe preeclampsia: Use of diuresis as a clinical parameter to determine the duration of postpartum therapy. Am J Obstet Gynecol, 2005; 192:1788-1794.

Gibbs RS, Infection after cesarean section. Clin Obstet Gynecol 1985; 28(4):697-710.

Gibbs RS, Dinsmoor NJ, Newton ER, Ramamurthy RS. A randomized trial of intrapartum versus immediate postpartum treatment of women with intraamniotic infection. Obstet Gynecol 1988; 72:823-828.

Gillen-Goldstein J, Lockwood CJ. Abruptio placentae. Up To Date version 10.3, August 2002.

Goldenberg RL. The management of preterm labor. Obstet Gynecol Nov 2002; 100(5) Pt 1:1020-1037.

Gonen R, Hannah ME, Milligan JE. Does prolonged preterm premature rupture of membranes predispose to abruptio placentae? Obstet Gynecol 1989; 74:47-50.

Guinn DA, Goepfert AR, Owen J, Brumfield C, Hauth JC. Management options in women with preterm contractions: A randomized clinical trial. Am J Obstet Gynecol 1997; 177:814-818.

Hall MH, Halliwell R, Carr-Hill R. Concomitant and repeated happening of complications of the third stage of labor. Br J Obstet Gynaecol 1985; 92:732-738.

Hamilton EF, Bujold E, McNamara H, Gauthier R, Platt RW. Dystocia among women with symptomatic uterine rupture. Am J Obstet Gynecol Mar 2001; 184(4):620-624.

Harding JE, Pang J, Knight DB, Liggins GC. Do antenatal corticosteroids help in the setting of preterm rupture of membranes? Am J Obstet Gynecol 2001; 184:131-139.

Hartfield VJ. Late effects of symphysiotomy. Trop Doct 1975; 5:76-78.

Hibbard BM, Jeffcoate TNA. Abruptio placentae. Obstet Gynecol 1966; 27:155.

Hikock DE, Gordon DC, Milberg JA, Williams MA. The frequency of breech presentation by gestational age at birth: a large population-based study. Am J Obstet Gynecol 1992; 166(3):851-852.

Hofmeyr GJ, Gulmezoglu AM. Maternal hydration for increasing amniotic fluid volume in oligohydramnios and normal amniotic fluid volume. Cochrane Database Syst Rev 2000; CD000134.

Hofmeyr GJ, Hannah ME. Planned cesarean section for term breech delivery. In: Cochrane database of systemic reviews, issue 3. Oxford: Update Software.

Hoskins IA, Friedman DM, Frieden FJ, et al. Relationship between antepartum cocaine abuse, abnormal umbilical artery Doppler velocimetry, and placental abruption. Obstet Gynecol 1991; 78:279.

Iams JK. Prediction and early detection of preterm labor. Obstet Gynecol 2003; 101(2):402-412.

Isler CM, Barrilleaux PS, Rinehart BK, Magann EF, Martin JN. Postpartum seizure prophylaxis: Using maternal clinical parameters to guide therapy. Obstet Gynecol 2003; 101:66-69.

Koonings PP, Paul RH, Campbell K. Umbilical cord prolapse. A contemporary look. J Reprod Med 1990; 35:690.

Kramer MS, Usher RH, Pollack R, et al. Etiologic determinants of abruptio placentae. Obstet Gynecol 1997; 89:221.

Langton J, Fishwick K, Kumar B, et al. Spontaneous rupture of an unscarred gravid uterus at 32 weeks gestation. Hum Repord 1997; 12:2066-2067.

Levy DL, Warsof SL. Oral ritodrine and preterm premature rupture of membranes. Obstet Gynecol 1985; 66:621-623.

Lopez-Llera M. Main clinical types and subtypes of eclampsia. Am J Obstet Gynecol 1992; 166:4.

Lurie S, Levy R, Ben-Arie A, Hagay Z. Shoulder dystocia: could it be deduced from the labor partogram? Am J Perinatol 1995; 12:61-62.

Magali R, Sepandj F, Liston RM, Dooley KC. Random protein-creatinine ratio for the quantification of proteinuria in pregnancy. Obstet Gynecol 1997; 90(6):893-895.

Mantel G, Buchmann E, Rees H, et al. Severe acute maternal morbidity: a pilot study of a definition of a near miss. BJOG 1998; 105:985-990.

Mark SP, Croughan-Minihane MS, Kilpatrick SJ. Chorioamnionitis and uterine function. Obstet Gynecol 2000; 95:909-912.

Mattar F, Sibai BM. Preeclampsia: Clinical characteristics and pathogenesis. Clinics in Liver Disease, Feb 1999; 3(1):15-29.

McShane PM, Heyl PS, Epstein MF. Maternal and perinatal morbidity resulting from placenta previa. Obstet Gynecol 1985; 65:176.

Menitove JE. In Cecil Textbook of Medicine, 21st ed, Goldman (ed), W.B. Saunders Co, Philadelphia, Pennsylvania, 2000.

Mercer B, Miodovnik M, Thurnau G, Goldenberg R, Das A, Merenstein G, et al. Antibiotic therapy for reduction of infant morbidity after preterm premature rupture of the membranes: A randomized controlled trial. JAMA 1997; 278:989-995.

Mercer BM. Preterm premature rupture of the membranes. Obstet Gynecol 2003 Jan; 101(1):178-193.

Mercer BM, Goldenberg RL, Moawad AH, Meis PJ, Iams JD, Das AF, et al. The preterm prediction study: Effect of gestational age and cause of preterm birth on subsequent obstetric outcome. National Institute of Child Health and Human Development Maternal-Fetal Medicine Units Network. Am J Obstet Gynecol 1999; 181:1216-1221.

Mitra AG, Whitten MK, Laurent SL, Anderson WE. A randomized, prospective study comparing once-daily gentamicin versus thrice-daily gentamicin in the treatment of puerperal infection. Am J Obstet Gynecol 1997; 177(4):786-792.

Naef RW 3rd, Allbert JR, Ross EL, Weber BM, Martin RW, Morrison JC. Premature rupture of membranes at 34-37 weeks gestation: Aggressive versus conservative management. Am J Obstet Gynecol 1998; 178:126-130.

Neithardt AB, Dooley SL, Borensztajn J. Prediction of 24-hour protein excretion in pregnancy with a single voided urine protein-to-creatinine ratio. Am J Obstet Gynecol 2002; 186:883-886.

Newton ER. Intraamniotic infection. Up To Date, December, 2002, version 11.1.

Norwitz ER. Eclampsia. Up To Date, August 2002, version 10.3.

Offenbacher S, Lieff S, Boggess KA, et al. Maternal periodontitis and prematurity. Part I: Obstetric outcome of prematurity and growth restriction. Ann Periodontol 2001; 6:164-174.

Oyelese Y, Scorza WE, Mastrolia R, Smulian JC. Postpartum hemorrhage. Obstet Gynecol Clin N Am 2007; 34:421-441.

Oyelese Y, Ananth C. Placental abruption. Obstet Gynecol 2006; 108(4):1005-1016.

Pearlman MD, Tintinalli JE. Evaluation and treatment of the gravida and fetus following traum during pregnancy. Obstet Gynecol Clin North Am 1991; 18:371.

Pearlman MD. Trauma in *Operative Obstetrics* 2nd edition, Gilstrap LC, Cunningham GF, Vandorsten JP eds, McGraw-Hill, NY, 2002.

Phelan JP, Ouzounian JG, Gherlam RB, et al. Shoulder dystocia and permanent Erb's palsy: the role of fundal pressure. Am J Obstet Gynecol 1997; 176:S138.

Postpartum Hemorrhage. ACOG Practice Bulletin #76, Oct 2006.

Premature rupture of membranes. ACOG Practice Bulletin, #80, Apr 2007.

Pritchard JA, Cunningham FG, Pritchard SA. The Parkland Memorial Hospital protocol for treatment of eclampsia: evaluation of 245 cases. Am J Obstet Gynecol 1984; 148:951.

Pritchard JA, Cunningham FG, Pritchard SA, Mason RA. On reducing the frequency of severe abruptio placentae. Am J Obstet Gynecol 1991; 165:1345.

Reyes-Ceja L, Cabrera R, Insfran E, Herrera-Lasso F. Pregnancy following previous uterine rupture. Study of 19 patients. Obstet Gynecol 1969; 34:387-389.

Ritchie EH. Pregnancy after rupture of the pregnant uterus. A report of 36 pregnancies and a study of cases reported since 1932. J Obstet Gynaecol Br Commonw, 1971; 78:642-648.

Roberts D, Dalziel S. Antenatal corticosteroids for accelerating fetal lung maturation for women at risk of preterm birth. Cochrane Database of Systemic Reviews 2006, Issue 3. Art. No:CD004454. DOI: 10.1002/14651858. CD004454.pub2.

Robinson JN, Regan JA, Norwitz ER. The epidemiology of preterm labor and delivery. Up To Date version 11.1, December, 2002.

Rochat RW, Koonin LM, Atrash AF, et al. Maternal mortality in the United States: report from the maternal mortality collaborative. Obstet Gynecol 1988; 72:91.

Rodriquez-Thompson D, Lieberman ES. Use of a random urine protein-to-creatinine ratio for the diagnosis of significant proteinuria during pregnancy. Am J Obstet Gynecol Oct 2001; 185(4).

Russo-Stieglietz K, Lockwood CJ. Placenta previa. Up to Date version 10.3, August 2002.

Scheer K, Nubar J. Variation of fetal presentation with gestational age. Am J Obstet Gynecol 1976; 125(2):269-270.

Seo K, McGregor JA, French JI. Preterm birth is associated with increased risk of maternal and neonatal infection. Obstet Gynecol 1992; 79:75-80.

Shiono PH, Klebanoff MA, Rhoads GG. Smoking and drinking during pregnancy. JAMA 1986; 255:82-84.

Shipp TD, Zelop CM, Repke JT, Cohen A, Lieberman E. Interdelivery interval and risk of symptomatic uterine rupture. Obstet Gynecol Feb 2001; 97(2):175-177.

Shoulder Dystocia. ACOG Practice Bulletin #40, November 2002b.

Sibai BM, el-Nazer A, Gonzalez-Ruiz A. Severe preeclampsia-eclampsia in young primigravid women: subsequent pregnancy outcome and remote prognosis. Am J Obstet Gynecol 1986; 155:1011.

Sibai BM, Mabie WC, Shamsa F, et al. A comparison of no medication versus methyldopa or labetalol in chronic hypertension during pregnancy. Am J Obstet Gynecol 1990; 162:960.

Sibai BM, Mercer B, Sarinoglu C. Severe preeclampsia in the second trimester: recurrence risk and long-term prognosis. Am J Obstet Gynecol 1991; 165:1408.

Sibai BM, Sarinoglu C, Mercer BM. Eclampsia. VII. Pregnancy outcome after eclampsia and long-term prognosis. Am J Obstet Gynecol 1992; 166:1757.

Silver R, Depp R, Sabbagha RE, Dooley SL. Placenta previa: aggressive expectant management. Am J Obstet Gynecol 1984; 150:15.

Simhan H, Caritis S. Inhibition of preterm labor. Up To Date, Version 11.1, Dec 2002.

Singla AK, Lapinski RH, Berkowitz RL, Saphier CJ. Are women who are Jehovah's Witnesses at risk of maternal death? Am J Obstet Gynecol. 2001 Oct;185(4):893-5.

Sperling RS, Newton E, Gibbs RS. Intraamniotic infection in low-birthweight infants. J Infect Dis 1988; 157:113-117.

Strong TH. Transfusion of blood components and derivatives in the obstetric intensive care patient. In *Obstetric Intensive Care: a practical manual.* Eds. Foley MR and Strong TH. W.B. Saunders, Philadelphia, PA, 1997.

Tucker JM, Goldenberg RL, Davis RO, Copper RL, Winkler CL, Hauth JC. Etiologies of preterm birth in an indigent population: Is prevention a logical explanation? Obstet Gynecol 1991; 77:343-347.

Vaginal birth after previous cesarean delivery. ACOG Practice Bulletin #54, Jul 2004.

Ventura SJ, Martin JA, Curtin SC, Mathews TJ, Park MM. Births: Final data for 1998. National Vital Statistics Reports; 48(3), Hyattsville, MD, National Center Health Statistics, 2000.

Wiener CP, Renk K, Klugman M. The therapeutic efficacy and cost-effectiveness of aggressive tocolysis for premature labor associated with premature rupture of the membranes. Am J Obstet Gynecol 1988; 159:216-222.

Wykes CB, Johnston TA, Paterson-Brown S, Johanson RB. Symphysiotomy: a lifesaving procedure. BJOG Feb 2003; 110(2):219-221.

Yla-Outinen A, Heinonen PK, Tuimala R. Predisposing and risk factors of umbilical cord prolapse. Acta Obstet Gynecol 1985; 64:567.

Medication Database

Every effort has been made to ensure the accuracy of the information and dosing regiments for the medications included in this text. It is, however still the provider's responsibility to use clinical judgment and consult with the pharmacy or other appropriate sources regarding dosage and contraindications based on the clinical situation because dosage recommendations may change over time and inadvertent errors in the text can occur and the author cannot be held responsible for any errors found in this book.

Analgesics

Percocet

Other Names:	N/A
Indications:	Postoperative pain relief
Contraind:	Known allergy, respiratory depression
Dosage:	1-2 tablets (2.5mg oxycodone/325mg acetaminophen)
Dosage Interval:	Q4-6 hours
Route of Admin:	PO
Adverse Rxns:	Pruritis, nausea, emesis
Breastfeeding:	Compatible with breastfeeding with minimal risk for adverse effects during nursing. Recommended that infants be monitored for sedation or changes in feeding patterns.

Notes: This medication is commonly used for post-cesarean pain control when the patient is tolerating a regular diet.

Mechanism of action: This medication is a mixture of acetaminophen and oxycodone. The oxycodone is an opiate receptor agonist. There are different strengths that may be carried on formulary with the most common being Percocet 2.5/325 or 5/325 which mean that each tablet contains either 2.5mg or 5mg of oxycodone and 325mg of acetaminophen respectively.

Morphine

Other Names:	N/A
Indications:	Pain relief during latent labor
Contraind:	Known allergy, respiratory depression
Dosage:	2-5mg (IV), 10mg (IM)
Dosage Interval:	Q 4 hours
Route of Admin:	IV/IM

Adverse Rxns: Pruritis, respiratory depression, decreased FHR variability, nausea, emesis

Breastfeeding: Compatible with breastfeeding, but studies indicate that a significant amount of narcotics may be transferred to the infant.

Notes: The onset of analgesia from IV morphine is approximately 5 minutes, and 30-40 minutes from an IM dose. The half-life of the drug in the neonate is approximately 7 hours.

Mechanism of action: This medication is an opiate receptor agonist.

Meperidine

Other Names: Demerol
Indications: Pain relief during latent labor
Contraind: Known allergy, respiratory depression
Dosage: 25-50mg IV, 50-100mg IM
Dosage Interval: Q1-2 hours (IV), Q2-4 hours (IM)
Route of Admin: IM/IV
Adverse Rxns: Pruritis, respiratory depression, decreased FHR variability, nausea, emesis
Breastfeeding: This is not usually given in the postpartum period.

Notes: The onset of action of meperidine is 5 minutes (IV) and 30-45 minutes (IM). The neonatal half-life is extremely long (up to 63 hours) for active metabolites. Because of this, extreme caution should be used in administering this medication during latent labor as one study reported that the chance of a neonate requiring naloxone treatment increased four-fold after high doses of meperidine when compared to an epidural (Sharma, 1997).

Mechanism of action: This medication is an opiate receptor agonist.

Fentanyl

Other Names: Sublimaze
Indications: Analgesia in labor, pain control postpartum for some procedures (i.e. manual extraction of placenta)
Contraind: Known allergy, respiratory depression
Dosage: 50-100 mcg
Dosage Interval: Q 1-2 hours
Route of Admin: IV/IM

Adverse Rxns: Respiratory depression (less likely than with morphine), mild bradycardia

Breastfeeding: This medication is generally not given in the postpartum period.

Notes: This medication is nearly one hundred times more potent than morphine, but is less likely to result in respiratory depression, although is complication may still occur. Its onset of action is almost immediate when given IV.

Mechanism of action: This medication is an opiate receptor agonist.

Nalbuphine

Other Names: Nubain
Indications: Pain relief during latent labor
Contraind: Known allergy
Dosage: 10mg
Dosage Interval: Q 3-4 hours
Route of Admin: IV or IM
Adverse Rxns: Pruritis, respiratory depression, decreased FHR variability, sedation, nausea, emesis.
Breastfeeding: Generally used only in the antepartum period.

Notes: This medication takes effect within minutes when administered intravenously, and within 15 minutes when given IM. It has a half-life in the neonate of around 4 hours.

Mechanism of action: This medication is a partial opiod agonist.

Butorphanol

Other Names: Stadol
Indications: Pain relief during latent labor
Contraind: Known allergy
Dosage: 1-2mg
Dosage Interval: Q 4 hours
Route of Admin: IV or IM
Adverse Rxns: Pruritis, respiratory depression, decreased FHR variability, increased BP, nausea, emesis.
Breastfeeding: This medication is not usually given in the postpartum period.

Notes: The onset of action of this medication is within minutes when given IV. When administered IM, the onset of analgesia is usually within 30 minutes. It has been reported to increase blood pressure and should not be administered to patients with hypertension or preeclampsia. A 2 mg dose of butorphanol is equivalent to approximately 10mg of morphine (PDR, 2003).

Mechanism of action: This medication is a mixed opiod agonist-antagonist.

Ketorolac

Other Names:	Toradol
Indications:	Postpartum or postoperative pain control
Contraind:	Known allergy to ketorolac or NSAIDs, actively bleeding ulcer
Dosage:	30mg IV/IM (with maxiumum 120mg/day), 10-20mg PO (with maximum 40mg/day)
Dosage Interval:	Q 6 hours (IV/IM), Q4-6 hours (PO)
Route of Admin:	IV/IM/PO
Adverse Rxns:	Gastrointestinal distress or bleeding, tinnitis
Breastfeeding:	This medication is compatible with breastfeeding.

Notes: This medication is a nonsteroidal anti-inflammatory (NSAID) agent that is very helpful with postoperative pain management as it may be given parenterally and you do not have to wait for the patient's bowel function to return.

Mechanism of action: This medication is an NSAID that inhibits cyclooxygenase and therefore, prostaglandin synthesis.

Antibiotics

Ampicillin

Other Names:	N/A
Indications:	Chorioamnionitis, endometritis
Contraind:	Known allergy
Dosage:	2 grams
Dosage Interval:	Q 6 hours
Route of Admin:	IV
Adverse Rxns:	Anaphylaxis, Urticaria, GI upset
Breastfeeding:	Compatible with breastfeeding, although potential for modification of infant bowel flora, allergic response, and interference with infant culture results if required.

Notes: This antibiotic is part of the first line treatment for chorioamnionitis (See Chapter 14). It is also added to the standard antibiotic regiment for postpartum endometritis after 24 hours if the patient remains febrile in order to provide coverage for enterococcus.

Mechanism of action: The amino side group allows this drug to penetrate gram negative organisms. It then inhibits the crosslinking of bacteria cell wall components.

Clindamycin

Other Names:	Cleocin
Indications:	Treatment of postpartum endometritis (in addition to gentamycin)
	Third-line treatment choice for Group B streptococcus
Contraind:	Allergy to clindamycin
Dosage:	900 mg
Dosage Interval:	Q8 hours
Route of Admin:	IV
Adverse Rxns:	Abdominal cramps, diarrhea, elevation of liver function tests, pseudomembranous colitis
Breastfeeding:	Considered safe in breastfeeding.

Notes: This medication covers Gram-positive organisms, and most anaerobes. It does not penetrate the CSF, but it is actively transported into abscesses.

Mechanism of action: This drug binds to the 50s ribosomal subunit interface of bacteria and causes abnormal reading of mRNA, and therefore defective bacterial proteins.

Dicloxicillin

Other Names:	Dynapen
Indications:	Treatment of mastitis, superficial nipple infections
Contraind:	Allergy to PCN
Dosage:	500mg
Dosage Interval:	Q 6 hours
Route of Admin:	PO
Adverse Rxns:	Hypersensitivity reactions
Breastfeeding:	Considered safe.

Notes: This is the first choice of antibiotics for the treatment of mastitis.

Mechanism of action: The amino side group allows this class of drugs to penetrate gram negative organisms, then it inhibits crosslinking of bacteria cell wall components.

Gentamycin

Other Names:	Garamycin
Indications:	Treatment of chorioamnionitis and postpartum endometritis
Contraind:	Allergy to Gentamycin, renal failure (must reduce dosage)
Dosage:	5 mg/kg Q24 hours (*ONLY FOR POSTPARTUM USE) Or 1.5mg/kg Q8 hours (for antepartum or postpartum use)
Dosage Interval:	This may be given either Q8 hours or Q24 hours as above
Route of Admin:	IV
Adverse Rxns:	Neurotoxicity, ototoxicity, vertigo, nephrotoxicity
Breastfeeding:	Considered safe. Small amounts of the medication are excreted into breast milk.

Notes: In the postpartum period, 24-hour dosing regiment may be used. Prior to delivery, the Q8 hour dosing should be used. This medication is an amnioglycoside which covers gram negative bacteria.

Mechanism of action: The antibiotic binds at the 30s/50s interface and causes incorrect reading of mRNA and defective bacterial proteins.

Penicillin G

Other Names:	N/A
Indications:	First line treatment for GBS prophylaxis in labor
Contraind:	Allergy to PCN
Dosage:	5 million units initially, then 2.5 million units with subsequent doses
Dosage Interval:	Q4 hours
Route of Admin:	IV
Adverse Rxns:	Hypersensitivity reactions, rare neurologic toxicity, neutropenia, nephrotoxicity
Breastfeeding:	Considered safe. Small amounts are excreted into breast milk. No adverse effects reported.

Notes: This is the first line therapy for GBS prophylaxis in labor because it is not as broad spectrum as other antibiotics commonly used, such as Ampicillin.

Mechanism of action: B-lactam binds penicillin binding proteins and prevents crosslinking of bacterial cell wall components.

Antivirals

Acyclovir

Other Names:	Zovirax
Indications:	Active Herpes simplex virus (HSV I or HSV II)
Contraind:	Allergy to acyclovir, renal failure
Dosage:	Primary outbreak: 200mg Q4 hours x 10 days
	Recurrent outbreak: 200mg Q4 hours x 5 days
	Chronic treatment: 400mg Q12 hours
	Or
	200mg 3-5x/day up to 12 months
Dosage Interval:	See above
Route of Admin:	IV or PO
Adverse Rxns:	Skin irritation, crystalline nephropathy possible if given rapidly IV
Breastfeeding:	Considered safe.

Notes: This medication is used for the treatment of both primary and secondary HSV outbreaks as well as for prophylaxis against recurrence.

Mechanism of action: This medication is metabolized to a triphosphate analog that inhibits DNA polymerase. It binds to viral thymidine kinase as well.

Zidovudine

Other Names:	Retrovir, (formerly known as AZT)
Indications:	Given during labor in HIV + patients
Contraind:	Allergy to Zidovudine
Dosage:	2mg/kg IV bolus followed by infusion of 1mg/kg/hr until delivery
Dosage Interval:	continuous infusion
Route of Admin:	IV
Adverse Rxns:	Headaches, nausea, anemia, neutropenia, myalgias
Breastfeeding:	This medication is excreted in high enough concentrations into breastmilk to decrease the viral load, but breastfeeding in HIV positive women is generally not encouraged in the US.

Notes: This medication is used during labor to decrease the risk of HIV transmission from the mother to the fetus.

Mechanism of action: This is a thymidine analog which is a reverse transcriptase inhibitor.

Valacyclovir

Other Names:	Valtrex
Indications:	Herpes simplex virus (HSV 1 or 2)
Contraind:	Can interact with nephrotoxic medications
Dosage:	Primary outbreak 1 gram Q12 hours
	Secondary outbreak 500mg Q12 hours
	Suppression therapy 1 gram Q24 hours
Dosage Interval:	See above
Route of Admin:	PO
Adverse Rxns:	GI upset, headaches, hemolytic uremic syndrome or thrombotic thrombocytopenic purpura are possible at very high doses.
Breastfeeding:	Considered safe.

Notes: This medication is used both for the treatment of herpes outbreaks as well as for prophylaxis during pregnancy to prevent outbreaks near term which would preclude a vaginal delivery.

Mechanism of action: This medication is metabolized to acyclovir.

Seizure Prophylaxis/Treatment

Ativan

Other Names:	Lorazepam
Indications:	Status epilepticus, eclampsia (for the acute seizure)
Contraind:	Acute narrow-angle glaucoma
Dosage:	4mg IV (dilute first) over 2 minutes
Dosage Interval:	May repeat after 10-15 minutes if needed
Route of Admin:	IV/IM
Adverse Rxns:	Ataxia, CNS depression, respiratory depression
Breastfeeding:	Effects are unknown. American Academy of Pediatrics states effects may be concerning if prolonged use occurs.

Notes: This is a benzodiazepine. The onset of action is rapid (i.e. < 5 minutes). It is metabolized in the liver. Diazepam (valium) is similar to lorazepam, but has a longer half-life.

Mechanism of action: This medication enhances GABA-mediated chloride influx, which results in neuronal inhibition. The exact mechanism by which it exerts its anticonvulsant effects is not clear.

Dilantin

Other Names:	Phenytoin
Indications:	Seizure prophylaxis, eclampsia
Contraind:	Heart block, sinus bradycardia, anticonvulsant hypersensitivity syndrome
Dosage:	10-15 mg/kg (slow IV infusion, not greater than 50 mg per minute)
	Followed by maintenance doses of 100 mg IV Q 6-8 hours
Dosage Interval:	Q 6-8 hours
Route of Admin:	IV
Adverse Rxns:	Nystagmus, ataxia, bone marrow suppression, hepatotoxicity, CNS depression, arrythmias, hypotension
Breastfeeding:	There are conflicting reports on the safety of phenytoin with breastfeeding, but at least one source does not recommend breastfeeding as low concentrations of the drug are secreted into human milk (Mosby, 2003).

Notes: This medication is metabolized in the liver. It has a many drug interactions, which should be checked as soon as possible. This medication is not as effective as magnesium sulfate in the prevention of eclamptic seizures and should only be used for this when magnesium is not available or contraindicated.

Mechanism of action: Dilantin reduces the flux of sodium, calcium, and potassium across neuronal membranes.

Magnesium Sulfate

Other Names:	N/A
Indications:	Seizure prophylaxis with pre-eclampsia, treatment of eclampsia
Contraind:	Myasthenia gravis
Dosage:	Prophylaxis = 4-6 gram bolus over 15-20 minutes, then 2 gm/hour

Eclampsia = 6 grams over 15-20 minutes followed by 2 gm/hr as a continuous infusion

Dosage Interval: prophylaxis = Continuous infusion

Eclampsia = continuous infusion

Route of Admin: IM/IV

Adverse Rxns: Respiratory depression, CNS depression, hypotension, muscle weakness.

(See Chapter 14—Magnesium Sulfate Toxicity)

Breastfeeding: Compatible with breastfeeding

Notes: See Chapter 14 for a discussion of preeclampsia/eclampsia. If given IV, the onset of action is within seconds, if IM the onset is approximately 1 hour. Because of this, the medication is rarely given IM. For seizure prophylaxis, in the very rare situation that IV access is not continuously available, the following regiment may be given:

10 grams of a 50% magnesium sulfate solution into the buttocks

(5 grams into each buttocks)

Then

5 grams of a 50% magnesium sulfate solution into the buttocks every 4 hours after the initial IM doses.

Mechanism of action: Magnesium sulfate decreases neuromuscular conduction as well as the release of acetylcholine, and results in vasodilation as well. It is thought that its anticonvulsant properties are a result of a direct action on the cerebral cortex.

Hemorrhage

Carboprost

Other Names:	Hemabate, PGF-2alpha
Indications:	Postpartum hemorrhage due to uterine atony
Contraind:	Asthma
Dosage:	0.25mg
Dosage Interval:	0.25mg Q 15 minutes up to 8 doses
Route of Admin:	IM/into myometrium
Adverse Rxns:	Bronchoconstriction, fevers, chills, nausea, vomiting, diarrhea, pulmonary vasoconstriction
Breastfeeding:	This medication is generally used for the acute treatment of postpartum hemorrhage and is not usually continued after this.

Notes: This medication may be given after either a vaginal delivery or during a cesarean section for uterine atony. It may also be injected directly into the myometrium during a cesarean section. It is important to not administer this drug to patients with asthma as it may result in significant respiratory distress from bronchoconstriction.

Mechanism of action: This medication is 15-methyl-prostaglandin F2 alpha, which is a synthetic prostaglandin that stimulates the uterus to contract.

Methylergonovine

Other Names:	Methergine
Indications:	Postpartum hemorrhage
Contraind:	Hypertension, Preeclampsia/Eclampsia
Dosage:	0.2mg
Dosage Interval:	Q2-4 hours
Route of Admin:	IM
Adverse Rxns:	Hypertension, can cause fatal poisoning in patients sensitive to ergot alkaloids, chest pain, dizziness, tinnitus, diarrhea, palpitations, headache.
Breastfeeding:	May be used during breastfeeding. Small amount of the drug appears in the milk, but no adverse effects have been reported.

Notes: Remember not to give this to preeclamptics/hypertensive patients as it will increase blood pressure and may precipitate a hypertensive crisis or stroke. It should not be given as an IV bolus.

Mechanism of action: This medication induces uterine smooth muscle contractions, which allows the uterus to clamp down if it is atonic and hemorrhaging.

Misoprostol

Other Names:	Cytotec
Indications:	Postpartum hemorrhage, labor induction (SEE NEXT SECTION)
Contraind:	Asthma (causes bronchoconstriction), VBAC
Dosage:	Postpartum hemorrhage = 400-1000 mcg
Dosage Interval:	x 1 dose
Route of Admin:	per rectum for postpartum hemorrhage, (can be per vagina, but if there is significant bleeding it will come out too quickly)
Adverse Rxns:	Diarrhea, abdominal pain, nausea, fevers, chills
Breastfeeding:	Contraindicated per manufacturer instructions secondary to the potential for severe diarrhea in the infant.

Notes: This medication is a prostaglandin E analog that is given when uterine atony is the presumed cause of a postpartum hemorrhage.

Mechanism of action: This medication will is a prostaglandin E analog that stimulates uterine contractions.

Pitocin

Other Names:	Oxytocin
Indications:	Postpartum hemorrhage due to uterine atony, labor induction/augmentation
Contraind:	Contraindications to labor augmentation/induction
Dosage:	See Chapter 7 for dosing regiments
Dosage Interval:	Continuous IV drip
Route of Admin:	IV
Adverse Rxns:	Uterine hyperstimulation (with fetal distress possible), water intoxication with large doses for a prolonged period of time, postpartum atony

Breastfeeding: Because the half-life is so short, and it is only administered immediately postpartum, usually after delivery of the placenta, it does not create issues with breastfeeding.

Notes: Pitocin is a synthetic form of oxytocin, a natural hormone in the body. If it seems odd that this medication is given for postpartum atony, and this is a potential complication of the medication, don't worry. A prolonged induction with pitocin is a risk factor for postpartum atony (remember that the uterus is a muscle that can fatigue like any other muscle). The pitocin will stimulate the uterus to contract, which will hopefully correct uterine atony and bleeding. If it does not, then other medications/interventions are required. (See Chapter 14) When given for atony, no more than 30-40 units are added to 1 liter of crystalloids.

Mechanism of action: Oxytocin receptors are present in the uterus near term, and stimulation of these will cause the uterus to contract.

Labor Induction/Augmentation

Dinoprostone

Other Names: Prostin E2, Cervidil
Indications: Cervical ripening
Contraind: Previous cesarean section, hypersensitivity to prostaglandins, contraindications to labor induction
Dosage: dinoprostone gel = 0.5mg / 2.5 ml syringe
                   Cervidil vaginal insert = 0.3 mg/hr released
Dosage Interval: Usually single dose (vaginal insert left in place for 12 hours, gel may be repeated Q 6 hours for a maximum of three doses.)
Route of Admin: Vaginal
Adverse Rxns: Nausea, emesis, fevers
Breastfeeding: This medication is used for labor induction and is not a factor for the postpartum period.

Notes: If the dinoprostone gel is used, then the fetus must be continuously monitored for at least two hours. If the vaginal insert is placed, then the fetus must be monitored for as long as it is left in. Pitocin should not be given until 6-12 hours after the dose is given.

Mechanism of action: This drug is a synthetic prostaglandin that stimulates uterine contractions as well as "softens" the cervix to prepare it for labor. (See Chapter 7)

Misoprostol

Other Names: Cytotech
Indications: Labor induction, postpartum hemorrhage
Contraind: Asthma (causes bronchoconstriction), VBAC
Dosage: Labor induction = 25-50 mcg
Dosage Interval: Q4-6 hours
Route of Admin: per vagina, (can be rectal during postpartum hemorrhage)
Adverse Rxns: Diarrhea, abdominal pain, nausea, uterine hyperstimulation (with fetal distress)
Breastfeeding: Contraindicated per manufacturer instructions secondary to the potential for severe diarrhea in the infant (Drugs in Pregnancy and Lactation)

Notes: This medication is a prostaglandin E analog. The most common dosing regiment for labor induction is 25 mcg Q4-6 hours. This lower dose regiment decreases the incidence of uterine hyperstimulation that can occur. Additional doses should generally not be given if the patient is contracting more than 3 times in 10 minutes.

Mechanism of action: This medication is a prostaglandin E analog that stimulates uterine contractions.

Pitocin

Other Names: Oxytocin
Indications: Labor induction/postpartum hemorrhage
Contraind: Contraindication to labor induction, fetal distress
Dosage: 1-40 mIU/min for labor (see Chapter 7 for low and high dose options)
Dosage Interval: Continuous IV drip
Route of Admin: IV
Adverse Rxns: Uterine hyperstimulation (with fetal distress possible), water intoxication with large doses for a prolonged period of time, postpartum atony
Breastfeeding: Because the half-life is so short, and it is only administered immediately postpartum, usually after delivery of the placenta, it does not create issues with breastfeeding.

Notes: Pitocin is a synthetic form of oxytocin, a natural hormone in the body. It takes approximately 40 minutes to reach a steady state concentration, however, the half-life of pitocin is only 3-5 minutes, which is important to remember if you turn off the infusion as an intervention for fetal distress.

Mechanism of action: Oxytocin receptors are present in the uterus near term, and stimulation of these will cause the uterus to contract.

Tocolytics

Indomethacin

Other Names:	Indocin
Indications:	Preterm labor at < 32 weeks gestation
Contraind:	Aspirin allergy, Gestational age > 32 weeks
Dosage:	50 mg loading dose, followed by 25mg doses
Dosage Interval:	Q6 hours
Route of Admin:	PO/PR
Adverse Rxns:	Oligohydramnios, fetal renal failure
Breastfeeding:	This medication is used for tocolysis and is not a factor for the postpartum period.

Notes: This medication is given for no more than 48-72 hours secondary to the potential for oligohydramnios and fetal effects.

Mechanism of action: This medication is a prostaglandin synthesis inhibitor. It is thought to stop uterine contractions by inhibiting the synthesis of prostaglandins, which are implicated in causing contractions.

Magnesium Sulfate

Other Names:	N/A
Indications:	Preterm labor, seizure prophylaxis with pre-eclampsia, treatment of eclampsia
Contraind:	Myasthenia gravis
Dosage:	4-6 gram bolus, followed by 2-4 grams/hour
Dosage Interval:	Continuous IV drip
Route of Admin:	IV for preterm labor
Adverse Rxns:	Respiratory depression, CNS depression, hypotension, muscle weakness (See Chapter 14—Magnesium Sulfate Toxicity)
Breastfeeding:	Compatible with breastfeeding

Notes: See Chapter 14 for a discussion of preeclampsia/eclampsia. If given IV, the onset of action is within seconds, if IM the onset is approximately 1 hour. (Magnesium is almost never given IM for preterm labor.) These patients must be closely monitored to ensure they have adequate urine output (as magnesium sulfate is excreted by the kidneys) and for evidence of pulmonary edema or cardiovascular toxicity. If the patient's serum creatinine is > 1.3 mg/dL, then the continuous infusion dose (usually 2-4 grams/hour) should be cut in half and serum magnesium levels monitored closely.

Mechanism of action: Magnesium sulfate decreases neuromuscular conduction, decreases the release of acetylcholine, and results in vasodilation as well.

Nifedipine

Other Names: Procardia
Indications: Preterm labor/preterm contractions
Contraind: Hypotension
Dosage: 10-20 mg
Dosage Interval: Q4-6 hours
Route of Admin: PO
Adverse Rxns: Hypotension, edema, dizziness, nausea, pulmonary edema, reflex tachycardia
Breastfeeding: This medication is used for tocolysis and should not be a factor for the postpartum period.

Notes: This medication is often used for preterm contractions in the same situation as terbutaline. The side effects of nifedipine are often better tolerated than the tachycardia and palpitations that may occur with terbutaline.

Mechanism of action: This is a calcium-channel blocker. The theory behind this drug as a tocolytic is that by blocking the influx of calcium into the uterine muscle cells, it will decrease contractions, which are dependent on the calcium.

Terbutaline

Other Names: Brethine, Bricanyl
Indications: Tocolysis, uterine hyperstimulation
Contraind: Cardiac arrhythmias, myocardial ischemia or chest pain, pulmonary edema, Poorly controlled hyperthyroidism, Poorly controlled diabetes
Dosage: 0.125-0.25mg (intermittent IV/SQ dosing)

315

5-10 mcg/min (continuous IV)
2.5-5.0mg (PO)

Dosage Interval: IV drip = continuous
SQ or IV intermittent = Q3-4 hours
PO = Q4-6 hours

Route of Admin: IV/SQ/PO

Adverse Rxns: Hypotension, tachycardia, arrythmias, pulmonary edema, nausea, tremor, headache, myocardial ischemia

Breastfeeding: This medication is used for tocolysis and is not a factor for the postpartum period.

Notes: This medication is most often given SQ or IV for the initial evaluation of preterm labor or while intervening for fetal distress caused by uterine contractions, which can be stopped for a short period of time with this drug. It can also be given PO for maintenance tocolysis. It is not used as a continuous drip in many hospitals at this time. Sometimes a subcutaneous pump is used to delivery a more constant dose to patients requiring long-term tocolysis. The risk of pulmonary edema must always be kept in mind, especially with multiple gestations.

The SQ or IV doses of 0.125mg-0.25mg are used during labor when uterine hyperstimulation is present and immediate relaxation of the uterus is required because of fetal distress. In these cases, the IV route is preferred as the onset of action is much faster.

Mechanism of action: This is a B2 adrenergic agonist that decreases smooth muscle contractions through these actions. Although this medication is selective for the B2 receptors, B1 receptors in the heart are also stimulated which causes the tachycardia seen with its administration.

References:

Drugs in Pregnancy and Lactation: A reference guide to fetal and neonatal risk. 5th edition, Briggs GG, Freeman RK, Yaffe SJ eds, Lippincott Williams & Wilkins, 1998.

Goldenburg, RL. The management of preterm labor. Obstet Gynecol, Nov 2002; 100(5):1020-1037.

Mosby's Drug Consult. Nissen D, ed. Elsevier Science Company, 2003, www.mdconsult. com.

Prescribing reference for Obstetricians and Gynecologists, Fall-Winter 2002-2003, Murphy JL ed. Prescribing Reference, Inc. *www.PrescribingReference.com.*

Sharma SK, Sidawi JE, Ramin SM, Lucas MJ, Leveno KJ, Cunningham FG. Cesarean delivery: A randomized trial of epidural versus patient-controlled meperidine analgesia during labor. Anesthesiology 1997; 87:487-494.

Simhan H, Caritis S. Inhibition of preterm labor. Up To Date, Version 11.1, Dec 20.

Appendix A

Common Terms & Abbreviations

ACOG—American College of Obstetricians and Gynecologists

AROM—Artificial rupture of membranes

BPP—Biophysical profile

C/S—Cesarean section

CST—Contraction stress test

DIC—Disseminated intravascular coagulation

EBL—Estimated blood loss

EDC—Estimated date of confinement

EDD—Estimated date of delivery

FHR—Fetal heart rate

FHRT—Fetal heart rate tracing

FKC—Fetal kick counts

FM—Fetal movement

FSE—Fetal scalp electrode

Hydrocephalus—An increased amount of cerebrospinal fluid in the fetal brain

IM—Intramuscular

IUGR—Intrauterine growth restriction

IV—Intravenous

IUPC—Intrauterine pressure catheter

LF—Low forceps

LOA—Left occiput anterior

LOP—Left occiput posterior

LR—Lactated Ringers

Multiparous—Having previously delivered at least one baby.

MVUs—Montevideo units (used to determine strength/adequacy of contractions.)

Myomectomy—An operation during which myomas, or fibroids, are removed from the uterus. These can be subserosal, intramural, or submucosal.

NKDA—No known drug allergies

NRFHRT—Non—reassuring fetal heart rate tracing

NS—Normal Saline

NST—Non—stress test

NTTP—Non—tender to palpation

Nullipara—A gravid patient who has never delivered a baby.

OA—Occiput anterior

OF—Outlet forceps

OP—Occiput posterior

PRN—as needed

PROM—Premature rupture of membranes (occuring before the onset of labor)

PPROM—Preterm premature rupture of membranes (occuring before 37wks gestation)

RNST—Reactive NST

ROA—Right occiput anterior

ROM—Rupture of membranes

ROP—Right occiput posterior

SQ—Subcutaneous

SROM—Spontaneous rupture of membranes

SSE—Sterile speculum exam

STAT—Urgent priority

SVD—Spontaneous vaginal delivery

SVE—Sterile vaginal exam

VAC—Vacuum delivery

VTE—Venous Thromboembolic Event

WNL—Within normal limits

Appendix B

Sample Notes and Orders Notes

- Basic Principles
- Notes
    - Admission H&P
    - Cesarean Counseling Note
    - Delivery Note
        - Shoulder Dystocia Note
    - Labor Progress Note
    - Labor Intervention Note
    - Magnesium Sulfate Note
    - Operative Note (for Cesarean Section)
    - Postpartum Note
        - SVD
        - Cesarean Section
    - Vaginal Birth After Cesarean (VBAC) Counseling Note
- Orders
    - Admission Orders
    - Magnesium Sulfate Orders
    - Oxytocin Orders
    - Postoperative Orders
    - Postpartum Orders
    - Additional Orders for 3rd/4th Degree lacerations
- Dictation
    - Cesarean Section Dictation

SAMPLE NOTES

BASIC PRINCIPLES

1. Always label your notes with the date and time they are written. If you need to add any information later, always start a new note and notate the date and time. Do not go back in the chart to change information, it gives the appearance of hiding something, even when that is not the intention.
2. Write legibly. Nothing is defensible if it cannot be read.
3. Sign your name at the end of the note. If your signature is not legible, then print your last name after your signature.

Notes are generally in the **SOAP** format, which includes the following:

Subjective: This entails how the patient is feeling and what complaints or symptoms they are experiencing.

Objective: This is where you record the vital signs, fetal heart rate and contraction information, as well as laboratory data.

Assessment: Make an assessment on the condition of the fetus/maternal condition in a few sentences.

Plan: Outline a clear plan for each condition that needs to be addressed.

This format will give you an outline to clearly and consistently relay the maternal and fetal condition and what, if any, additional interventions need to occur.

In the notes contained here, when there are multiple options in parentheses, choose the most appropriate for the situation.

L&D Triage: Most hospitals have a standard form on which to triage patients who present to labor and delivery. The format will vary depending on the hospital forms. A triage note is essentially a mini-history and physical and your main goal is determine first if the patient and fetus are stable, and secondly, does the patient need to be admitted to the hospital. Always make sure that you have asked the following FOUR QUESTIONS:

- Are you having any **BLEEDING?**

- Are you having any **CONTRACTIONS?** (include time of onset/frequency/intensity)
- Do you feel like your broke you **WATER?** (include time/color of fluid)
- Have you felt your baby **MOVING?** (if not, then how long since the baby moved?)

You will insert the answers to these questions into your note. An example of this is shown in the Admission H&P note.

1. **Admission H&P:** Every patient that is admitted to L&D will need a complete history and physical exam. If you cannot locate the patient's regular chart, which happens all too often, you can get most everything you need by just talking to the patient. An exception to this is prenatal laboratory tests, which you will need and can obtain either by locating the chart or from the computer system if you hospital has one.

Basic Outline

S: The patient is a ____ y/o G__ P ____ at ____ wks by (Sure LMP/Unsure LMP/1st trimester US/2nd trimester US). She presents with a chief complaint of _____. (Contractions /ROM/Bleeding/etc.) She reports (Put answers to the **FOUR QUESTIONS** here).

Her prenatal course has been complicated by: _____.

PMH:
PSH:
OB:
GYN:
ALL:
SOC:
FAM:
MED: (include doses)

O: Pulse-   BP-   Temp-   RR-

FHRT- Baseline = ____ 's (130's, 150's, etc) with (increased/average/minimal/absent) variability and (accelerations/decelerations).

The FHRT is overall (reassuring/nonreassuring/ominous)

TOCO- Contractions are every _____ minutes and occurring (regularly/irregularly)

HEENT:
LUNGS:
HEART:
ABD:
EXT:
GU: V/V(vulva/vagina) -
    CVX (cervix)   - ___ / ___ / ___ (Effacement / Dilation / Station)

    EFW: _____ gms by (Leopold maneuvers/ultrasound)

    PRESENTATION: (Vertex/Breech/Transverse) by (Leopolds/ultrasound)

    Pelvis is (Adequate/Inadequate) by clinical pelvimetry

PRENATAL LABS: Hct-   Hgb-   Plt-
                Sickdex*-   UA-   GC/Chlam-
                HIV-   Hep B-   Blood Type-
                Rubella-   GBS*-   Antibody screen-
                Amnio*-   PAP-

                Rhogam given*: _____ (gestational age)

                *(include if applicable)

US EXAMS: Date: _____ GA by US = _____ GA by LMP = _____
                EFW = _____   Abnormalities = _____

A: Pt is a ___ y/o G___P___ at ___ + ___ weeks with the following issues:

    1) _____ (List diagnoses, such as, Latent labor, Active labor, presents for)
    2) _____ (labor induction, with preeclampsia, etc.)

P: 1) Admit to labor and delivery

2) Continuous fetal monitoring

3) _____ (address each diagnosis above here. See example note)

Admission H&P Example

S: The patient is a 25 y/o G4P2012 at 38+2 wks by sure LMP and 1st trimester US. She presents with a chief complaint of regular uterine contractions since 0600 this morning

She reports RUC's every 5 minutes

She denies any vaginal bleeding

She denies any ROM

She reports good FM.

Her prenatal course has been complicated by her Rh negative status and mild asthma for which she was treated with Proventil inhalers prn this pregnancy without problems.

PMH: Asthma since age 14, no history of intubations/hospitalizations.

PSH: Appendectomy at age 12, D&C at age 21.

OB: 1996—SVD at term, 7lb 8oz male, uncomplicated

1998—first trimester SAB with a D&C

2000—SVD at term, 8lb 0oz female, uncomplicated

2002—current pregnancy

GYN: Reg menses since age 13, No history of STD/PID, No abnormal PAPs

ALL: Percocet (Nausea/Vomiting/Hives)

SOC: Denies tobacco/ETOH/illicit drug use

FAM: No family h/o DM/HTN/Cancer

MED: PNV 1 Tab QD

Proventil MDI Q4hr prn (has only required this approximately 1x/month)

O: Pulse—77   BP—125/87   Temp—98.7F   RR—12

FHRT—Baseline = 140's with average variability and accelerations. RNST.

The FHRT is overall reassuring

TOCO—Contractions are every 3-4 minutes and regular.

HEENT: WNL

LUNGS: CTA B with no expiratory wheezes noted.
HEART: RRR with normal S1/S2
ABD: Gravid, Uterus is NTTP
EXT: NTTP, 1+ bilateral pedal edema with no cords palpable
GU: V/V(vulva/vagina) : Normal vaginal discharge, no lesions noted.
CVX (cervix) : 75/4/-1

EFW: 3800 gms by Leopold maneuvers
PRESENTATION: Vertex by Leopolds

PRENATAL LABS: Hct—33.5%   Hgb—11.0   Plt—256
Sickdex—n/a   UA—neg   GC/Chlam—neg
HIV—neg   Hep B—neg   Blood Type—A neg
Rubella—immune   GBS—neg   Antibody screen—neg
Amnio—n/a

Rhogam given: 28+2 weeks

US EXAMS: Date: 1/3/02 GA by US = 11+3wks GA by LMP = 11+0wks
EFW = n/a   Abnormalities = none

Date: 3/7/02 GA by US = 20+1wks GA by LMP = 20+0wks
EFW = 330gms   Abnormalities = none

A: The patient is a 25 y/o G4P2012 at 38+2 wks with the following issues:

1. Patient is in active labor
2. Reassuring FHRT
3. Asthma—well-controlled this pregnancy with prn inhalers and no history of prior intubations or hospitalizations for this.

P: 1. Labor

- Admit to labor and delivery
- Manage labor, no augmentation required at this time.

2. Continuous fetal monitoring
3. Asthma

- Check pulse ox now
- Use proventil MDI as needed
- Will ensure no hemabate given for uterine atony.

2. **Cesarean counseling note:**

   Basic outline

   The patient was counseled by me regarding our recommendation to proceed with a cesarean section for the following indication: _____.

   Risks and benefits of the procedure were discussed. These included, but were not limited to:

   - Hemorrhage with the need for transfusion of blood products
   - Risk of adverse reaction or infection from blood products, should they be required, including adverse reaction to the transfusion or infection with HIV/Hepatitis/other infections
   - Infection after the procedure requiring intravenous antibiotics
   - Damage to bowel, bladder, or other abdominal organs with need for further surgery to repair/remove damaged organs
   - *Need to remove the uterus if severe bleeding encountered which would preclude any future childbearing
   - Risk of maternal death

   The patient and her spouse verbally acknowledged that they understood the indication for the procedure, as well as the risks and benefits.

   The consent form was signed, witnessed, and placed on the chart.

   * Note: This sounds extreme, and the last part probably even obvious, but needs to be spelled out clearly in case there are complications.

3. **Delivery note:** If you think of a delivery note as a narrative of how the delivery occurred, it will be easier to remember all the essential elements. This note should be written after every vaginal delivery (both spontaneous and operative).

Basic Outline

The patient progressed to C/C/+____ (+1/+2/+3 or at whatever station they began to push) and with good maternal effort delivered a liveborn (male/female) infant over an (intact perineum/midline episiotomy/mediolateral episiotomy) with APGARS of ____/____.

The infant presented in the (OA/OP/LOA/LOP/ROA/ROP) position. After delivery of the head, the mouth was (bulb suctioned/Delee suctioned) and allowed to spontaneously restitute.

No nuchal cord was present/A loose nuchal cord was manually reduced/A tight nuchal cord was surgically reduced.

The anterior then posterior shoulders delivered without difficulty (or if there is a shoulder dystocia, see the example below for how to document this). The rest of the body delivered easily and the normal 3-vessel cord was clamped x 2 and cut and the infant (placed on the maternal abdomen/handed to the nurses/pediatricians for baby care).

The placenta delivered (spontaneously/by manual extraction) and inspection of the placenta demonstrated that it was (intact/fragmented). The cord insertion appeared (normal, velamentous, circumvallate, etc).

The uterus was cleared of all clots and debris. The cervix was inspected and (lacerations/no lacerations) were noted. The sidewalls were inspected and (lacerations/no lacerations) were noted. The perineum was inspected with findings of (describe any lacerations or extension of the episiotomy here).

Describe how each laceration, if any, was repaired including the type of suture used.

Uterine tone was noted to be (adequate/poor) after delivery. Pitocin was administered as per protocol and the patient required (no additional uterotonics/list specific medications if required) after delivery. The patient remained stable during and after the delivery.

EBL for the delivery was _____ cc.

Delivering physicians: _____ (Staff), _____ (Resident)

Delivery Note Example

The patient progressed to C/C/+2 and with good maternal effort delivered a liveborn male infant over a midline episiotomy with APGARS of 8/9.

The infant presented in the OA position. After delivery of the head, the mouth was bulb suctioned and allowed to spontaneously restitute.

A loose nuchal cord x 1 was manually reduced without difficulty.

The anterior then posterior shoulders delivered without difficulty. The rest of the body delivered easily and the normal 3-vessel cord was clamped x 2 and cut and the infant was placed on the maternal abdomen.

The placenta delivered spontaneously and inspection of the placenta demonstrated that it was intact. The cord insertion appeared normal.

The uterus was cleared of all clots and debris. The cervix was inspected and no lacerations were noted. The sidewalls were inspected and no lacerations were noted. The perineum was inspected with findings of extension of the midline episiotomy into the anal sphincter with no evidence of involvement of the rectal mucosa.

The anal sphincter was repaired with figure-of-eight sutures of 2-0 vicryl without difficulty. The remaining laceration was repaired in the standard fashion also using 2-0 vicryl suture. A digital rectal exam after the repair demonstrated no sutures in the rectum.

Uterine tone was noted to be adequate after delivery. Pitocin was administered as per protocol and the patient required no additional uterotonics. The patient remained stable during and after the delivery.

EBL for the delivery was 400 cc.

Delivering physicians: Joe Smith (Staff), Josephine Smith (Resident)

Shoulder Dystocia Example Addendum*:

*(insert this after the part of the note describing the delivery of the fetal head. Insert a description of additional maneuvers as needed. *Make sure* you indicate which shoulder was anterior and how long it took to deliver the shoulder.)

After delivery of the fetal head, which presented in the _____ position, and bulb-suctioning of the mouth and nares, with appropriate downward traction in the standard fashion, the anterior shoulder (left shoulder/right shoulder) did not deliver spontaneously. At this time, additional staff, including pediatrics, was requested, and McRoberts position employed, along with suprapubic pressure. With these maneuvers, the anterior shoulder delivered, followed by the posterior shoulder and the rest of the infant. The normal 3-vessel cord was clamped x 2 and cut and the infant handed to pediatrics. The infant was noted to be moving both arms and had no bruising noted. The time from delivery of the fetal head to delivery of the shoulders was 30 seconds.

4. **Labor progress note:** This is a note that you will write whenever you check on a patient during labor to determine how they are progressing.

Basic Outline

S: Patient reports feeling _____ with (adequate/marginal/inadequate) pain control.

O: Pulse-   BP-   Temp-   RR-

FHRT- Baseline = _____ 's (130's, 150's, etc) with (increased/average/minimal/absent) variability and (accelerations/decelerations).

The FHRT is overall (reassuring/nonreassuring/ominous)

TOCO- Contractions are every _____ minutes and occurring (regularly/irregularly)

Cervical Exam: ___/___/___ (Effacement/Dilation/Station)

Fetal head position is: ____ (OA/OP/ROA/ROP/LOA/LOP)

Medications: Pitocin is at ____ miu/min (if patient is on pitocin)
Antibiotics (i.e. Ampicillin 2gm IV Q6)
Other medications

A: ____ y/o G__P_____ at ____ + ____ weeks in labor.

Labor is (progressing appropriately/protracted)

The FHRT is (reassuring/nonreassuring/ominous)

P: Continue to monitor labor progress and intervene as needed. (or list intervention if not progressing appropriately)

Continue to monitor FHRT (or list intervention is not reassuring) and anticipate SVD.

Labor Progress Example

S: Patient reports feeling well with adequate pain control.

O: Pulse—95   BP—130/75   Temp—98.8F   RR—10

FHRT—Baseline = 140's with average variability and intermittent mild variable decelerations with spontaneous recovery

The FHRT is overall reassuring.

TOCO—Contractions are every 5 minutes and occurring regularly

Cervix—90%/5/-1

Fetal head position = LOA

Medications: Pitocin is at 6 miu/min
PCN G 2.5million units IV Q4

A: 27 y/o G3P1011 at 38 + 2 weeks in active labor.

Labor is progressing appropriately

The FHRT is overall reassuring with mild variable decelerations.

P: Continue to monitor labor progress and continue with pitocin.

Will place IUPC and start amnioinfusion for variable decelerations.

Continue to monitor FHRT and anticipate SVD.

5. Labor/Fetal Intervention note:

Basic Outline

S: Went to see patient secondary to _____ (FHR decelerations, bradycardia, complaint of SROM, complaint of increasing pain)

O: Pulse-   BP-   Temp-   RR-

FHRT: Baseline = _____ 's (130's, 150's, etc) with (increased/average/minimal/absent) variability and (accelerations/decelerations).

The FHRT is overall (reassuring/nonreassuring/ominous)

TOCO—Contractions are every ____ minutes and occurring (regularly/ irregularly)

Cervical Exam: ____/____/____ (Effacement/Dilation/Station)

Fetal head position is: _____ (OA/OP/ROA/ROP/LOA/LOP)

*Interventions taken: AROM performed with clear fluid/thin meconium/ moderate meconium/thick meconium.

Internal monitors placed (IUPC/FSE)
Terbutaline 0.25mg IV given x 1
O2 by facemask administered to mother
Maternal position changed to side, knee-chest, etc

FHR recovered after _____ minutes.

A: ____ y/o G__P_____ at ____ + ____ weeks in labor with the following issues:

Labor is (progressing appropriately/protracted)

FHRT is overall reassuring/nonreassuring/ominous with

Variable decelerations/Late decelerations/accelerations/ and

Increased/average/decreased/absent variability.

P: Continue to monitor labor progress and intervene as needed.

Continue to monitor FHRT (if overall reassuring)

Labor/Fetal Intervention for Distress Example

S: Went to see patient secondary to FHR deceleration to the 80's.

O: Pulse-   100   BP-   110/78   Temp—99.0F   RR—12

FHRT: Baseline = 130's with average variability prior to deceleration.

TOCO—Contractions are every 2 minutes and occurring regularly

Cervical Exam: C/6/0

Fetal head position is: ROA

Interventions taken: -   Pitocin (prev at 10miu/min) stopped.
                        -    AROM performed with clear fluid noted.
                        -    Internal monitors placed (IUPC/FSE)
                        -    Terbutaline 0.25mg IV given x 1
                        -    O2 by facemask administered to mother
                        -    Maternal position changed to side, knee-chest, etc

With the above interventions, the FHR recovered back to a baseline of 120's-130's and average variability.

A: 22 y/o G1P0 at 37 + 0 weeks in labor with the following issues:

Labor is progressing appropriately.

S/P variable deceleration which responded to conservative measures. FHRT is currently reassuring.

P: Continue to monitor labor progress and intervene as needed. Will continue to hold pitocin at this time and monitor. Consider restarting in approximately 30 minutes if FHRT continues to be reassuring.

Continue to closely monitor FHRT.

Labor/Fetal Intervention for Pain Control Example

S: Went to see patient secondary to complaint of feeling increased pain with contractions. Patient requesting additional pain relief.

O: Pulse—105   BP—114/88   Temp—98.9F   RR—14

FHRT: Baseline = 120's with average variability and no decelerations

The FHRT is overall reassuring.

TOCO—Contractions are every 4-5 minutes and occurring regularly

Cervical Exam: C/5/0

Fetal head position is: LOA

A: 32 y/o G3P2002 at 40 + 2 weeks in labor with the following issues:

- Labor is progressing appropriately.
- FHRT is overall reassuring.
- Increased pain with contractions.

P: After discussing options for pain control with patient, she desires an epidural. Will contact anesthesia to see patient.

Continue to monitor labor progress and intervene as needed.

Continue to monitor FHRT (if overall reassuring)

6. **Magnesium Sulfate Note:** In general, when patients are on magnesium sulfate, it will be for either tocolysis because of preterm labor, or for seizure prophylaxis for preeclampsia. It is important to check on these patients approximately every 2-3 hours to ensure that they do not have signs/sx of magnesium toxicity and good urine output (since it is excreted by the kidneys).

Basic Outline

S: The patient reports feeling _____. She denies any (bleeding/ROM) She also denies any (Shortness of breath/Chest pain/Nausea/Vomiting/Visual changes/Blurry vision) Pt does currently complain of (Shortness of breath/Chest pain/Nausea/Vomiting/Blurry vision)*

O: Pulse-   BP-   Temp-   RR-

Urine output = ____ cc/hour over the past 2 hours

FHRT: Baseline = _____ 's (130's, 150's, etc) with (increased/average/minimal/absent) variability and (accelerations/decelerations).

The FHRT is overall (reassuring/nonreassuring/ominous)

TOCO—Contractions are every ____ minutes and occurring (regularly/ irregularly)

LUNGS: (check for evidence of pulmonary edema, crackles)
HEART: (ensure regular rate, rhythm)
EXT: (check DTR's in upper/lower extremities)

Cervix: (only perform if the patient is in labor. It is not necessary for patients on magnesium sulfate for PTL to check their cervix with every 2-hour note.)

Current Mag dose: _____ grams/hour

Mag level: _____ at _____ (time)

A: ____ y/o G__P_____ at ____ + ____ weeks receiving magnesium sulfate at ____ gms/hour for (seizure prophylaxis/preterm labor) currently (with/without) evidence of magnesium toxicity.

P: (If stable without signs of toxicity) Continue magnesium sulfate at current dose and continue to monitor.

(If unstable or with signs of toxicity then take appropriate measures such as decreasing or stopping the infusion and/or administering calcium gluconate. See Chapter 14)

* Note: It is important to know what the normal side effects of magnesium sulfate are, as well as those that are potential signs of toxicity. See Chapter 14. Also, for patients who are being treated for preeclampsia, it is important to ask the following questions, which can be signs of worsening disease:

- Do you have a headache?
- Do you have any right upper quadrant pain?
- Are you seeing any flashing lights?

Magnesium Sulfate Note Example

S: The patient reports feeling relatively well. She denies any bleeding/ROM. She also denies any Shortness of breath/Chest pain/Nausea/Vomiting. Pt does currently complain of some blurry vision and hot flushes.

O: Pulse—80   BP—120/68   Temp—98.5F   RR—10

Urine output = 60cc/hour over the past 2 hours

FHRT: Baseline = 140's with decreased variability, no decels, and accelerations.

The FHRT is overall reassuring.

TOCO—Contractions are every 10 minutes and occurring irregularly. They have decreased in frequency over the past two hours.

LUNGS: CTA B
HEART: RRR with normal S1/S2
EXT: DTR's 2+ upper and lower extremities

Current Mag dose: 3 grams/hour

A: 38 y/o G2P0010 at 32+2 weeks receiving magnesium sulfate at 3 gms/hour for preterm labor currently without evidence of magnesium toxicity.

P: Will continue magnesium sulfate at current dose and continue to monitor closely for signs/symptoms of toxicity. If contractions continue to decrease, will consider decreasing dose of magnesium sulfate.

7. **Operative note:** An operative note is done after a cesarean delivery. Make sure that under procedure, you specify the type of uterine incision, i.e. low transverse

cesarean section, low vertical cesarean section, classical cesarean section, as these all have implications for future deliveries. (See Chapter 10)

Basic Outline

*(memory aid: P^3 SSAAFFE UDC^3)

Preop Dx:
Postop Dx:
Procedure:
Surgeons: _____ (Staff), _____ (Resident), _____ (Med Student)
Specimens:
Anesthesia:
Antibiotics:
Findings:
Fluids:
EBL:
UO:
Drains:
Complications:
Condition:
Count:

Cesarean Section Example

Preop Dx: Term IUP at 37+5 weeks, Arrest of Dilation
Postop Dx: SAA
Procedure: LTCS
Surgeons: _____ (Staff), _____ (Resident), _____ (Med Student)
Specimens: Placenta to pathology, Cord gases
Anesthesia: Epidural
Antibiotics: Cefazolin 2gm IV at cord clamp
Findings: Liveborn male infant w/APGARS 8/9, WT = 3560gms
Fluids: 1200cc LR
EBL: 850cc
UO: 400cc clear, yellow urine
Drains: Foley to gravity
Complications: None
Condition: Stable to recovery room
Count: Sponge, needle, instrument count correct x 2

8. Postpartum Notes:

Basic Outline

S: The patient reports feeling _____ this morning. She has had (minimal/ average/heavy) lochia overnight using approximately one pad every ____ hours. She describes her pain as (well-controlled, marginally controlled, poorly controlled.) She denies any (nausea/vomiting/fevers/chills) overnight and tolerated a (regular/clear liquid) diet. She (is/is not) able to urinate with minimal discomfort and (has/has not) ambulated overnight.

    The patient is (breastfeeding/bottle-feeding) and the infant is feeding (well/poorly) and otherwise doing (well/having issues being addressed by the pediatricians.*)

O: Pulse-   BP-   Tcurr-   Tmax-   RR-

HEART:
LUNGS:
BREASTS: (Lactating/engorged/note any erythema or infection)
ABD: Uterus is (firm/soft) at U (+/- 1, 2, 3 . . . See Chapter 2)
GU: (This is generally only if there is a specific complaint or the patient had a significant laceration and repair.)
EXT:
Labs: (note if any labs drawn)
Meds: (note medication/dosage/route/schedule)
Rubella: (immune/nonimmune)
Rh: (positive/negative)

A: ____ y/o G__P_____ postpartum day # ____ with the following issues:

- Lochia is currently (appropriate/heavy)
- Pain control is currently (adequate/inadequate)
- (Note other issues such as fevers, nausea, etc)

P: - Continue to monitor lochia (or order a CBC if it is extremely heavy)
      - Continue current medications for pain (or additional meds as needed)

- Continue routine postpartum care
- (Address other issues here)

* Note: If the baby is having problems, note exactly what these issues are in the chart.

Postpartum SVD Note Example

S: The patient reports feeling well this morning. She has had average lochia overnight using approximately one pad every 4-5 hours. She describes her pain as well-controlled on ibuprofen. She denies any nausea/vomiting/fevers/chills overnight and tolerated a regular diet without difficulty. She is able to urinate with minimal discomfort and has ambulated overnight.

The patient is breastfeeding and the infant is feeding well and being seen by the pediatricians for some mild jaundice.

O: Pulse—90   BP—127/87   Tcurr—98.7F   Tmax—99.0F   RR—12

HEART: RRR
LUNGS: CTA B
BREASTS: Lactating with no evidence of infection
ABD: Uterus is firm at U—1
GU: Episiotomy repair intact without erythema or evidence of infx
EXT: NTTP, trace bilateral LE edema

Labs: none pending

Meds: Ibuprofen 800mg PO Q8

Rubella: nonimmune
Rh: positive

A: 21 y/o G1P1001 postpartum day # 2 with the following issues:

- Lochia is currently appropriate
- Pain control is currently adequate
- Patient is rubella non-immune
- Pt is currently doing well

P: - Continue to monitor lochia
         - Continue current medications for pain
         - Continue routine postpartum care
         - Ensure patient receives rubella vaccine prior to discharge

Postpartum Cesarean Note Example

S: The patient reports feeling well this morning. She has had minimal lochia overnight using approximately one pad every 6 hours. She describes her pain as marginally controlled at this time. She has taken one percocet overnight for pain. She denies any nausea, vomiting, fevers, or chills and tolerated ice chips overnight. She currently has a foley catheter in place. She also denies any lightheadedness/dizziness. She has not been up to ambulate yet.

The patient is bottle-feeding and the infant is doing well.

O: Pulse—88   BP—124/76   Tcurr—99.0F   Tmax—99.2F   RR—12

Urine output = 800 cc overnight (='s 66cc/hr)

HEART:	RRR
LUNGS:	CTA B
BREASTS:	Lactating without any erythema or evidence of infection
ABD:	Uterus is firm at U, incision is C/D/I without erythema or drainage
	Abdomen is nondistended and appropriately tender to palpation with no rebound/guarding. Normoactive bowel sounds.
GU:	Deferred
EXT:	NTTP

Labs:	Preop Hct = 34.6 Postop Hct = 27.8

Meds:	Percocet 1-2 tab PO Q4-6 hours prn
	Motrin 800mg PO Q8 hours

Rubella:	immune
Rh:	positive

A: 36 y/o G3P2012 postop day # 1 with the following issues:

- Lochia is currently appropriate
- Patient is hemodynamically stable (adequate UO, stable VS, approp Hct)
- Pain control is currently poor, but patient has not taken full doses of her current meds.
- No evidence of infection at this time.

P: - Continue to monitor for bleeding/infection
- D/C foley catheter, will check DTV in 4-6 hours
- Continue current medications for pain, giving two additional percocet now, and then ensure patient takes ibuprofen on schedule and does not get behind on her pain control.
- Continue routine postoperative care.
- Pt to ambulate today with assistance
- Advance diet to clears/regular as tolerated.

9. VBAC Counseling Note:

The patient is a ___y/o G_P_ at ___wks by ___. She had a previous cesarean section for ___ and this was documented as a ___ (low transverse cesarean section/low vertical cesarean section). She currently desires to attempt a vaginal delivery with this pregnancy.

Patient was counseled regarding the potential risks and complications of a VBAC to include but not limited to uterine rupture with fetal distress and the need for an emergent cesarean section. Risks of this complication include bleeding, transfusion, hysterectomy, and poor fetal outcome. She also understands that there is a chance she will require a cesarean section during labor for normal obstetric indications. The patient verbalized understanding that she has the option to have a repeat cesarean section at this time and that she understands the potential risks and desires to proceed with VBAC attempt.

VBAC Counseling Note Example:

The patient is a 34y/o G2P1 at 38+0wks by LMP and 8wk sonogram who presents with SROM that occurred at approximately 0530 today. She had a previous cesarean section for a breech presentation and this was documented as a low transverse cesarean section. She currently desires to attempt a vaginal delivery with this pregnancy.

Patient was counseled regarding the potential risks and complications of a VBAC to include but not limited to uterine rupture with fetal distress and the need for an emergent cesarean section. Risks of this complication include bleeding, transfusion, hysterectomy, and poor fetal outcome. She also understands that there is a chance she will require a cesarean section during labor for normal obstetric indications. The patient verbalized understanding that she has the option to have a repeat cesarean section at this time and that she understands the potential risks and desires to proceed with VBAC attempt.

SAMPLE ORDERS

1. **Admission orders:** Anytime a patient is admitted to labor and delivery, they will require orders so the nurses know what you want done for them.

   *(memory aid: ADC VAN DIMFL)

   - Admit: Admit to labor and deliver. Attending is _____
   - Diagnosis: (Term IUP in labor/PTL/PROM/SROM/etc)
   - Condition: (Stable/Unstable/Critical)
   - Vital signs: As per protocol
   - Allergies: Specify allergies (NKDA if none)
   - Nursing: Notify MD for Temp > 100.4F
     - SBP > 140 < 90
     - DBP > 90 < 50
     - Pulse > 105
   - Diet: (NPO/Clear liquids/Regular diet/etc)
   - IVF: LR or NS at 125cc/hr (if the patient is NPO)
   - I/O's: (This is not usually required for most patients unless they are on magnesium sulfate or postop)
   - Medications: Antibiotics if GBS positive, evidence of chorioamnionitis, or other indications.
   - Fetal Monitoring: (Continuous FHR monitoring/Continuous TOCO)
   - Labs: Type and Screen, CBC

   Sample Admission orders:

   - Admit: Admit to labor and deliver. Attending is Dr. Smith
   - Diagnosis: Term IUP in labor
   - Condition: Stable
   - Vital signs: As per protocol
   - Allergies: Clindamycin—Hives
   - Nursing: Notify MD for Temp > 100.4F
     - SBP > 140 < 90
     - DBP > 90 < 50
     - Pulse > 105
   - Diet: Clear liquids
   - IVF: Heplock
   - I/O's: N/A
   - Medications: Penicillin G 5 million units IV now, then 2.5 million units IV

Q4 hours during labor for GBS prophylaxis.
- Fetal Monitoring: Continuous FHR monitoring/Continuous TOCO
- Labs: Type and Screen, CBC

2. Magnesium Sulfate orders

For preeclampsia:

- Start magnesium sulfate infusion now with 6 grams IV over 20 minutes followed by continuous infusion of 2 grams/hour.
- Please place foley catheter
- Strict I/O's
- Notify M.O. for urine output of < 30cc/hour
- VS as per protocol
- Continuous fetal monitoring

For tocolysis:

- Start magnesium sulfate infusion now with (4 or 6) grams IV over 20 minutes followed by continuous infusion of (2-4) grams/hour.
- Please place foley catheter
- Strict I/O's
- Notify M.O. for urine output of < 30cc/hour
- VS as per protocol
- Continuous fetal monitoring

3. Pitocin orders

Low-dose protocol:

- Please start pitocin at 1mU/min, may increase dose by 2 mU/min every 30 minutes to a maximum of 40mU/min.
- If uterine hyperstimulation or fetal distress present, notify physician and stop pitocin infusion.
- Continuous FHR monitoring
- Continuous TOCO monitoring

High-dose protocol:

- Please start pitocin at 6mU/min, may increase dose by 6 mU/min every 20 minutes to a maximum of 42mU/min.

- If uterine hyperstimulation or fetal distress present, notify physician and stop pitocin infusion.
- Continuous FHR monitoring
- Continuous TOCO monitoring

Resuming high-dose pitocin after uterine hyperstimulation

- May restart pitocin at half of dose it was being given when stopped.
- May increase pitocin dose by 3mU/min every 20-40 minutes to a maximum of 42mU/min.
- If uterine hyperstimulation or fetal distress present, notify physician and stop pitocin infusion.

4. **Postoperative orders**

- Admit: Transfer to recovery
- Diagnosis: S/P Cesarean section
- Vital signs: As per protocol
- Allergies: Specify allergies (NKDA if none)
- Nursing: Foley catheter to gravity
                  Strict I/O's
- Diet: NPO
- IVF: Lactated Ringers at _____ cc/hr (normal rate is approx 125cc/hr)
- Meds: (antibiotics, pain medications*)
- Labs: CBC in AM

- Notify M.O. for: Temp > 100.4F
                     SBP >140 < 90
                     DBP > 90 < 50
                     Pulse > 105
                     Urine Output < 30cc/hr

* Note: Pain medication immediately postop will usually either be covered by the anesthesiologist with a longer-acting medication in an epidural, or with a PCA (patient-controlled anesthesia) device. Check with your institution as far as whose responsibility it is to order PCAs.

5. **Postpartum orders**

- Admit: Transfer to postpartum when stable
- Diagnosis: S/P SVD

- Vital signs: As per protocol
- Allergies: Specify allergies (NKDA if none)
- Nursing: Foley catheter to gravity (if in place)
   Strict I/O's
- Diet: NPO
- IVF: Lactated Ringers at _____ cc/hr (normal rate is approx 125cc/hr)
- Meds:
- Labs: CBC in AM
- Notify M.O. for: Temp > 100.4F
   SBP >140 < 90
   DBP > 90 < 50
   Pulse > 105
   Urine Output < 30cc/hr

6. **Additional orders for patients with 3rd/4th degree lacerations**

- Ice pack to perineum x 24-48 hours
- Stool softeners (see what your hospital carries, commonly colace)
- Sitz baths BID

DICTATION

Cesarean section dictation: It is important to dictate the operative note on a cesarean section as soon after the procedure as possible so that you remember exactly what you did, especially if anything was out of the ordinary routine.

Always start the dictation by stating your name (spelling it if necessary) and the patient's name and identification number:

"This is Dr. _____ dictating an operative report for patient _____, medical record number_____."

The rest of dictation, include the following information

Date of operation:
Preoperative diagnosis:
Postoperative diagnosis:
Procedure performed:
Surgeons:
Staff:
Anesthesia:
Estimated blood loss:
Intravenous fluids:
Urine output:

Fetal sex/weight:
Apgars
Antibiotics given:

Indications for procedure:

Procedure: This is where you will describe the procedure in detail.

After informed consent was obtained from the patient, she was taken to the operating room where an epidural/spinal/general anesthetic was administered. The FHR in the operating room was ＿＿ bpm prior to procedure. A foley catheter was then placed and the patient prepped and draped in the normal, sterile fashion. After anesthesia was determined to be adequate, a Pfannenstiel skin incision was made using a scalpel and the incision carried down to the underlying fascia, which was incised in the midline. The fascia was then incised in a curvilinear fashion on either side using mayo scissors. Two Kocher clamps were then used to grasp the anterior edge of the fascia and the rectus muscles were separated both sharply and bluntly from the fascia. The Kocher clamps were then placed on the inferior edges of the fascia and the muscles again dissected away from the fascia. The rectus muscles were then split bluntly in the midline and the peritoneum grasped between two Kelly clamps superiorly with care taken to avoid the bladder and bowel. After ensuring that the peritoneal window was clear, it was incised using Metzenbaum scissors and the abdomen entered. The peritoneal incision was sharply/bluntly extended and the bladder blade placed to provide exposure of the lower uterine segment. The vesicouterine fold was elevated using pickups and incised using Metzenbaum scissors. This incision was extended in a curvilinear manner in each direction. The bladder flap was then created bluntly without difficulty. A low transverse/low vertical/classical uterine incision was then made with a new scalpel and carried down in layers until the uterine cavity was entered. The incision was then extended bluntly/sharply with bandage scissors. The fetus presented in the vertex/breech/transverse position. The fetal vertex/buttocks was brought through the incision with appropriate fundal pressure and the infant was bulb-suctioned, the rest of the infant delivered and then the umbilical cord doubly clamped and cut and the infant handed off to pediatrics. APGARS were ＿＿ / ＿＿. The placenta was then manually removed/spontaneously expressed and the uterus cleared of all clots and debris. Good uterine tone was noted and the patient received prophylactic antibiotics. The uterus was exteriorized and the incision was repaired in one/two layers with 0-vicryl suture without difficulty and good hemostasis was noted. The uterus, fallopian tubes, and ovaries were visualized and were normal in appearance. The uterus was then replaced into the abdomen and the gutters cleared of all clots and debris. (*If the bladder flap or peritoneum is closed, then note this here) The uterine incision was again visualized and noted to be hemostatic. The fascia was then closed with two running sutures of 0-vicryl/PDS without difficulty. The subcutaneous tissue was then irrigated and good hemostasis obtained. The skin was then closed with staples/subcutaneous sutures using

4-0 vicryl/monocryl/etc. The incision was covered with a sterile dressing and all clots were expressed from the uterus. The patient was taken to the recovery room in stable condition. Sponge, needle, and instrument counts were correct x 2.

Example:

This is Dr. Jon Smith dictating operative report on patient Jane Doe, medical record 123-45-6789.

Date of operation: 12/12/02
Preoperative diagnosis: Intrauterine pregnancy at 39+5 weeks. Arrest of dilation
Postoperative diagnosis: Same as above
Procedure performed: Primary low transverse cesarean section
Surgeons: Jon Smith, Bill Smith (resident), Will Smith (medical student)
Staff: Jon Smith
Anesthesia: Epidural
Estimated blood loss: 1000cc
Intravenous fluids: 1500cc LR
Urine output: 400cc
Fetal sex/weight: Male/3500gms
Apgars: 9/9
Antibiotics given: Ancef 2gm

Indications for procedure: Pt is a 25y/o G1P0 at 39+5wks gestation who presented to labor and delivery in active labor. She progressed to C/7/0 and despite greater than 2 hours of adequate contractions as documented by an intrauterine pressure catheter, failed to make any further cervical change. The patient was counseled regarding conservative management versus a cesarean delivery, including the risks of bleeding, transfusion, infection, damage to the bowel/bladder, hysterectomy, and death and she and her partner verbalized understanding.

Procedure: After informed consent was obtained from the patient, she was taken to the operating room where an epidural was administered. The FHR in the operating room was 150 bpm without evidence of decelerations prior to procedure. A foley catheter was then placed and the patient prepped and draped in the normal, sterile fashion. After anesthesia was determined to be adequate, a Pfannenstiel skin incision was made using a scalpel and the incision carried down to the underlying fascia, which was incised in the midline. The fascia was then incised in a curvilinear fashion on either side using mayo scissors. Two Kocher clamps were then used to grasp the anterior edge of the fascia and the rectus muscles were separated both sharply and bluntly from the fascia. The Kocher clamps were then placed on the inferior edges of the fascia and the muscles again dissected away from the fascia. The rectus muscles were then split bluntly in the midline and the peritoneum grasped between two Kelly clamps superiorly with care taken to avoid the bladder and bowel. After ensuring that the peritoneal window was clear, it was incised using Metzenbaum scissors and the abdomen entered. The peritoneal incision was sharply extended and the bladder blade placed to provide exposure of the lower uterine segment. The vesicouterine fold was elevated using pickups and incised using Metzenbaum scissors. This incision was extended in a curvilinear manner in each direction. The bladder flap was then created bluntly without difficulty. A low transverse uterine incision was then made with a new scalpel and carried down in layers until the uterine cavity was entered. The incision was then extended bluntly. The fetus presented in the vertex position. The fetal vertex was brought through the incision with appropriate fundal pressure and the infant was bulb-suctioned and then the umbilical cord doubly clamped and cut and the infant handed off to pediatrics. APGARS were 8/9. The placenta was then spontaneously expressed and the uterus cleared of all clots and debris. Good uterine tone was noted and the patient received prophylactic antibiotics. The uterus was exteriorized and the incision was repaired in two layers with 0-vicryl suture without difficulty and good hemostasis was noted. The uterus, fallopian tubes, and ovaries were visualized and were normal in appearance. The uterus was then replaced into the abdomen and the gutters cleared of all clots and debris. The uterine incision was again visualized and noted to be hemostatic. The fascia was then closed with two running sutures of 0-vicryl without difficulty. The subcutaneous tissue was then irrigated and good hemostasis obtained. The skin was then closed with staples. The incision was covered with a sterile dressing and all clots were expressed from the uterus. The patient was taken to the recovery room in stable condition. Sponge, needle, and instrument counts were correct x 2.

Appendix C

Cesarean "Talk-through"

While you will probably assist on many cesarean sections before performing one, it is imperative that you know, without hesitation, the steps involved and how to perform each of them so that you are prepared when you do get the chance. When starting to learn about the procedure, it is helpful to "talk through" the operation in sequence, asking for instruments and verbalizing what steps you are taking. This will help engrain the procedure in your mind, make your staff more comfortable in the OR when they hear you say what you are going to do, and will make the operative dictation much easier.

If you pay attention to your attending in the OR before you do the procedure, you will find there are always some small variations, such as different sutures, or different ways to close certain layers. Make mental notes of these for when you operate with them. Do what your attending is comfortable with and, as you become more senior, decide what you think works best and incorporate it into your practice. The following is a practice walk-through in which you call for instruments and say what steps you are taking. (The bold lines are where you call for instruments. The italics indicate what you are saying and what you are doing.)

Please refer to the section at the end of this Appendix for figures of the common instruments used during a cesarean section.

* NOTE: The primary surgeon stands on the patient's right side by convention.

The patient is lying on the OR table with a left hip roll and the abdomen is prepped and the patient is draped. Before starting, check the following:

1. Bovie (electrocautery) is functioning and the patient has a grounding pad on her thigh.
2. The suction is on the field and functioning
3. Foley catheter is in place
4. Antibiotic prophylaxis has been ordered
5. The lights are focused on the area where the incision will be made
6. All necessary personnel (nurse, pediatricians, anesthesia, husband) are present or standing by.

- **"Allis clamp"**

- *"Testing anesthesia level"*: Clamp the skin at the planned incision line and by the umbilicus. If the patients anesthesia is adequate, this will not hurt. If it is not adequate, she will let the anesthesiologist know and you wait for them to correct this problem.

- **"Two laps"**   Place one laparotomy tape above the planned incision site and one below to provide traction and counter-traction as you make you incision.

- **"Scalpel"**   This will usually be a # 10 Blade

- *"Start time"*   Say this as you make your incision so the nurse can note it

- *"Making incision to fascia"*   After getting through the skin, concentrate on the middle 6-8cm of the incision and go down to the fascia

- *"Scoring fascia"*   Score the fascia on either side of the midline so you can see the rectus muscles

- **"Pickups w/teeth & Mayo scissors"**

- *"Extending fascial incision"*   Do this by lifting up with your pickups, then incising with your Mayo scissors (tips up!)

- **"Two Kocher clamps"**

- *"Placing clamps on*   Place one clamp on the superior edge of the fascia *anterior fascia"*   on either side of the midline and lift up for exposure.

- **"Mayo scissors"**

- *"Dissecting fascia from rectus"* This can be done both bluntly and with the Mayo scissors, incising the rectus muscle where it is attached in the midline to the fascia.

- *"Placing clamps on inferior fascia"* Place clamps on inferior edge of fascia, one on each side of midline

- *"Dissecting fascia*   Again, do this bluntly and sharply down to the pubic
  from rectus"   Symphysis, ask for Mayo scissors if needed.

- *"Removing clamps"*   Remove Kocher clamps and give them back to OR tech

- **"Two hemostats and Metzenbaum scissors"**

- *"Identify peritoneum"*   Identify peritoneum in midline, above the bladder, place the hemostats approximately 1cm apart and elevate them to ensure there is no bowel, bladder, or anything else below the area you are going to incise!

- *"Incising peritoneum"*   Make small incision in peritoneum with Metzenbaum scissors

- *"Extending peritoneal*   This can be done bluntly by stretching, or with
  incision"   Metzenbaum scissors

- **"Bladder blade and**   A Rich may also be called a Richardson retractor.
  large Rich retractor"

- *"Placing bladder*   Place the bladder blade so you can see the
  blade & Rich"   lower uterine segment and the large Rich superiorly so you have adequate visualization.

- **"Pickups and**   You should be more specific on the pickups
  Metzembaum Scissors" depending on what your institution carries. Either Russian or Debakey pickups are appropriate.

- *"Identifing bladder flap"* Identify the vesico-uterine fold where the bladder reflection is and elevate the serosa just above this in the midline. Make a curvilinear incision in both directions with scissors

- **"Kelly clamp"**

- *"Making bladder flap"* Clamp the Kelly onto the inferior edge of the incision and, with your fingers always on the uterus, push gently down to push the bladder away from the uterus

- *"Replacing bladder blade"* Place the bladder blade in between the bladder and the uterus, using the Kelly clamp for exposure

- *"Removing clamp"* Remove the Kelly clamp and hand back to the scrub tech

- *"Palpating uterus"* Palpate the uterus to determine if it is rotated significantly and find the midline where you will make your incision.

- **"Scalpel"**

- *"Uterine incision"* Make a small incision in the lower uterine segment above your bladder flap. After the first pass, palpate the incision and use suction to visualize the area. Make successive passes with care to NOT CUT THE BABY!. If you are going layer by layer, often the membranes will push out at some point.

- *"Extending uterine incision."* Extend the uterine incision superior-laterally in a curvilinear fashion by one of two methods:

  1) Call for "bandage scissors" and place your left hand inside the uterus between the scissors and the baby and extend the incision superiorly and laterally.
  2) Insert the index fingers at each corner and pull upwards in the same direction as you would cut with bandage scissors.

- *"Placing hand in uterus"*   Place your right hand into the uterus and grasp the infant's head.

- *"Remove bladder blade"*   Your assistant will remove the bladder blade to allow you more room for the fetal head.

- *"Fundal pressure"*   With this, your assistant will provide fundal pressure which will allow you to deliver the baby. You may also apply the fundal pressure with your left hand rather than your assistant. At the same time as fundal pressure is applied, elevate the fetal head through the incision with the right hand. Make sure and do not flex your wrist significantly during delivery as this can cause an unwanted extension of the uterine incision.

- **"Bulb suction"**

- "Suctioning baby"   Suction out the infants mouth and nares

- **"Kelly clamps x 2"**

- *"Clamping and cutting the cord."*   Doubly clamp and ligate the umbilical cord as you would during a vaginal delivery.

      * NOTE: This is the time to obtain an additional portion of the umbilical cord for gases if the situation warrants. i.e.—the cesarean was done for fetal distress or the fetus is very premature

- *"Baby to peds"*   Hand the infant to the waiting pediatrician.

- *"Delivering placenta"*   Provide moderate traction on the umbilical cord with the remaining Kelly clamp to deliver the placenta. If this does not work, then the placenta can be manually removed by inserting one hand into the uterus and finding the plane between the membranes and the uterus.

- **"Ring forceps"**

- *"Removing membranes"*   As the placenta comes out of the uterus, the membranes will trail and you will use the ring forceps to grasp them and help remove them.

- **"Wet and Dry lap"**

- *"Exteriorizing uterus"*   Grasp the fundus with the thumb and fingers of one hand and exteriorize the uterus. Wrap the fundus with the wet lap and use your left hand to provide traction.
  (See Chapter 10 for a discussion of this technique)

- *"Removing clots from uterus"*   Use the dry lap to clean out the interior of the uterus to make sure there are no membranes or clots left in the cavity.

- *"Checking uterine tone"*   As you clean out the uterus, ensure it clamps down appropriately so that hemorrhage from uterine atony does not occur. If the uterus will not firm up, you must take action to prevent hemorrhage. See Chapter 14.

- *"Please give pitocin"*   This lets the anesthesiologist know you would like pitocin, usually 20-30 units, placed into the patient's IV fluids to help with uterine tone.

- **"Bladder blade"**   Replace the bladder blade to keep the bladder away from your sutures as you repair the uterine incision.

- **"Ring Forceps"**
  or
  "Pennington clamp"   Use these to grasp each lateral angle of the incision. You may also use them to clamp off bleeding areas of the incision until you can incorporate them with your suture. You can also use an allis clamp for the angles

- *"Inspecting incision"*   Look at the incision to make sure you do not have an extension laterally into the uterine vessels or inferiorly into the cervix.

- **"Suture, 0-vicryl*"**   *This is a common suture used for uterine closure. Your staff may prefer chromic or another suture.

354

- *"Repairing uterine incision"* — Begin at the opposite side and close the incision sewing towards yourself. With the first bite, make sure you have palpated with your fingers laterally to where you are placing the suture to ensure you do not accidentally incorporate the uterine artery or ureter. This is a running, locked suture.

- **"Suture, 0-vicryl*"** — *Again, your staff may prefer chromic or another suture, and some staff do not place a second layer, although there is now data that suggests this is helpful and decreases the risk of uterine rupture.

- *"Placing imbrication layer"* — This is a method by which the initial uterine incision is oversewn and it can be done in either a horizontal or vertical fashion.

- *"Inspecting incision"* — After the uterine incision is closed, observe it to check for obvious bleeding. If there is significant bleeding from an area, call for a suture and repair it. If not, then proceed to the next step.

- *"Inspecting cul-de-sac" and anatomy."* — Push the uterus forwards and look into the cul-de-sac look for clots and debris. If there is a significant amount either, then use a lap to remove it. Look at the exterior of the uterus, ovaries, and fallopian tubes for any abnormalities that will need to be dictated in the operative report.

- *"Inspecting incision"* — Look again at the uterine incision to ensure there is no active bleeding. If there is, then call for a suture and repair it, otherwise, proceed to the next step.

- *"Replacing uterus"* — Remove the bladder blade, then turn the uterus at a slight angle and then place it back into abdominal cavity.

- **"Bladder blade"** — Replace the bladder blade and look at the incision again.

- **Medium Rich retractor, clean lap tape and** — Place the retractor at one corner of the incision under the peritoneum and retract upwards. The other person will then use either a clean lap,

irrigation"	irrigation, or both and clean out the lateral gutter on that side of the uterus. This is then repeated on the opposite side.
- *"Inspecting incision"*	Look one last time at your incision, especially the lateral angles, to ensure there is no significant bleeding.
- **"Medium Rich retractor, pickups with teeth, and 0-vicryl suture."**	Insert the retractor at one corner of the incision above the fascia and visualize the corner of the fascial incision. Use the pickups to grasp the angle and place your suture there. This is generally a simple running suture. Continue until you are approximately halfway then stop and tie. At this point, your assistant (the staff) will call for another suture and do the same on the opposite side.
- **"Irrigation and clean lap"**	Irrigate the subcutaneous tissue then place the lap sponge in the incision. As you remove the lap, look for bleeding in the subcutaneous tissue. If there is any, cauterize the area using your bovie.
- *"Is the count correct?"*	Ask this question as your circulating nurse should have either completed or at least started to recount all instruments, lap sponges, and needles that were placed on the field during the operation. If the count is incorrect, you must locate any missing items!
- **"Staples and two Adson pickups or 4-0 vicryl suture and Adson pickups"**	You will ask for either of these depending on your staff's preference for closing the skin. Staples are generally used in obese patients or in patients who have chorioamnionitis, although this is not a hard and fast rule. Also, other sutures than vicryl may be used. If you do use suture, you will usually place steri-strips afterwards.
- **"Sterile towel"**	Place the sterile towel over the closed incision.
- *"Taking down drapes"*	Hold the towel on the incision as you remove the drapes.

- **"Wet and dry laps"** Clean off any remaining prep from the abdomen, taking care not to rub so hard as to open the incision.

- **"Sterile bandage and tape"** Place the bandage on the incision and then cover with tape.

- *"Evacuating clots"* Place one hand on the abdomen and palpate the fundus and the other into the vagina after moving the patients legs. Check uterine tone and evacuate clots from the vagina.

- **"Wet and dry towel"** Use these to clean the perineum and remove the clots you expressed.

When you have completed the operation, remove your gown, put on non-sterile gloves, and assist the nurses in taking the patient to the recovery room. After doing this, talk with the anesthesiologist and ask about the following information for your operative report:

Estimated blood loss
Urine output
Fluids given during the procedure

Next, talk to your nurse and ask her for these items:
APGARS
Birth weight
Infant gender (if you do not remember)

For an example of how to dictate an operative note, please refer to Appendix B: Sample Notes and Orders.

Instruments for Cesarean Section:

Scalpel

Bovie electrocautery

Needle driver

Clamps:

Kocher

Kelly

Mosquito

Pennington

Ring forceps

Pickups:

Adson

Bonney

De Bakey

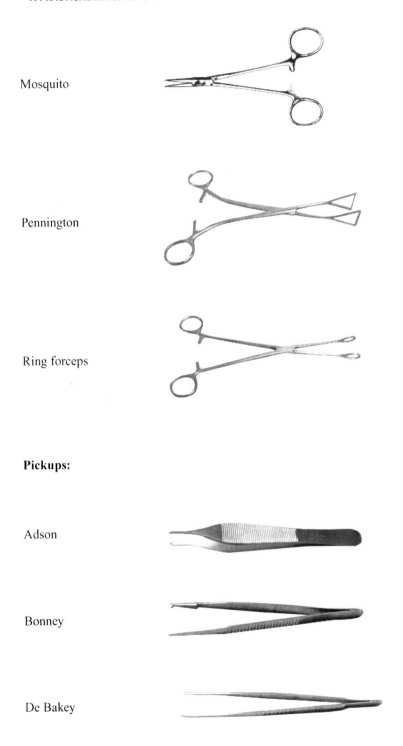

Ferris Smith

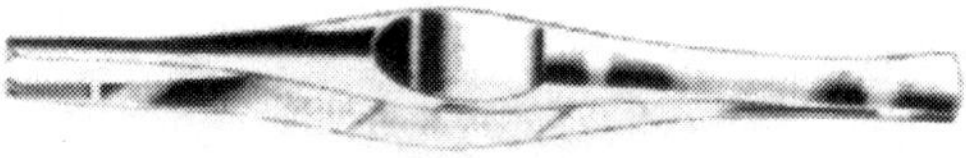

Rat tooth

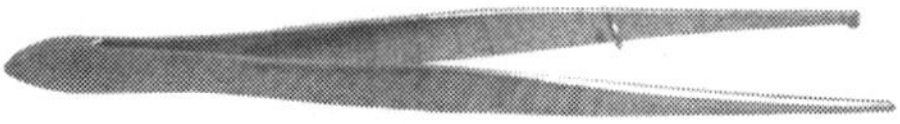

Russian

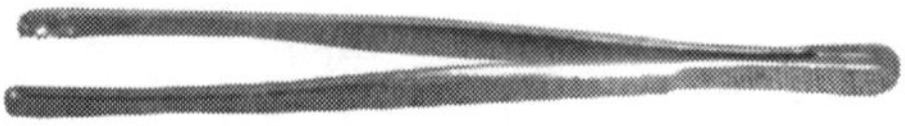

Retractors:

Bladder blade

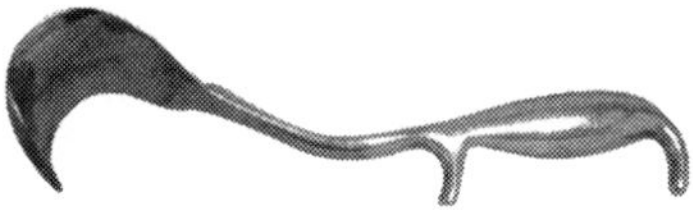

Richardson-Eastman

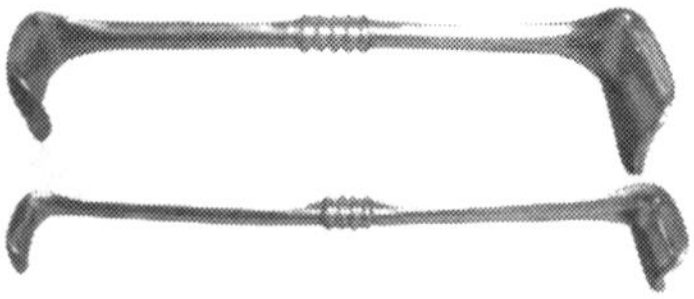

Scissors:

Bandage

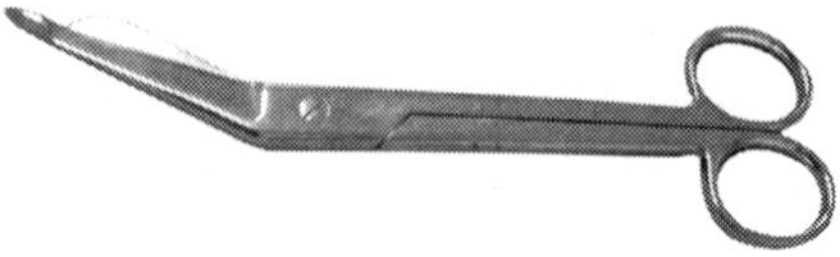

Mayo

Metzenbaum

Suction devices:

Yankauer

Pool

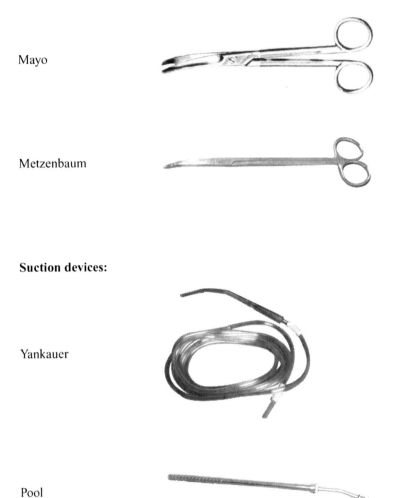

Index

A

U

ultrasound 23, 26, 29, 31, 40, 43, 48-9,
  58-63, 65-6, 86-8, 91, 118-19, 121,
  125, 236-7, 248-52
umbilical cord 7, 11, 31, 45-6, 60, 63, 77,
  111, 116-18, 120, 179-80, 221-3, 225,
  285-7, 291-2, 353
umbilical cord prolapse 11, 45, 71, 107, 165,
  185, 244, 265, 286-7, 291-2, 295, 299
urinalysis 27, 92, 237
uterine hyperstimulation 47-8, 68, 72, 74-8,
  80-1, 127, 129-32, 221, 311, 313, 315-
  16, 343-4
uterine hypertonus 44
uterine rupture 11, 124-5, 127, 129, 132,
  134, 171, 180, 186, 190-4, 196-7, 244,
  288-90, 294, 297-8, 341
uteroplacental insufficiency 72, 78, 221, 266

V

vaginal birth after cesarean *see* VBAC
vaginal bleeding 29, 89, 249-51, 279, 326
Valsalva 42, 90
vasa previa 29, 46, 107, 124, 165, 186
VBAC (Vaginal Birth After Cesarean) 156,
  160-1, 164-5, 190-2, 209, 239, 341
VBAC (vaginal birth after cesarean), benefits
  190
VBAC, attempting 190, 192-3
vertical incision 176-7, 181, 188
  infraumbilical 176
  low 170-1, 180

W

water intoxication 130-1, 311, 313
Woods screw maneuver 284

370

LaVergne, TN USA
10 February 2010
172580LV00004B/389/P